# *Protocols for Infectious Diseases in Obstetrics and Gynecology*

*Second Edition*

**Series:**
***Protocols in Obstetrics and Gynecology***

**Series Editor:**
John T. Queenan, MD
Professor and Chairman
Department of Obstetrics and Gynecology
Obstetrician and Gynecologist-in-Chief
Georgetown University School of Medicine
Washington, DC

**Other Titles in the Series:**
*Protocols for High-Risk Pregnancies*
John T. Queenan, John C. Hobbins

*Protocols for Office Gynecologic Surgery*
Philip D. Darney, Abner Korn, and Nicolette S. Horbach

# Protocols for Infectious Diseases in Obstetrics and Gynecology

*Second Edition*

*Edited by*

**Philip B. Mead, MD**
Professor and Chair
Department of Obstetrics and Gynecology
University of Vermont College of Medicine
Burlington, Vermont

**W. David Hager, MD**
Professor
Department of Obstetrics and Gynecology
Consultant in Infectious Diseases
Albert B. Chandler Medical Center
University of Kentucky College of Medicine
Lexington, Kentucky

**Sebastian Faro, MD, PhD**
John M. Simpson Professor and Chairman
Department of Obstetrics and Gynecology
Rush Medical College
Chicago, Illinois

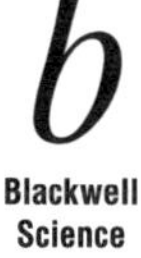


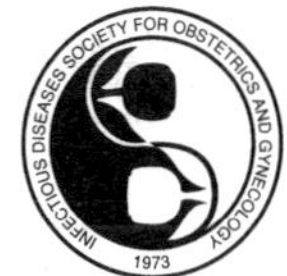

*Editorial Offices:*
Commerce Place, 350 Main Street, Malden, Massachusetts 02148, USA
Osney Mead, Oxford OX2 0EL, England
25 John Street, London WC1N 2BL, England
23 Ainslie Place, Edinburgh EH3 6AJ, Scotland
54 University Street, Carlton, Victoria 3053, Australia

*Other Editorial Offices:*
Blackwell Wissenschafts-Verlag GmbH, Kurfürstendamm 57, 10707 Berlin, Germany
Blackwell Science KK, MG Kodenmacho Building, 7–10 Kodenmacho Nihombashi, Chuo-ku, Tokyo 104, Japan

**Distributors:**

*USA*
Blackwell Science, Inc.
Commerce Place
350 Main Street
Malden, Massachusetts 02148
(Telephone orders: 800-215-1000 or 781-388-8250; fax orders: 781-388-8270)

*Canada*
Login Brothers Book Company
324 Saulteaux Crescent
Winnipeg, Manitoba, R3J 3T2
(Telephone orders: 204-224-4068)

*Australia*
Blackwell Science Pty, Ltd.
54 University Street
Carlton, Victoria 3053
(Telephone orders: 03-9347-0300; fax orders: 03-9349-3016)

*Outside North America and Australia*
Blackwell Science, Ltd.
c/o Marston Book Services, Ltd.
P.O. Box 269
Abingdon
Oxon OX14 4YN
England
(Telephone orders: 44-01235-465500; fax orders: 44-01235-465555)



*Acquisitions:* Chris Davis
*Production:* Erin Whitehead
*Manufacturing:* Lisa Flanagan
Cover design by Colour Mark
Typeset by Graphicraft Limited, Hong Kong
Printed and bound by Edwards Brothers, Inc.

Printed in the United States of America

99 00 01 02 5 4 3 2 1



**Library of Congress Cataloging-in-Publication Data**
Protocols for infectious diseases in obstetrics and gynecology / edited by Philip B. Mead, W. David Hager, Sebastian Faro. — 2nd ed.
p. cm. — (Protocols in obstetrics and gynecology)
Rev. ed. of: Infection protocols for obstetrics and gynecology. c1992.
Includes bibliographical references and index.
ISBN 0–632–04324–5
1. Generative organs, Female—Infections Handbooks, manuals, etc. 2. Communicable diseases in pregnancy Handbooks, manuals, etc. I. Mead, Philip B., 1937– . II. Infection protocols for obstetrics and gynecology. III. Series.
[DNLM: 1. Pregnancy Complications, Infectious. 2. Bacterial Infections. 3. Communicable Diseases. 4. Genital Diseases, Female. WQ 256 P967 2000]
RG218.I52 2000
618—dc21
DNLM/DLC
for Library of Congress

99–30332
CIP

To Ann, Linda, and Sharon

**Notice:** The indications and dosages of all drugs in this book have been recommended in the medical literature and conform to the practices of the general community. The medications described and treatment prescriptions suggested do not necessarily have specific approval by the Food and Drug Administration for use in the diseases and dosages for which they are recommended. The package insert for each drug should be consulted for use and dosage as approved by the FDA. Because standards for usage change, it is advisable to keep abreast of revised recommendations, particularly those concerning new drugs.

# *Contents*

# Contributors

**Lindsay S. Alger, MD**
Professor, Department of Obstetrics, Gynecology, and Reproductive Sciences
Associate Director
Division of Maternal-Fetal Medicine
University of Maryland Medical Center
Baltimore, Maryland

**H. H. Allen, MD**
Professor of Obstetrics and Gynecology
University of Western Ontario
London, Ontario, Canada

**Marvin S. Amstey, MD**
Professor, Department of Obstetrics and Gynecology
University of Rochester School of Medicine and Dentistry
Director of Residency Education
The Genesee Hospital
Rochester, New York

**Joseph J. Apuzzio, MD**
Professor of Obstetrics and Gynecology
Director, Division of Maternal-Fetal Medicine
Department of Obstetrics and Gynecology
University of Medicine and Dentistry of New Jersey-New Jersey Medical School
Newark, New Jersey

**David A. Baker, MD**
Director, Division of Infectious Diseases
Professor of Obstetrics, Gynecology, and Reproductive Medicine
School of Medicine
State University of New York at Stony Brook
Stony Brook, New York

**Roger Bawdon, PhD**
Associate Professor, Department of Obstetrics and Gynecology
University of Texas Health Science Center
Dallas, Texas

**Jorge D. Blanco, MD**
Medical Director, Sacred Heart Women's Hospital
Clinical Professor and Associate Chairman
Department of Obstetrics and Gynecology
University of Florida College of Medicine
Pensacola, Florida

**Noelle C. Bowdler, MD**
Associate Professor, Department of Obstetrics and Gynecology
University of Iowa Hospitals and Clinics
Iowa City, Iowa

**Zane A. Brown, MD**
Professor of Obstetrics and Gynecology
University of Washington School of Medicine
Seattle, Washington

**Walter Chaim, MD**
Department of Obstetrics and Gynecology
Soroka Medical Center
Faculty of Health Sciences
Ben-Gurion University of the Negev
Beer Sheva, Israel

**Penny Clark, PhD**
Research Scientist and Director of the Research
Microbiology Laboratory
Department of Obstetrics and Gynecology
University of Florida College of Medicine
Gainesville, Florida

**William R. Crombleholme, MD**
Professor and Vice Chair for Clinical Affairs
Department of Obstetrics, Gynecology, and Reproductive Sciences
University of Pittsburgh
Magee-Women's Hospital
Pittsburgh, Pennsylvania

**Mara J. Dinsmoor, MD**
Associate Professor, Department of Obstetrics and Gynecology
Medical College of Virginia Commonwealth University
Richmond, Virginia

**Geraldo Duarte, MD**
Associate Professor
Department of Gynecology and Obstetrics of Medicine School of Ribeiro Preto
Sao Paulo University
Ribeiro Preto-Sao Paulo, Brazil

**Patrick Duff, MD**
Professor of Obstetrics and Gynecology
Division of Maternal-Fetal Medicine
Residency Program Director
University of Florida College of Medicine
Gainesville, Florida

**Nancy L. Eriksen, MD**
Associate Professor
Department of Obstetrics and Gynecology and Reproduction Sciences
University of Texas Health Science Center
Houston, Texas

**J. M. Ernest, MD**
Associate Professor
Department of Obstetrics and Gynecology
Division of Maternal-Fetal Medicine
The Bowman Gray School of Medicine
Winston-Salem, North Carolina

**David A. Eschenbach, MD**
Professor of Obstetrics and Gynecology
University of Washington School of Medicine
Seattle, Washington

**Sebastian Faro, MD, PhD**
John M. Simpson Professor and Chairman
Department of Obstetrics and Gynecology
Rush Medical College
Chicago, Illinois

**Stephen J. Fortunato, MD**
Director, Perinatal Research Center
Women's Hospital at Centennial Medical Center
Nashville, Tennessee

**Rudolph P. Galask, MD**
Professor, Department of Obstetrics and Gynecology
University of Iowa Hospitals and Clinics
Iowa City, Iowa

**Stanley A. Gall, MD**
Professor and Chairman of Obstetrics and Gynecology
University of Louisville School of Medicine
Louisville, Kentucky

**Ronald S. Gibbs, MD**
E. Stewart Taylor Professor and Chairman
Department of Obstetrics and Gynecology
University of Colorado Health Sciences Center
Denver, Colorado

**Mark Gibson, MD**
Professor and Chair
Department of Obstetrics and Gynecology
West Virginia University Health Center
Morgantown, West Virginia

**Larry C. Gilstrap III, MD**
Emma Sue Hightower Professor and Chairman
Department of Obstetrics, Gynecology, and Reproductive Sciences
University of Texas-Houston Health Sciences Center
Houston, Texas

**Paulo C. Giraldo, MD**
Professor of Gynecology and Obstetrics
University of Campinas
Sao Paulo, Brazil

**Bernard Gonik, MD**
Professor and Associate Chairman
Department of Obstetrics and Gynecology
Wayne State University School of Medicine
Chief, Department Obstetrics and Gynecology
Sinai-Grace Hospital
Detroit, Michigan

**Michael G. Gravett, MD**
Associate Professor
Director, Maternal-Fetal Medicine
Department of Obstetrics and Gynecology
Oregon Health Sciences University
Portland, Oregon

**John H. Grossman III, MD, PhD, MPH**
Professor of Obstetrics and Gynecology, Microbiology and Immunology, and Prevention and Public Health
Acting Dean
School of Medicine and Health Sciences
George Washington University
Washington, District of Columbia

**Hope K. Haefner, MD**
Assistant Professor of Obstetrics and Gynecology and Surgery
University of Michigan Medical Center
Ann Arbor, Michigan

**W. David Hager, MD**
Professor, Department of Obstetrics and Gynecology
Consultant in Infectious Diseases
Albert B. Chandler Medical Center
University of Kentucky College of Medicine
Lexington, Kentucky

**James H. Harger, MD**
Professor of Obstetrics and Gynecology
University of Pittsburgh School of Medicine
Pittsburgh, Pennsylvania

**David L. Hemsell, MD**
Professor of Obstetrics and Gynecology
University of Texas Southwestern Medical Center at Dallas
Dallas, Texas

**Gale B. Hill, PhD**
Professor, Department of Obstetrics and Gynecology
Associate Professor, Department of Microbiology
Duke University Medical Center
Durham, North Carolina

**Michael K. Hill, MD**
Clinical Associate Professor of Medicine
Section of Infectious Diseases
Department of Medicine
Louisiana State University School of Medicine
New Orleans, Louisiana

**Sharon L. Hillier, PhD**
Associate Professor of Obstetrics, Gynecology, and Reproductive Sciences
University of Pittsburgh School of Medicine
Director of Reproductive Infectious Disease Research
Magee-Women's Research Institute
Pittsburgh, Pennsylvania

**Udo B. Hoyme, MD**
Professor of Obstetrics and Gynecology
Klinikum Erfurt GmbH
Klinik fur Frauenheilkunde und Geburtshilfe
Erfurt, Germany

**Mahmoud A. Ismail, MD**
Associate Professor
Department of Obstetrics and Gynecology
University of Chicago
Pritzker School of Medicine
Chicago, Illinois

**David C. Kmak, MD**
Assistant Professor, Department of Obstetrics and Gynecology
Wayne State University School of Medicine
Hutzel Hospital
Detroit, Michigan

**Abner P. Korn, MD**
Associate Clinical Professor
Department of Obstetrics and Gynecology and Reproductive Sciences
University of California
Director of Gynecology, San Francisco General Hospital
San Francisco, California

**A. Karen Kreutner, MD**
Private Practice
Charleston, South Carolina

**Marijane A. Krohn, PhD**
Associate Professor
Department of Obstetrics and Gynecology and Reproductive Sciences
University of Pittsburgh School of Medicine
Pittsburgh, Pennsylvania

**Daniel V. Landers, MD**
Associate Professor
Department of Obstetrics, Gynecology, and Reproductive Sciences
Director, Division of Infectious Diseases and Immunology
University of Pittsburgh
Magee-Women's Hospital
Pittsburgh, Pennsylvania

**Bryan Larsen, PhD**
Dean for University Research
Professor, Department of Obstetrics and Gynecology and Microbiology
University of Osteopathic Medicine and Health Sciences
Des Moines, Iowa

**John W. Larsen, Jr., MD**
Oscar I. and Mildred S. Dodek Professor and Interim Chairman
Department of Obstetrics and Gynecology
Director, Wilson Genetics Center
The George Washington University Medical Center
Washington, District of Columbia

**William L. Ledger, MD**
Chairman, Department of Obstetrics and Gynecology
Weill Medical College of Cornell University
New York, New York

**Charles H. Livengood III, MD**
Associate Professor of Obstetrics and Gynecology
Director, Chlamydia Laboratory
Duke University Medical Center
Durham, North Carolina

**Maurizio Maccato, MD**
Assistant Professor
Departments of Pediatrics, Microbiology, and Immunology
Baylor College of Medicine
Houston, Texas

**Mark G. Martens, MD**
Professor and Vice Chairman
Department of Obstetrics and Gynecology
University of Minnesota School of Medicine
Chairman, Department of Obstetrics and Gynecology
Hennepin County Medical Center
Minneapolis, Minnesota

**Eli Maymon, MD**
Department of Obstetrics and Gynecology
Soroka Medical Center
Faculty of Health Sciences
Ben-Gurion University of the Negev
Beer Sheva, Israel

**William M. McCormack, MD**
Professor of Medicine and of Obstetrics and Gynecology
SUNY Health Science Center
Brooklyn, New York

**Robert S. McDuffie, Jr., MD**
Chief of Perinatology, Department of Obstetrics and Gynecology
Kaiser Permanente St. Joseph Hospital
Denver, Colorado

**James A. McGregor, MD, CM**
Senior Technical Physician, Denver Health Medical Center
Professor of Obstetrics and Gynecology
University of Colorado School of Medicine
Denver, Colorado

**S. Gene McNeeley, Jr., MD**
Director, Department of Obstetrics and Gynecology
Wayne State University School of Medicine
Hutzel Hospital
Detroit, Michigan

**Philip B. Mead, MD**
Professor and Chair, Department of Obstetrics and Gynecology
University of Vermont College of Medicine
Burlington, Vermont

**R. David Miller, MD**
Private Practice
Tustin, California

**Howard L. Minkoff, MD**
Chairman, Department of Ob/Gyn
Maimonides Medical Center
Professor, Department of Obstetrics and Gynecology
SUNY Health Science Center
Brooklyn, New York

**Gilles R. G. Monif, MD**
Assistant Dean
Creighton University School of Medicine
Omaha, Nebraska

**Walter J. Morales, MD, PhD**
Florida Perinatal Associates (Private Practice)
Division of Maternal-Fetal Medicine
Tampa, Florida

**Edward R. Newton, MD**
Professor and Chairman, Department of Obstetrics and Gynecology
East Carolina University School of Medicine
Greenville, North Carolina

**Paul Nyirjesy, MD**
Associate Professor, Department of Obstetrics and Gynecology and Reproductive Sciences
Division of Infectious Diseases
Department of Medicine
Temple University School of Medicine
Philadelphia, Pennsylvania

**Newton G. Osborne, MD, PhD**
Professor and Chair
Department of Obstetrics and Gynecology
Howard University College of Medicine
Washington, District of Columbia

**Bryan T. Oshiro, MD**
Department of Perinatology
McKay Dee Hospital
Ogden, Utah

**Joseph G. Pastorek II, MD**
Private Practice
Metairie, Louisiana

**Mark D. Pearlman, MD**
Vice Chair and Associate Professor of Obstetrics and Gynecology
University of Michigan Health System
Ann Arbor, Michigan

**Charles V. Sanders, MD**
Edgar Hull Professor and Chairman
Department of Medicine
Louisiana State University School of Medicine
New Orleans, Louisiana

**N. J. Scaglione, WHNP**
Women's Heath Nurse Practitioner
Women Now Health Care
Milwaukee, Wisconsin

**Richard H. Schwarz, MD**
Chairman
Department of Obstetrics and Gynecology
New York Methodist Hospital
Professor of Obstetrics and Gynecology
Weill Medical College of Cornell University
New York, New York

**John L. Sever, MD, PhD**
Professor of Pediatrics, Obstetrics and Gynecology, and Microbiology and Immunology
George Washington University Medical Center
Children's National Medical Center
Washington, District of Columbia

**Neil S. Silverman, MD**
Medical Director
Inpatient Obstetric Services
Division of Maternal-Fetal Medicine
Cedars-Sinai Medical Center
Associate Professor of Obstetrics and Gynecology
UCLA School of Medicine
Los Angeles, California

**David E. Soper, MD**
Professor and Director
Department of Gynecology and Obstetrics
Medical University of South Carolina
Charleston, South Carolina

**Michael R. Spence, MD, MPH**
Medical Officer
Department of Public Health and Human Services
State of Montana
Helena, Montana

**Rhoda Sperling, MD**
Associate Professor and Director
Division of Obstetric and Gynecologic Infectious Diseases
Department of Obstetrics, Gynecology, and Reproductive Science
Mount Sinai Medical Center
Mount Sinai School of Medicine
New York, New York

**Richard L. Sweet, MD**
Professor and Chair
Department of Obstetrics and Gynecology and Reproductive Sciences
University of Pittsburgh
Magee-Women's Hospital
Pittsburgh, Pennsylvania

**Jessica L. Thomason, MD**
Clinical Professor of Obstetrics and Gynecology
University of Wisconsin School of Medicine
Medical Director, Women Now Health Care
Milwaukee, Wisconsin

**Gael P. Wager, MD, MPH**
Private Practice
Flagstaff, Arizona

**Cheryl K. Walker, MD**
Assistant Professor
Department of Obstetrics and Gynecology
University of California, Irvine
College of Medicine
Orange, California

**D. Heather Watts, MD**
Pediatric, Adolescent, Maternal AIDS Branch
CRMC/ NICHD/ NIH
Bethesda, Maryland

**George D. Wendel, Jr., MD**
Professor
Department of Obstetrics and Gynecology
University of Texas Southwestern Medical School
Dallas, Texas

**Steven S. Witkin, PhD**
Professor of Immunology and
Director, Division of Immunology
and Infectious Diseases
Department of Obstetrics and Gynecology
Weill Medical College of Cornell University
New York, New York

**Pål Wölner-Hanssen, MD, PhD**
Associate Professor, Department of Obstetrics and Gynecology
University of Lund
Lund, Sweden

**M. Lynn Yonekura, MD**
Medical Director, Perinatal Services
California Medical Center
Los Angeles, California

# *Preface*

First published in 1992, *Infection Protocols for Obstetrics and Gynecology* was patterned after the popular *Protocols for High-Risk Pregnancies*, conceived and edited by Dr. John Queenan and Dr. John Hobbins. It was designed to provide a concise but thorough discussion of the common and not so common infections encountered in the practice of obstetrics and gynecology. This new edition, now titled *Protocols for Infectious Diseases in Obstetrics and Gynecology, Second Edition*, has the same goal: to put all essential material for diagnosis and management of any given infection at the busy clinician's fingertips. The question may come during office hours from a pregnant patient worried about chickenpox exposure or it may come at 3AM from a resident in the hospital ER needing to know about antibiotic therapy for a cephalosporin-allergic pregnant woman with suspected gonococcal infection. In either case, the answer is to be found in this book, an authoritative, easily accessible addition to your medical library.

While keeping the same format as the first edition, all chapters in this book have been revised and updated. In addition, 13 new chapters have been added on topics such as hepatitis C and vulvodynia that have grown in importance since the first edition. The most recent (1998) CDC Guidelines for Treatment of Sexually Transmitted Diseases have been incorporated throughout. Even the dimensions of the book have been modified so that it can be carried more easily in the clinic or at the bedside.

Acknowledgments are in order to the many people who helped bring this book to light. First, Dr. John Queenan's encouragement and wise counsel are, as always, deeply appreciated. Next, we're grateful to Jim Swan, Editorial Director of *Contemporary OB/GYN* at Medical Economics Company, for the many extra hours he spent working with authors and guiding the editorial process. Two *Contemporary OB/GYN* publishers, Tom Pizor and Barbara Pritchard, have provided strong support for this project since it started 10 years ago. We also appreciate the support of Chris Davis, Erin Whitehead, and their colleagues at Blackwell Science, who have encouraged and facilitated the reediting of this book and shown their determination to get updated information to clinicians in the most expeditious way possible.

Finally, our greatest thanks go to our authors, the members of the Infectious Diseases Society for Obstetrics and Gynecology. These individuals are devoting their professional lives to improving our understanding and treatment of infections of women. Their knowledge, experience, and enthusiasm are evident on each page, making this, we think, a unique publication.

Philip B. Mead, MD
Burlington, Vermont

W. David Hager, MD
Lexington, Kentucky

Sebastian Faro, MD, PhD
Chicago, Illinois

PART 1

# *Obstetrics*

CHAPTER

# 1

# *The Relationship Between Lower and Upper Genital Tract Infection in Pregnancy*

*Sharon L. Hillier*

## Background and Incidence

Most of the microorganisms that cause upper genital tract infections in pregnancy are derived from the vagina or cervix. Therefore, the organisms that have been recovered most frequently from the amniotic fluid of pregnant women with intact fetal membranes or from the chorioamnion are those that colonize the vagina. In the past, the cervical mucus plug was thought to be an important barrier to upper genital tract invasion. A more contemporary view holds that organisms from the lower genital tract can ascend to cause infections of the decidua, chorioamnion, and amniotic fluid. Historically, it was also believed that organisms residing in the lower genital tract could not invade the amniotic fluid unless the membranes were ruptured. When amniotic fluid has been sampled by transabdominal amniocentesis, however, several organisms that typically reside in the vagina can be detected, suggesting that these organisms may invade intact membranes and thereby cause upper genital tract infections during pregnancy.

The prevalence of symptomatic intra-amniotic infection, as defined by fever during labor and other clinical signs, ranges from 1.4% among women with the most normal vaginal microflora to a high of 3.7% among women with a bacterial flora consistent with bacterial vaginosis (BV). The prevalence of amniotic fluid bacteria among women in preterm labor with intact fetal membranes has been estimated at 10% to 20%, with the highest prevalence of amniotic fluid invasion observed among women at earlier gestational ages. Similarly, the incidence of chorioamnion invasion by genital organisms has ranged from 20% to 60%, with the highest prevalences seen at earlier gestational ages.

## BV as a Risk Factor for Upper Tract Infections in Pregnancy

BV is characterized by a shift in the vaginal microflora from one in which lactobacilli predominate to one with higher concentrations of obligately anaerobic gram-negative rods, genital mycoplasmas, and *Gardnerella vaginalis* (see Chapter 39). Many of the microorganisms associated with BV produce virulence factors such as sialidase, mucinases, proteases, and endotoxin. For example, an elevated level of protease in the vaginal fluid has been associated with preterm labor and was noted in nearly half of women who had preterm premature rupture of membranes. Sialidases or neuraminidases are enzymes that can alter the host response to bacterial infections. Organisms present in the vagina that produce sialidase include some strains of *G. vaginalis* and most strains of *Prevotella bivia*. Women with BV have higher vaginal levels of these organisms.

Mucinase is another type of enzyme produced by vaginal bacteria that is found more frequently among women with BV. The production of mucinase may partly explain how the organisms associated with BV bypass the mucous barrier in the cervix to invade the upper genital tract and cause chorioamnion infection, amnionitis, or postpartum endometritis. Mucinases have been reported in nearly half of women with BV and about one-fourth of women without this syndrome.

A number of studies have evaluated the relationship between BV-associated organisms and amniotic fluid infection. Silver and coworkers reported a higher incidence of amniotic fluid infection in women with abnormal vaginal flora, as assessed by Gram's stain. These women also were more likely to have *G. vaginalis* or *Mycoplasma hominis* recovered from their amniotic fluid. In addition, BV has been shown to increase the risk of clinical amnionitis nearly fourfold among women undergoing cesarean section.

Perhaps the most compelling evidence suggesting that the presence of BV in the vagina is a risk factor for amniotic fluid infection comes from studies that evaluated fluid obtained by transabdominal amniocentesis from women in preterm labor. Gravett and coworkers reported that BV was diagnosed in 5 of 5 women whose amniotic fluid contained organisms associated with BV, but in only 14 of 39 women whose amniotic fluid was sterile. The author's group evaluated 225 women with intact fetal membranes who were admitted for preterm labor at less than 34 weeks' gestation. Once again, amniotic fluid was obtained by transabdominal amniocentesis. Of the 43 women in this group who had BV, 10 (23%) had bacteria recovered from the amniotic fluid, compared with 13 (10%) of 126 women with normal vaginal flora. The primary organisms present in the amniotic fluid of women with BV in preterm labor were *Fusobacterium nucleatum,* anaerobic gram-negative rods, *G. vaginalis*, and the genital mycoplasmas. These studies clearly show that BV-associated microorganisms can penetrate cervical mucus, invade the placental membrane, and cause infections of the amniotic fluid even when the membranes remain intact.

Women with BV are nearly three times as likely to have histologic evidence of chorioamnionitis and about three times as likely to have organisms recovered from the chorioamnion as are women with normal vaginal flora. Although *Ureaplasma urealyticum* can frequently be isolated from the amniotic fluid or placental membranes, the recovery of this organism alone does not appear to be associated with preterm delivery. By comparison, the recovery of obligately anaerobic gram-negative rods—such as *F. nucleatum, Bacteroides ureolyticus, P. bivia*, and anaerobic gram-positive cocci—is associated with both preterm birth and histologic evidence of chorioamnionitis.

A third type of upper tract infection observed more frequently among women with BV than in those who have normal vaginal flora is postpartum endometritis. Women having BV at the time that they undergo cesarean section are approximately four times as likely to develop postpartum endometritis as are women with normal vaginal flora. The failure of antibiotic prophylaxis to prevent postpartum infection in these women is likely due to a combination of factors, including improper choice of an antibiotic, preexisting deep-seated infection, and/or failure to administer an appropriate antibiotic so as to prevent infection.

Some research—from longitudinal studies in which women were enrolled early in pregnancy—supports the view that the organisms associated with BV can move into the upper genital tract relatively early during pregnancy. At least three studies have reported a threefold increased incidence of second-trimester pregnancy loss among women with BV compared with those having normal vaginal microflora. These data are widely interpreted as meaning that the organisms associated with BV can initiate chronic upper genital tract infections during pregnancy and that these infections sometimes can lead to spontaneous abortion or late miscarriage in the second trimester of pregnancy. Although a few randomized clinical trials have suggested that treatment of BV can reduce the incidence of preterm delivery, additional studies will be needed to assess whether earlier treatment of BV can lead to a reduced incidence of miscarriage and preterm delivery.

## Association of STD Pathogens with Upper Genital Tract Infections in Pregnancy

Cervical infection with *Neisseria gonorrhoeae* or *Chlamydia trachomatis* has been recognized as a risk factor for preterm delivery. In addition, recent reports from the Vaginal Infections and Prematurity (VIP) study suggest that *Trichomonas vaginalis* infection is another risk factor for preterm low-birthweight delivery, even after accounting for coexistent BV or concomitant infection with *C. trachomatis* or *N. gonorrhoeae*. Because screening for *C. trachomatis* and *N. gonorrhoeae* has become a standard part of prenatal care, documented episodes of invasive upper genital tract infection by these pathogens during pregnancy are rare. Nevertheless, *N. gonorrhoeae* has been found to invade the chorioamnion and induce histologic chorioamnionitis. Because *C. trachomatis* is an obligate intracellular parasite, it would not be found free in the amniotic fluid. It is uncertain how frequently *C. trachomatis* can ascend to cause upper tract infection during pregnancy. The finding in case reports using polymerase chain amplification methods—namely, that upper tract invasion by these organisms may occur—supports the view of many researchers that both gonococcal and chlamydial infection should be rigorously investigated and treated during pregnancy.

Numerous attempts have been made to detect *T. vaginalis* in the amniotic fluid of women with intact fetal membranes and in the chorioamnion of the placenta after delivery. Nevertheless, little evidence exists to suggest that *T. vaginalis* ascends to cause upper genital tract infection frequently during pregnancy.

## Respiratory Pathogens and Upper Genital Tract Infection During Pregnancy

Respiratory pathogens can be transmitted to the genital tract through oral–genital contact or by autoinoculation from a patient's mouth to her genital area. As noted earlier, *F. nucleatum* is one of the microorganisms most frequently recovered from the amniotic fluid of women with intact fetal membranes. Although in some cases this organism originates in the genital tract, it is also part of the normal oral flora. *Haemophilus influenzae*, a common respiratory pathogen that has also been associated with pelvic inflammatory disease (PID), has been noted to be an etiologic agent of amniotic fluid infection in the presence of intact fetal membranes. *Actinomyces*, an anaerobic gram-positive organism that has been associated with PID among women with intrauterine devices (see Chapters 62 and 63), similarly has been shown to cause chorioamnionitis in some patients. It is likely that some microorganisms can cause amnionitis directly by disseminated spread through the bloodstream. *Listeria monocytogenes* is one such organism.

## Uropathogens and Upper Genital Tract Infections During Pregnancy

Asymptomatic bacteriuria in pregnancy has long been recognized as a risk factor for preterm birth. Furthermore, clinical and epidemiologic evidence indicates that antibiotic treatment can effectively reduce the occurrence of delivery of preterm, low-birthweight infants of women with asymptomatic bacteriuria. *Escherichia coli* is the most common uropathogen found in the vaginas of pregnant women; it appears in 10% to 25% of vaginal samples from women seeking prenatal care. Although it has long been recognized that *E. coli* is an important cause of neonatal sepsis, the idea that this organism could ascend to cause chorioamnion infection and preterm birth has only recently been acknowledged. One study showed that the recovery of *E. coli* from the chorioamnion was significantly associated with delivery of an infant before 34 weeks' gestation. In addition, large epidemiologic studies have suggested that highdensity vaginal colonization with *E. coli* is associated with a twofold increased risk of very low-birthweight delivery (less than 1500 g).

## Group B *Streptococcus* in the Vagina and Upper Genital Tract Infection

Like *E. coli*, group B *Streptococcus* (GBS) is a normal part of the vaginal flora of 20% to 35% of pregnant women seeking prenatal care. GBS can also invade the chorioamnion. This capability is thought to be one mechanism by which GBS causes preterm delivery. In one study of 212 women delivering at less than 34 weeks' gestation, GBS was recovered from 7% of chorioamnion cultures versus 2% of chorioamnion cultures in women delivering at more than 34 weeks' gestation. Further, two-thirds of the women having GBS in the chorioamnion showed histologic evidence of chorioamnionitis.

Numerous studies have documented the ability of GBS to invade intact fetal membranes and cause an acute amnionitis, which often results in preterm delivery. Both amnionitis and preterm delivery are recognized risk factors for GBS sepsis occurring in the first seven days of life (see Chapter 5). Because most infants with early-onset GBS sepsis become ill within the first few hours after delivery, the current hypothesis is that many of these infants become infected in utero rather than during their passage through the birth canal. This method of infection is especially prevalent among infants born preterm who develop GBS sepsis.

GBS colonization has been evaluated as a risk factor for clinically diagnosed amniotic fluid infection in a number of studies. In one study, clinically diagnosed amnionitis occurred 3.5 more times frequently among women colonized by GBS even after adjusting for duration of membrane rupture, duration of internal monitoring, and numbers of vaginal examinations in a multivariate model. Not surprisingly, the risk of developing amniotic fluid infection increased with each level of increasing density of colonization. Women having very high-density vaginal colonization by GBS (3+) had a threefold increased incidence of amnionitis, whereas women with lower-density colonization (1+ to 2+) had an approximately twofold increased risk of amnionitis. In the same study, women with vaginal GBS infection were somewhat more likely to deliver preterm, although this association was not statistically significant after multivariate adjustment. Although the need for intrapartum penicillin prophylaxis to GBS-colonized women is well recognized as part of an effort to prevent early-onset neonatal sepsis due to GBS, additional studies are urgently needed to better define the association between lower genital tract GBS and upper tract infection.

## Utility of Vaginal Cultures for Assessing Risk of Upper Tract Infection Among Women in Preterm Labor

Although many vaginal microorganisms can ascend into the upper genital tract to cause chorioamnion infection, amnionitis, and postpartum endometritis, the utility of vaginal cultures for assessing the etiology of these infections remains unclear. Because many women carry potential pathogens as part of their normal flora, routine assessment of genital pathogens for predicting upper tract infection is not warranted. All pregnant women should be screened at their first visit for *N. gonorrhoeae* and *C. trachomatis.* When women present with preterm contractions or have a history of prior preterm delivery, it may be advisable to determine whether BV is present. In addition, a vaginal/rectal swab culture to detect GBS is clearly warranted at 35 to 37 weeks' gestation to direct intrapartum antibiotic prophylaxis so as to prevent early-onset GBS sepsis. Because few data as yet suggest that antibiotic intervention can decrease sequelae related to high-density vaginal *E. coli* colonization, there is probably no advantage in requesting additional cultures for *E. coli.*

## Suggested Readings

Abadi MA, Abadi J. *Actinomyces* chorioamnionitis and preterm labor in a twin pregnancy: a case report. Am J Obstet Gynecol 1996;175:1391–1392.

Gravett MG, Hummel D, Eschenbach DA, et al. Preterm labor associated with subclinical amniotic fluid infection and with bacterial vaginosis. Obstet Gynecol 1986;67:229–237.

Hillier SL, Krohn MA, Cassen E, et al. The role of bacterial vaginosis in amniotic fluid infection in women in preterm labor with intact fetal membranes. Clin Infect Dis 1995;20(suppl 2):S276–S278.

Hillier SL, Krohn MA, Kiviat NB, et al. Microbiologic causes and neonatal outcomes associated with chorioamnion infection. Am J Obstet Gynecol 1991;165:955–961.

Hillier SL, Martius J, Krohn MA, et al. A case-control study of chorioamnionic infection and histologic chorioamnionitis in prematurity. N Engl J Med 1988;319:972–978.

Krohn MA, Hillier SL, Nugent RP, et al. The genital flora of women with intraamniotic infection. J Infect Dis 1995;171:1475–1480.

Krohn MA, Thwin SS, Rabe LK, et al. Vaginal colonization by *Escherichia coli* as a risk factor for very low birthweight delivery and other perinatal complications. J lnfect Dis 1997;175:606–610.

Llahi-Camp JM, Rai R, Ison C, et al. Association of bacterial vaginosis with a history of second trimester miscarriage. Hum Reprod 1996; 11:1575–1578.

Pao CC, Kao SM, Wang HC, et al. Intraamniotic detection of *Chlamydia trachomatis* deoxyribonucleic acid sequences by polymerase chain reaction. Am J Obstet Gynecol 1991;164:1295–1299.

Silver HM, Sperling RS, St. Clair PJ, et al. Evidence relating bacterial vaginosis to intraamniotic infection. Am J Obstet Gynecol 1989; 161:808–812.

Smith LG Jr, Summers PR, Miles RW, et al. Gonococcal chorioamnionitis associated with sepsis: a case report. Am J Obstet Gynecol 1989;160:573–574.

Watts DH, Krohn MA, Hillier SL, et al. Bacterial vaginosis as a risk factor for post-cesarean endometritis. Obstet Gynecol 1990; 75:52–58.

Winn HN, Egley CC. Acute *Haemophilus influenzae* chorioamnionitis associated with intact amniotic membranes. Am J Obstet Gynecol 1987;156:458–459.

Yancey MK, Duff P, Clark P, et al. Peripartum infection associated with vaginal group B streptococcal colonization. Obstet Gynecol 1994;84:816–819.

CHAPTER

# 2

# *Intra-amniotic Infection*

*Jorge D. Blanco*

## Background and Incidence

Confusion exists over the meaning of the term "chorio-amnionitis," also called amnionitis. To the clinician, it is the clinically evident infection of the fetus, amniotic cavity, and mother; to the pathologist, it is the leukocytic infiltration of the placenta. As histologic findings may occur without any evidence of clinical infection, the two entities are not totally synonymous. In this chapter, for the sake of clarity, the term "intra-amniotic infection" (IAI) will be used to mean the clinical entity.

Intra-amniotic infection occurs in approximately 0.5% to 1% of all pregnancies, and the rate may increase with extended time from rupture of membranes (ROM) until delivery. Although the majority of infected persons have ROM, on rare occasions the infection also may occur with intact membranes.

## Etiology

In the woman with intact membranes, microorganisms such as *Listeria monocytogenes* and group A streptococci can infect the fetus transplacentally by hematogenous spread from the mother. In women with ROM or those with intact membranes but in labor, the usual culprit is ascending infection by organisms from the cervical microflora. Creatsas and coworkers concluded that untreated endocervical infections are an etiologic factor for IAI. The microbiology in these women includes the usual genital tract pathogens, including anaerobes (especially the *Bacteroides* group, *Prevotella* sp., and the peptostreptococci), the group B streptococci, and the aerobic gram-negative bacilli (especially *Escherichia coli*).

In the majority of women, the etiology of IAI is polymicrobial. Although the role of the genital mycoplasmas remains unclear, they do not appear to be prominent in this infection. Likewise, the role of *Chlamydia trachomatis*—if any—is not well delineated. Bacterial vaginosis has been shown to represent a risk factor for the development of IAI.

## Diagnosis

Diagnosis of IAI often proves difficult, because it relies on exclusion. The clinical signs and symptoms are neither sensitive nor specific. Common findings include ROM and fever. Maternal tachycardia, fetal tachycardia, uterine tenderness, and malodorous amniotic fluid are seen less often. Table 2-1 suggests diagnostic criteria for this condition.

Clinical factors associated with an increased risk of IAI include the following:

- Number of vaginal examinations during labor (6 or more)
- Duration of labor (greater than 12 hours)
- Duration of ROM before labor (24 hours or longer)
- Maternal colonization with group B streptococci
- Meconium-stained amniotic fluid

**Table 2-1.** Diagnostic Criteria for Intra-amniotic Infection

Fever (≥37.8 °C)
Rupture of membranes
Two or more of the following:

- Maternal tachycardia (pulse > 100)
- Fetal tachycardia (fetal heart tones > 160)
- Uterine tenderness
- Malodorous amniotic fluid
- Peripheral leukocytosis (WBC > 15,000)
- No other site of infection

Source: Loof JD, Hager WD. Management of chorioamnionitis. Surg Gynecol Obstet 1984;158:161–166.

Certain laboratory tests may also assist in the diagnosis. An elevated peripheral leukocyte count is common, but care should be exercised in interpreting the peripheral white blood cell (WBC) count, as labor itself may elevate these levels. Urinalysis and culture will rule out a urinary tract infection. Cultures of the amniotic fluid may help isolate the organisms involved in the infection. For culture, an amniocentesis specimen is ideal, but in many women—especially those with ROM—this type of sample is difficult to obtain.

An adequate specimen may be acquired transcervically by means of an intrauterine pressure catheter. The first 3 to 5 mL aspirated through the catheter should be discarded, with the next 2 to 3 mL being sent for culture. Because bacteria gain entry to the amniotic cavity after ROM and because labor itself may result in the finding of amniotic fluid leukocytes, interpret Gram's stain results with care. A finding of no leukocytes or bacteria can be useful in ruling out IAI. Vaginal pool aspirates have little use for culture or for the diagnosis of infection.

Various studies have recently demonstrated elevated levels of cytokines such as interleukin-6 (IL-6) in the amniotic fluid and serum of infected women. The difficulty of performing such tests for cytokines, however, has prevented their widespread use for diagnosis. Although glucose levels are low in the amniotic fluid of infected women, the test for amniotic fluid glucose is not accurate enough to warrant its clinical use. Another rapid marker employed on a research-only basis for diagnosing IAI is the granulocyte colony-stimulating factor.

## Treatment

Management of IAI consists of prompt initiation of antibiotic therapy and progression to delivery. Administering antibiotics as soon as the diagnosis is made will limit the extent of infection in the mother and neonate. Because of this infection's polymicrobial etiology and its potential severity, administration of potent broad-spectrum antibiotic agents is indicated.

Because the results of large, comparative studies of antibiotics for IAI are not available, the majority of regimens are used on an empiric basis. Some studies support the use of IV penicillin G, 5000 U every 6 hours, combined with gentamicin, 1 to 1.5 mg/kg IV every 8 hours. Other studies support the use of ampicillin, 1 g IV every 6 hours, plus gentamicin, 1.5 mg/kg IV every 8 hours, which theoretically may have some benefit because the ratio of transplacental transmission is better for ampicillin than for penicillin. Neither of these combinations, however, provides adequate coverage for anaerobes such as *Bacteroides* sp. Therefore, patients undergoing cesarean section should receive clindamycin, 900 mg IV every 8 hours, in addition to ampicillin and gentamicin. For patients who deliver vaginally, a penicillin–gentamicin or ampicillin–gentamicin regimen is adequate.

An alternative may involve the use of a broad-spectrum third-generation cephalosporin, such as cefoxitin, cefotetan, and ceftizoxime, or an extended-spectrum penicillin, such as the ampicillin–sulbactam combination. Such agents have a good safety record, and many are well transmitted to the fetus. Most provide the required broad-spectrum coverage, and recent studies support their efficacy in treating IAI.

The timing of antibiotic administration is as critical to success as the choice of the antibiotic used. Several studies show clear neonatal benefits from immediate initiation of antibiotics. A delay in instituting therapy, even when delivery is imminent, may markedly increase perinatal morbidity and mortality. Maternal antibiotic treatment results in transplacental treatment of the fetus with an improved outcome. Equally important is prompt progression to delivery. Drainage of the uterine cavity is essential. Although no arbitrary or absolute time limit has been identified after which the risks for mother and fetus increase, efforts to effect delivery should begin as soon as the diagnosis is made.

Intra-amniotic infection is not necessarily an indication for cesarean section. In fact, because of the lower maternal morbidity, a vaginal delivery is preferred. Many patients, however, may need cesarean sections for obstetric reasons. Duff and coworkers have found that these patients more frequently require oxytocin for induction of labor and more frequently have arrest of labor leading to cesarean section for failure to progress.

## Sequelae

Although maternal morbidity is increased with IAI, maternal mortality is extremely rare. Women treated aggressively with antibiotics and delivered promptly will usually do well. Approximately 10% to 12% will exhibit bacteremia, and 40% to 50% will need cesarean section because of unsatisfactory progression in labor.

With appropriate intrapartum and neonatal treatment, the infected term baby will do well. As many as 20% of these neonates may have pneumonia on chest X ray, and 8% to 10% may have documented bacteremia. Several small studies, however, revealed that the mortality rate for these babies was not increased.

Unfortunately, outcomes for preterm infants are not as good. Perinatal mortality and morbidity are significantly higher for preterm neonates born to infected mothers than for those born to uninfected mothers. The combination of prematurity and IAI is ominous, and the addition of respiratory distress syndrome may have devastating consequences.

## Suggested Readings

Creatsas GC, Charalambidis VM, Zagotzidou E, et al. Untreated cervical infections, chorioamnionitis, and prematurity. Int J Gynaecol Obstet 1995;49:1–7.

Duff P. Antibiotics in treatment of chorioamnionitis. Am J Obstet Gynecol 1989;160:271.

Duff P, Sanders R, Gibbs RS. The course of labor in term patients with chorioamnionitis. Am J Obstet Gynecol 1983;147:391–395.

Gauthier DW, Meyer WJ. Comparison of Gram stain, leukocyte esterase activity, and amniotic fluid glucose concentrations in predicting amniotic fluid culture results in preterm premature rupture of membranes. Am J Obstet Gynecol 1992;167:1092–1095.

Gibbs RS, Dinsmoor MJ, Newton ER, et al. A randomized trial of intrapartum versus immediate postpartum treatment of women with intra-amniotic infection. Obstet Gynecol 1988;72:823–828.

Gibbs RS, Duff P. Progress in pathogenesis and management of clinical intra-amniotic infection. Am J Obstet Gynecol 1991;164: 1317–1326.

Greig PC, Ernest JM, Teot L, et al. Amniotic fluid interleukin-6 levels correlate with histologic chorioamnionitis and amniotic fluid cultures in patients in premature labor with intact membranes. Am J Obstet Gynecol 1993;169:1035–1044.

Hoskins IA, Zandieh P, Schatz F, et al. Amniotic fluid granulocyte colony stimulating factor levels: a rapid marker for diagnosing chorioamnionitis. Am J Reprod Immunol 1997;38:286–288.

Loof JD, Hager WD. Management of chorioamnionitis. Surg Gynecol Obstet 1984;158:161–166.

Newton ER, Piper J, Peairs W. Bacterial vaginosis and intra-amniotic infection. Am J Obstet Gynecol 1997;176:672–677.

Seaward PG, Hannah ME, Myhr TL, et al. International Multicentre Term Prelabor Rupture of Membranes Study: evaluation of predictors of clinical chorioamniotis and postpartum fever in patients with prelabor rupture of membranes at term. Am J Obstet Gynecol 1997;177:1024–1029.

Sperling RS, Newton ER, Gibbs RS. Intra-amniotic infection in low-birthweight infants. J Infect Dis 1988;157:113–117.

Yoder ER, Gibbs RS, Blanco JD, et al. A prospective, controlled study of maternal and perinatal outcome after intra-amniotic infection at term. Am J Obstet Gynecol 1983;145:695–701.

CHAPTER

# 3

# *Antibiotic Use for Preventing Preterm Birth*

*Ronald S. Gibbs*

## BACKGROUND

Traditionally, prevention of preterm birth has relied on the use of tocolytic drugs. These agents have proved to have only marginal efficacy, however, because their administration is not based on the pathophysiology of preterm labor. Hence, it is not surprising that the prematurity rate in the United States has not decreased, even with the widespread use of tocolytic agents. As evidence has accumulated showing that infection and inflammation may cause 20% to 40% of preterm births, attention has turned to the use of antibiotics to prevent prematurity.

This chapter summarizes indications for use of antibiotics to prevent preterm births in three clinical situations: (1) during prenatal care, (2) in preterm labor with intact membranes, and (3) after preterm premature rupture of the membranes (PPROM).

## ANTIBIOTICS DURING PRENATAL CARE

During prenatal care, screening for and treating certain infections may be warranted to prevent preterm birth. The following are steps to consider.

### Sexually Transmitted Disease

In accordance with standard treatment recommendations, screen and treat patients for infections by *Neisseria gonorrhoeae* and *Chlamydia trachomatis* to prevent spread to the newborn or to sexual partners. Some nonrandomized trials suggest that this practice may have the additional benefit of reducing the risk of prematurity.

## Bacteriuria

To prevent pyelonephritis, also screen and treat pregnant women for bacteriuria. One meta-analysis concluded that bacteriuria is directly associated with preterm birth.

Asymptomatic group B streptococcal (GBS) bacteriuria, in particular, has been associated with preterm birth. Given that a treatment trial of patients with GBS bacteriuria showed a decrease in preterm delivery, it is recommended that this infection be treated as soon as recognized. Note, however, that no consistent association has been identified between maternal genital tract GBS colonization and adverse pregnancy outcome. In the Vaginal Infections and Prematurity (VIP) study, heavy GBS colonization—but not low-level colonization—was associated with increased low-birthweight preterm delivery. A concurrent randomized trial of colonized women, on the other hand, did not show a reduction in low-birthweight preterm delivery. Because of these conflicting reports, treatment of maternal genital tract colonization is not currently recommended during the antepartum period.

## Mycoplasma Colonization

Numerous studies have failed to establish a relationship between mycoplasma colonization of the genital tract and adverse pregnancy outcome. In the VIP study, which involved nearly 5,000 patients, no association was found between maternal genital tract colonization with *Ureaplasma urealyticum* and any major pregnancy outcome. In a concurrent multicenter trial of more than 900 patients, use of erythromycin to treat patients with *U. urealyticum* had no effect on adverse pregnancy outcomes. Accordingly, screening for or treating infection with *U. urealyticum* is not recommended for the specific purpose of preventing preterm birth.

## Bacterial Vaginosis

Defined by either clinical or clinical-plus-laboratory criteria, bacterial vaginosis (BV) has been consistently associated with preterm birth or low-birthweight pregnancies in numerous studies involving a variety of populations. In addition, two recent randomized clinical trials and a historically controlled trial showed a beneficial effect in prenatal treatment of women with BV who were at high risk for preterm birth (that is, patients who had a previous preterm pregnancy or certain other demographic factors).

No published trials support treatment of BV in women at low risk.

## *Trichomonas Vaginalis* Infection

Screen for and treat *Trichomonas vaginalis* infection in patients at high risk for preterm birth. This recommendation is based upon the significant association between *T. vaginalis* and adverse pregnancy outcome in some studies and the safety of treatment after the first trimester. No published trials support treatment of *T. vaginalis* as a means of preventing preterm birth.

# Antibiotics with Preterm Labor and Intact Membranes

Women who begin preterm labor with intact membranes should be given antibiotic prophylaxis to prevent neonatal GBS sepsis. In addition, use of antibiotics has been investigated for prolongation of pregnancy. Most trials of this treatment have been small and of limited statistical power. A meta-analysis of seven clinical trials involving 795 women concluded that treatment with antibiotics did not prolong pregnancy. Only two of the seven trials showed a significant delay in delivery. Furthermore, antibiotics did not significantly decrease the rate of chorioamnionitis, endometritis, maternal infection, neonatal death, neonatal sepsis, neonatal pneumonia, or necrotizing enterocolitis. Thus routine use of antibiotics to prolong pregnancy is not recommended in patients who have preterm labor but intact membranes.

Nevertheless, treatment should be provided for patients who have BV or *T. vaginalis* infection. This opinion is based on extrapolation of data from treatment during prenatal care.

## Antibiotics After PPROM

In cases of preterm premature rupture of the membranes, prescribe antibiotic prophylaxis to prevent neonatal GBS sepsis. Evidence published in the past three years from several trials also supports routine use of additional broad-spectrum antibiotic therapy to prolong pregnancy and to decrease complications in patients with PPROM. This recommendation is based on two meta-analyses and the recent Maternal–Fetal Medicine Network Trial published in 1997. In aggregate, these data demonstrate a significant reduction in delivery within 7 days as well as reductions in clinical chorioamnionitis, neonatal sepsis, neonatal pneumonia, intraventricular hemorrhage, and postpartum infections. Because broad-spectrum antibiotics have the potential to cause adverse effects, however, prescribe this therapy only for patients with PPROM between 24 and 32 weeks and for no more than 7 days. Antibiotic therapy might consist of ampicillin–amoxicillin plus erythromycin, as was used in the Maternal–Fetal Medicine Network trial. If BV is present, use clindamycin by itself or as a substitute for erythromycin for 7 days or less.

## Adverse Effects of Antibiotics

Some 15% to 30% of all pregnant women are now candidates for intrapartum prophylaxis to prevent GBS neonatal sepsis. Therefore, if these recommendations are implemented, a large percentage of pregnant women are likely to receive intrapartum antibiotic therapy. To date, major adverse effects associated with such treatment have been few. Nevertheless, it is essential to maintain close surveillance to monitor emergence of antibiotic-resistant bacteria and serious infections caused by these bacteria.

## Suggested Readings

Carey JV, Blackwelder WC, Nugent RP, et al. Antepartum cultures for *Ureaplasma urealyticum* are not useful in predicting pregnancy outcome. Am J Obstet Gynecol 1991;164:728–733.

Egarter C, Leitich H, Husslein P, et al. Adjunctive antibiotic treatment in preterm labor and neonatal morbidity: a meta-analysis. Obstet Gynecol 1996;88:303–309.

Egarter C, Leitich H, Karas H, et al. Antibiotic treatment in preterm premature rupture of membranes and neonatal morbidity: a meta-analysis. Am J Obstet Gynecol 1996;174:589–597.

Eschenbach DA, Nugent RP, Rao AV, et al. A randomized placebo-controlled trial of erythromycin for the treatment of *Ureaplasma urealyticum* to prevent premature delivery. Am J Obstet Gynecol 1991;164:734–742.

Gibbs RS, Eschenbach DA. The use of antibiotics to prevent preterm birth. Am J Obstet Gynecol 1997;177:375–380.

Hauth JC, Goldenberg RL, Andrews WW, et al. Reduced incidence of preterm delivery with metronidazole and erythromycin in women with bacterial vaginosis. N Engl J Med 1995;333:1732–1736.

Klebanoff MA, Regan JA, Rao V, et al. Outcome of the Vaginal Infections and Prematurity study: results of a clinical trial of erythromycin among pregnant women colonized with group B streptococci. Am J Obstet Gynecol 1995;172:1540–1545.

McGregor JA, French JI, Parker R, et al. Prevention of premature birth by screening and treatment for common genital tract infections: results of a prospective controlled evaluation. Am J Obstet Gynecol 1995;173:157–167.

Mercer BM, Arheart KL. Antimicrobial therapy in expectant management of preterm premature rupture of the membranes. Lancet 1995;346:1271–1279.

Mercer B, Miodovnik M, Thurnau G, et al. Antibiotic therapy for reduction of infant morbidity after preterm premature rupture of the membranes. JAMA 1997;278:989–995.

Morales WJ, Schorr S, Albritton J. Effect of metronidazole in patients with preterm birth in preceding pregnancy and bacterial vaginosis: a placebo-controlled, double-blind study. Am J Obstet Gynecol 1994;171:345–349.

Regan JA, Klebanoff MA, Nugent RP, et al. Colonization with group B streptococci in pregnancy and adverse outcome. Am J Obstet Gynecol 1996;174:1354–1360.

CHAPTER

# 4

# *Screening Techniques for Group B Streptococcal Infection*

*Robert S. McDuffie, Jr.*

## Background

During the past two decades, considerable information has emerged on the epidemiology and pathophysiology of neonatal group B streptococcal (GBS) sepsis. In 1992 and 1993, the American College of Obstetricians and Gynecologists (ACOG) and the American Academy of Pediatrics (AAP) issued separate recommendations for prevention of this occurrence (1,2). Subsequently, pressure from both consumers and providers of health care mounted for a national consensus on guidelines for prophylaxis (3). In 1996, the Centers for Disease Control and Prevention (CDC), with input from ACOG and AAP as well as the Infectious Diseases Society of Obstetrics and Gynecology (IDSOG) and the American College of Nurse-Midwives (ACNM), recommended strategies based entirely on either clinical risk factors or late prenatal culture at 35 to 37 weeks' gestation (4).

As consensus on prophylactic strategies has now been reached, techniques to screen for GBS should now receive greater attention. Although culture for GBS remains the "gold standard" screening technique, rapid tests for detection are desirable and may prove helpful in certain clinical situations. This chapter reviews the available methods for screening and examines their sensitivity, specificity, predictive values, and relevance to clinical practice.

## CULTURE

*Streptococcus agalactiae* is a facultative gram-positive *Diplococcus* that grows readily on blood agar. Colonies are small, gray-white, flat, and mucoid, and the characteristic finding of ß-hemolysis occurs in more than 99% of GBS isolates. In the laboratory, these characteristics are used to select colonies for identification. Presumptive identification of GBS includes nonserologic methods such as Gram's stain, a negative catalase test, and the Christie–Atkins–Munch–Peterson (CAMP) test. In the CAMP test, group B streptococci and *Staphylococcus aureus* are plated together. If synergistic hemolysis occurs, it points to presumptive identification of GBS. Many laboratories use a latex agglutination test for definitive identification.

The site of culture is important in the isolation of GBS. The highest yield of GBS comes from cultures of the distal vagina and anorectum. The rectal portion is important, because the intestine presumably serves as the reservoir for GBS; taking such a sample increases the positive yield by 5% to 25%. The yield is lower from the cervix than from the distal vagina or rectum. Decisions regarding prophylaxis should be based on the presence of the organism anywhere in the anogenital tract. For convenience, most authorities recommend a single culture collected using paired swabs from the distal vagina and anorectum.

The technique of culture affects the yield of GBS. The traditional culture medium is 5% sheep blood agar, but many studies indicate that selective medium enhances the detection of GBS by approximately 50%. The preferred medium (recommended by the CDC and ACOG) is Todd–Hewitt broth with nalidixic acid plus gentamicin or colistin (for example, Lim or SBM broth). The addition of these antibiotics inhibits the growth of both normal lower genital tract flora and gram-negative Enterobacteriaceae that may interfere with recovery of GBS. The selective broth medium is inoculated with swabs from the distal vagina and anorectum. If selective broth medium is not available, swabs can be placed in transport media (for example, Amies) that will maintain GBS viability for as long as four days. After 18 to 24 hours of incubation in selective broth medium, an aliquot is plated onto 5% sheep blood agar.

After another 24 hours, potential GBS colonies are evaluated according to their morphology and the presence of hemolysis, as discussed earlier.

Urine cultures for GBS deserve special mention. In early pregnancy, many women undergo screening of urinary cultures. If GBS is cultured from her urine, a woman should be considered to be colonized in the genital tract. Because this colonization often is heavy, positive urinary tract cultures represent a risk factor for neonatal GBS sepsis. Hence, a woman with a positive result would be a candidate for prophylaxis in either the culture-based or risk-factor–based protocol. In addition, mothers who have urine cultures positive for GBS should receive treatment, because GBS infection can lead to cystitis or pyelonephritis. A follow-up culture should be performed after treatment ends.

Culture remains the gold standard against which other methods for detecting GBS are compared. Although use of a selective broth medium increases the yield of GBS, culture requires approximately 48 hours to complete. In the culture-based scheme suggested by the CDC, cultures are obtained prior to the onset of labor at 35 to 37 weeks' gestation. This schedule leaves adequate time for culture processing, notification of the provider, notification of the patient, and transmission of the information to the labor and delivery unit. In several other circumstances, however, rapid techniques for identification of GBS may prove helpful—for example, women presenting in labor without prenatal care and women presenting in labor prior to the return of culture results. Ultimately, development of a rapid screening technique with high sensitivity, specificity, and predictive value would be of great benefit in addressing this infection.

## Rapid Techniques

In any discussion of rapid techniques as screening tests for GBS detection, three points must be kept in mind. First, a comparison with a gold standard (here culture) must be made. Second, to be considered effective, a screening test must have high sensitivity, specificity, and predictive value. Third, predictive

**Table 4-1.** Rapid Tests for Detection of Group B Streptococci

| Test | Sensitivity | Positive Predictive Value | Comment |
|---|---|---|---|
| Gram's stain | 34%–100% | 13%–33% | Low positive predictive values due to the presence of other gram-positive organisms. |
| Starch serum medium | 45%–98% | 65%–98% | Requires 12-hour incubation. Lower sensitivity if performed by nurses than by laboratory personnel. |
| Immunofluorescent antibody | 33%–81% | 89% | Requires 6 to 18 hours. Higher sensitivity only if incubation exceeds 12 hours. |
| Coagglutination/ latex agglutination | 4%–100% | 15%–100% | Lower sensitivity with light colonization. |
| Enzyme immunoassay | 11%–74% | 24%–100% | Lower sensitivity with light colonization. |
| Nucleic acid probe | 8.3%–95% | 61%–100% | Higher sensitivity after incubation. |

values will change according to the prevalence of the organism in the population. In populations where GBS prevalence is low (5% to 10%), predictive values may be much lower than in those where the prevalence is higher (30%). Table 4-1 summarizes the rapid tests available for detection of GBS.

## Gram's Stain

Because Gram's stain is widely available and inexpensive, and the test is rapidly performed, investigators have considered its use for GBS detection. The Vaginal Infections in Prematurity (VIP) study group addressed this issue by comparing vaginal Gram's stain results with cervical vaginal culture in 7755 women in the late second trimester and 1452 parturients. The rates of GBS colonization in these groups were 18.4% and 14.9%, respectively. The sensitivity, specificity, positive predictive values, and negative predictive values of the Gram's stain were 28%, 69%, 17%, and 81%, respectively, in the late second trimester and 34%, 72%, 18%, and 86%, respectively, at delivery. Thus the low overall sensitivity and low positive predictive value of Gram's stain when used in conjunction with the lower genital tract limit its effectiveness as a screening tool for GBS infection.

## Rapid Identification from Culture

Because culture methods take 24 to 48 hours to yield results, investigators have pursued other techniques for identifying GBS rapidly after a short incubation period. These techniques include methods based on the starch serum medium and use of immunofluorescent antibodies.

The *starch serum medium* uses a colorimetric assay to detect GBS. This technique takes advantage of the fact that GBS are the only streptococci that produce the carotenoid pigment, which produces a color change (from white to orange) after 6 to 12 hours of incubation. Although several studies of this method indicate that it offers excellent sensitivity, specificity, and positive and negative predictive values (93% to 98%, 98% to 99%, 83% to 98%, and 98% to 99%, respectively), two important limitations remain. First, if the clinician uses this test during labor to determine whether a patient is a candidate for GBS prophylaxis, many women will have delivered by the time the result becomes available. Second, skilled laboratory personnel are needed to interpret the test, and they are not available 24 hours per day. (In a study that compared interpretations by microbiologic technicians with those by nurses, sensitivity and positive predictive values were 30% to 50% lower when tests were read by the nursing staff.)

In the *immunofluorescent antibody* test, an aliquot of selective broth medium is mixed with type-specific GBS antisera conjugated with a fluorescein dye. The technologist then identifies organisms under fluorescent microscopy. Comparisons of immunofluorescence testing with vaginal culture have demonstrated a sensitivity of only 49% after 6 hours or less of incubation in selective medium, although the sensitivity increases considerably with periods of incubation lasting as long as 18 hours. Again, the need for skilled technicians and the impracticality of longer incubation periods limit the usefulness of this test in laboring patients.

## Direct Antigen Detection

Other tests detect GBS antigen directly from clinical specimens of the anogenital tract. Antigen detection techniques from vaginal and cervical swabs using commercially available kits include those based on coagglutination, latex particle agglutination, and enzyme immunoassay. In these techniques, incubation has been studied as an adjunct to direct detection from clinical specimens. Although many tests are available, none appears to be superior to the others. Without incubation, the tests' sensitivities range from 4% to 88%. After incubation, sensitivities improve considerably (5).

These assays detect GBS before growth amplification occurs, and they work best in patients with heavy colonization. Indeed, every study that has addressed colonization found higher sensitivity in women with heavy colonization compared with the overall group. This issue of organism number is clinically relevant because an estimated 10% to 30% of cases of early-onset neonatal sepsis occur in mothers who are lightly colonized. Thus the ideal screening test for GBS must detect both heavily and lightly colonized patients.

## Nucleic Acid Probes

In the 1990s, the use of molecular biologic techniques for detection of infection increased significantly. The practical limitations of the aforementioned tests have led to the development of molecular biologic techniques for detection of GBS carriage.

Yancey and colleagues evaluated the use of a DNA probe complementary to a GBS RNA sequence to detect carrier status (6). While a 2.5-hour incubation period yielded a sensitivity of only 44%, sensitivity increased to 71% after 3.5 hours of growth (specificity 90%, positive predictive value 61%, and negative predictive value 94%).

Rosa compared a commercially available DNA-based kit with GBS culture on a selective agar plate (7). The sensitivity of this test for GBS from a lower vaginal perineal swab was 8.3% without incubation and 81% after 16 to 24 hours of growth.

Kircher recently examined another commercially available kit and compared results of vaginal and rectal swabs from 402 pregnant women during the third trimester with detection of GBS ribosomal RNA (rRNA) (8). While a 3-hour enrichment protocol produced a sensitivity of 73%, an 8-hour protocol achieved a sensitivity of 95%.

The need for specialized laboratory personnel and a significant incubation period to rule out light colonization preclude the use of nucleic acid probes for women in active labor. Thus a significant unmet needs remains—a sensitive and specific test that is not labor-intensive and can provide results to clinicians within one hour.

## Conclusion

Culture for GBS remains the gold standard screening technique. The use of selective broth medium enhances the rate of detection of GBS by nearly 50%. Both the distal vagina and anorectum should be swabbed.

As a group, rapid screening techniques applied after a short incubation period lack the consistent sensitivity and positive predictive values necessary to enable clinical decision making during labor. Furthermore, by the time results return, many multiparous women will have delivered. The inability of these tests to detect women with light colonization represents another major concern. With prolonged incubation, however, the sensitivity, specificity, and predictive values of some rapid tests improve greatly. Although the use of rapid tests remains problematic in labor, future analyses may determine whether these techniques can replace cultures with selective broth media in the outpatient setting.

### References

1. American College of Obstetricians and Gynecologists. Universal antepartum screening for maternal GBS not recommended. ACOG Newsletter 1993;37.

2. Committee on Infectious Diseases and Committee on Fetus and Newborn. Guidelines for prevention of group B streptococcal (GBS) infection by chemoprophylaxis. Pediatrics 1992;90:775–777.
3. Association of Trial Lawyers of America. Wake-up call for expectant parents. ATLA Alert Oct. 22, 1992.
4. Centers for Disease Control and Prevention. Prevention of perinatal group B streptococcal disease: a public-health perspective. MMWR 1996;46(RR-7):1–24.
5. Yancey MK, Armer T, Clark P, et al. Assessment of rapid identification tests for genital carriage of group B streptococci. Obstet Gynecol 1992;80:1038–1047.
6. Yancey MK, Clark P, Armer T, et al. Use of a DNA probe for the rapid detection of group B streptococci in obstetric patients. Obstet Gynecol 1993;81:635–640.
7. Rosa C, Clark P, Duff P. Performance of a new DNA probe for the detection of group B streptococcal colonization of the genital tract. Obstet Gynecol 1995;86:509–511.
8. Kircher SM, Meyer MP, Jordan JA. Comparison of a modified DNA hybridization assay with standard culture enrichment for detecting group B streptococci in obstetric patients. J Clin Microbiol 1996;34:342–344.

CHAPTER

# 5

# *Group B Streptococcal Infections in Pregnancy*

*John W. Larsen, Jr.*

## Background and Incidence

The group B *Streptococcus* (GBS) is the leading bacterial cause of neonatal sepsis, as well as a common cause of maternal peripartum infections. Approximately 8000 cases of early-onset neonatal sepsis occur in the United States each year. Some 10% to 30% of women carry GBS in their urogenital or lower gastrointestinal tracts. Usually, however, no clinical manifestations of GBS disease are noted prior to parturition.

Vertical transmission of colonization to the baby occurs at parturition in approximately 50% of cases. The overall attack rate of about 1.8/1000 live births increases to about 41/1000 if clinical risk factors such as prematurity, amniorrhexis, and maternal fever during labor are present. In its most severe form, early-onset neonatal GBS disease is a fulminant syndrome characterized by sepsis, pneumonia, and meningitis, with a high rate of fatality or residual damage.

Maternal disease usually takes a less severe form, appearing as chorioamnionitis, urinary tract infection (UTI), puerperal endometritis, or wound infection. Maternal GBS infections unrelated to UTI often are polymicrobial, involving other aerobic and anaerobic bacteria common to the pelvis.

## Diagnosis

Cultures should be performed in a manner that will produce the highest yield of positive results. For screening, sample the lower vagina and the anorectum—*not* the endocervix, as is done for gonococcal or chlamydial infection. Instruct the laboratory to use selective broth medium for 18 to 24 hours before plating onto blood agar (instead of using sheep blood agar or selective solid medium alone). This practice can increase the yield of screening cultures by as much as 50%.

Since studies have suggested that maternal genital colonization with GBS is an intermittent phenomenon, a culture-based strategy offers the best predictive value if sampling takes place within 5 weeks of parturition. The Centers for Disease Control and Prevention (CDC) recommends that screening cultures for GBS be performed at 35 to 37 weeks' gestation. This timing was selected to enhance the likelihood that results would be accurate and complete at the expected time of labor.

Several nonculture rapid tests for GBS have been devised. Current limitations of rapid methods are low sensitivity and low predictive value of a negative test, as compared with cultures in selective broth media. Nevertheless, a positive result of a rapid test is highly predictive and can be used as a basis for antibiotic treatment.

It is not necessary to perform screening cultures of the vagina and rectum for women who have previously given birth to a baby with GBS disease or women with previously demonstrated GBS bacteriuria. Both these groups should be considered to be GBS-positive and offered intrapartum antibiotic chemoprophylaxis.

Acceptable clinical practice is to evaluate the potential for GBS disease without screening cultures by implementing antibiotic chemoprophylaxis at the time of amniorrhexis or parturition, as indicated by clinical risk factors alone (Table 5-1). You should, however, honor requests of patients who ask for GBS testing.

## Management

The CDC, American Academy of Pediatrics, American College of Obstetricians and Gynecologists, and community

**Table 5-1.** Clinical Risk Factors for GBS Disease in Neonates*

| |
|---|
| Previous infant with invasive GBS disease |
| Temperature ≥ 38 °C (100.4 °F) |
| Amniorrhexis ≥ 18 hours |
| Delivery at < 37 completed weeks of gestation |
| Maternal history of GBS bacteriuria |

* If one or more of these factors is present, give penicillin or ampicillin intravenously at parturition (see Table 5-2).

groups have worked together to devise strategies for reducing the threat of perinatal GBS disease. All approaches have been keyed to optimizing antibiotic chemoprophylaxis or treatment of disease in its early stages. Giving penicillin or ampicillin intravenously during labor has been shown to be highly effective for preventing transmission of GBS from mother to baby and reducing the frequency of neonatal sepsis. Unfortunately, all antibiotic strategies have been hampered by an inability to eradicate GBS from a colonized mother before labor. The clinician managing obstetric patients must therefore select a strategy for GBS screening. Two approaches are acceptable:

- A strategy based on culture results at 35 to 37 weeks' gestation
- A strategy that bases the chemoprophylaxis decision on risk factors without culture

The following five scenarios represent the common clinical situations in GBS management:

1. ***Unknown maternal GBS status.*** Initiate intravenous antibiotics if one or more of the following clinical risk factors are present (Table 5-2):
   - Labor at less than 37 completed gestational weeks
   - Amniorrhexis at less than 37 completed weeks (treat for one week and reevaluate)*
   - GBS bacteriuria during pregnancy

* This recommendation goes beyond the current CDC guidelines and is based on the 1997 report of the Maternal–Fetal Medicine Units Network, which showed a benefit from antibiotic use for preterm amniorrhexis occurring between 24 and 32 weeks' gestation (JAMA 1997;278:989–995).

**Table 5-2.** Antibiotics for Intravenous Use Against GBS

| Agent | Comment |
|---|---|
| Penicillin G | Recommended for intrapartum chemoprophylaxis; give 5 million units IV to start, followed by 2.5 million units every 4 hours until delivery. |
| Ampicillin | May be used as an alternative for chemoprophylaxis and may be preferred for broader coverage based on clinical indications. Give 2 g IV to start, followed by 1 g every 4 hours until delivery. |
| Clindamycin or erythromycin | These drugs may be effective for penicillin-allergic patients; no data available directly support these agents' clinical effectiveness for this particular use. There is some concern that customary maternal doses may not achieve therapeutic levels in the baby.<br>*Clindamycin regimen*: 900 mg IV to start, followed by 900 mg every 8 hours until delivery.<br>*Erythromycin regimen*: 500 mg IV to start, followed by 500 mg every 6 hours until delivery. |

- Duration of amniorrhexis 18 hours or more before delivery
- Intrapartum temperature 38 °C or higher
- History of previous infant with invasive GBS disease

2. ***Prior newborn infected by GBS.*** Give intravenous antibiotic prophylaxis during labor or at the time of amniorrhexis (see Table 5-2). Further testing for GBS is unnecessary.
3. ***Positive maternal GBS test.*** Provide intravenous antibiotic prophylaxis during labor or at amniorrhexis if it occurs prior to labor (see Table 5-2). Antepartum oral antibiotics are not recommended for asymptomatic women with positive vaginal/rectal cultures. A urine culture that is positive for GBS indicates that treatment should be given at any time during pregnancy. If a GBS test was positive in a prior pregnancy, consider the patient to be still positive in the current pregnancy; additional GBS testing is therefore unnecessary. Note that this practice goes beyond the CDC guidelines on prevention of perinatal GBS disease so as to avoid missing patients who have false-negative tests.
4. ***Negative maternal GBS test.*** If the mother's intrapartum temperature during labor is 38 °C or higher and intrauterine

infection cannot be excluded, give intravenous antibiotics, presuming that amniotic fluid infection is present. Treat these patients with a broad-spectrum antibiotic that would cover GBS if the prior test for GBS was falsely negative.

5. ***Repeat cesarean section, no labor, membranes intact.*** In this case, no antibiotics are needed before the incision, even if the patient is known to be GBS-positive.

## Communication Issues

Effectiveness of management is enhanced by good communications among clinical caregivers, laboratory personnel, and patients. Specifically:

1. Laboratory results should be communicated to the obstetrician and hospital where the patient is expected to deliver.
2. Pediatricians should be informed about the mother's GBS status, whether she has been tested, and what antibiotics she has been given, if any.
3. Patients should be informed about their GBS status and the proposed intrapartum antibiotic regimen, if a culture-based strategy is used.

### Suggested Reading

American Academy of Pediatrics Committee on Infectious Diseases and Committee on Fetus and Newborn. Revised guidelines for prevention of early-onset group B streptococcal (GBS) infection. Pediatrics 1997;99:489–496.

Boyer KM, Gotoff SP. Prevention of early-onset neonatal group B streptococcal disease with selective intrapartum chemoprophylaxis. N Engl J Med 1986;314:1665–1669.

Centers for Disease Control and Prevention. Prevention of perinatal group B streptococcal disease: a public health perspective. MMWR 1996;45(RR-7):1–24.

Mercer BM, Miodovnik M, Thurnau GR, et al., for the National Institute of Child Health and Human Development Maternal-Fetal Medicine Units Network. Antibiotic therapy for reduction of infant mortality after preterm premature rupture of the membranes. JAMA 1997; 278:989–995.

Minkoff H, Mead P. An obstetric approach to the prevention of early-onset group B ß-hemolytic streptococcal sepsis. Am J Obstet Gynecol 1986;154:973–977.

Thomsen AC, Mørup L, Hansen KB. Antibiotic elimination of group B streptococci in urine in prevention of preterm labour. Lancet 1987;1:591–593.

Yancey MK, Schuchat A, Brown LK, et al. The accuracy of late antenatal screening cultures in predicting genital group B streptococcal colonization at delivery. Obstet Gynecol 1996;88:811–815.

CHAPTER

# 6

# *Prevention of Perinatal Septicemia*

*Gilles R. G. Monif*

## Background and Incidence

The term "neonatal septicemia" has been used to denote vascular invasion by a bacterial agent in the first 28 days of life. Bacteriologically proven neonatal septicemia is a rare event, occurring in one to five cases per 1000 live births (1,2). Although the incidence of proven newborn bacterial septicemia is low, the resultant mortality ranges from 30% to 50% (2,3).

Prior to 1986, cases of neonatal bacterial septicemia occurring in the first week of life were termed "early-onset." The pathogenesis of early-onset disease is associated primarily with maternal factors such as prolonged rupture of fetal membranes, chorioamnionitis, maternal urinary tract infection, or maternal fever in labor. Septicemia occurring after the first seven days of life (late-onset disease) primarily results from nosocomial disease occurring in debilitated, mechanically damaged, or anatomically compromised babies (3–6). Subsequent analysis of cases occurring in the first seven days of life has demonstrated an intermixing of these diverging pathogeneses.

To define a more homogeneous group for which more rigorous prevention guidelines could be formulated, the term "perinatal septicemia" was introduced. Perinatal septicemia identifies cases of septicemia occurring in the first 24 to 36 hours of life. With the exception of cases caused by hematogenous dissemination, the pathogenesis of this entity is tightly correlated with maternal factors that result in amniotic fluid colonization or infection. The pathogenesis of cases of infectious seticemia occurring after 36 hours is related to maternal factors, although the majority have a nosocomial origin. This relative homogeneity of pathogenesis has allowed better elucidation of prime etiologic agents and potential therapeutic intervention points.

## Epidemiology

The epidemiology of perinatal septicemia has significantly changed with time. In the 1960s and 1970s, most neonatal bacterial septicemia occurred in the first week of life. In recent years, however, technological advances in neonatology and neonatal intensive care have enabled more low-birthweight, anatomically compromised babies to survive. Consequently, the prevalence of disease has shifted into the late-onset group.

Prior to the 1980s, the predominant cause of perinatal septicemia was the Enterobacteriaceae. As screening for asymptomatic bacteriuria has diminished the prevalence of cases due to *Escherichia coli*, *Klebsiella pneumoniae*, *Proteus mirabilis*, and *Enterobacter* species, group B streptococci (GBS) have emerged as the major cause of this infection.

## Bacteriology

Table 6-1 lists the principal endogenous and exogenous bacteria isolated from septicemic infants in the first 36 hours after birth (1–7). More than 80% of isolates in cases of perinatal septicemia come from the endogenous group (1–7).

With the exception of *Neisseria gonorrhoeae*, the exogenous perinatal pathogens share an ability to induce a sustained maternal septicemia. Hematogenous dissemination to the products of conception has been documented for *Listeria monocytogenes*, *Haemophilus influenzae*, *Salmonella typhi*, other *Salmonella* species, and *Streptococcus pneumoniae.* For exogenous bacteria, hematogenous involvement of the products of conception is as valid a mechanism as ascending infection.

The group B streptococci and the Enterobacteriaceae account for approximately 85% of the cases of perinatal septicemia

**Table 6-1.** Bacteria Associated with Perinatal Septicemia

| |
|---|
| **Endogenous** |
| *Bacteroides* species |
| *Enterobacter* species |
| *Escherichia coli* |
| *Gardnerella vaginalis* |
| Group B, G, and D streptococci |
| *Klebsiella pneumoniae* |
| *Proteus mirabilis* |
| **Exogenous** |
| Group A and group G streptococci |
| *Haemophilus influenzae* |
| *Listeria monocytogenes* |
| *Neisseria gonorrhoeae* |
| *Salmonella typhi* |
| *Salmonella* species |
| *Streptococcus pneumoniae* |

due to endogenous bacteria. These organisms are present as constituents of the bacterial flora of the female genital tract in 14% to 28% and 18% to 35% of women, respectively; nevertheless, perinatal septicemia due to these organisms remains rare, with incidences of one in 250 to 300 deliveries and one in 450 to 600 deliveries, respectively. What ultimately governs the incidence of disease in a given institution are the obstetric management and prenatal monitoring protocols used for GBS and asymptomatic bacteriuria.

## Pathogenesis

### Amniotic Fluid Infection

The principal mechanism for the induction of perinatal septicemia involves amniotic fluid replication, ascending infection, or both. With rupture of the fetal membranes or effective cervical dilatation via labor, the probability of amniotic fluid colonization is directly correlated with the duration of one or both of these events. At the end of 24 hours following rupture of the fetal membranes, 65% or more of amniotic fluid specimens obtained by amniocentesis will yield one or more species of bacteria. Infection of the amniotic fluid is a relatively common phenomenon, but clinically overt chorioamnionitis appears in only a small percentage of these women.

A somewhat similar disassociation exists between amniotic fluid infection and perinatal septicemia. If one does a back-titration from cases of perinatal septicemia and analyzes the obstetric factors prevalent in these cases, the overwhelming majority of infants are found to have been born to women whose membranes had been ruptured for more than eight hours. The variability introduced by strain virulence and level of bacterial replication within amniotic fluid are presumed to account for the relative lack of correlation between colonization and the induction of disease. When present within amniotic fluid, exogenous pathogenic bacteria are much more likely to induce disease than are the more common constituents of the female genital tract (other than GBS and the Enterobacteriaceae).

## Asymptomatic Bacteriuria

The association of asymptomatic bacteriuria and with septicemia is more inferential than documented. The ability to attach the uroepithelial cells has been demonstrated to be a marker of virulence. The same organism isolated from urine invariably appears in the bacterial flora of the female genital tract. Ensuing neonatal disease is most probable when GBS causes asymptomatic bacteriuria. Asymptomatic bacteriuria is the factor most closely correlated with maternal gram-negative septicemia in the immediate perinatal period following spontaneous vaginal delivery. The same O or K and flagella types present in urine can be demonstrated in the corresponding endometrial and blood samples (8, 9).

## Maternal Infection

Maternal parturitional infection acts as a strong marker for potential perinatal septicemia. In 2586 deliveries taking place within a two-year period, eight cases of perinatal septicemia occurred—all to mothers who had experienced prolonged rupture of the fetal membranes. Four of these eight mothers had clinically overt chorioamnionitis. These four cases represented 22% of the progeny of women with clinically overt chorioamnionitis in these timeframes. Maternal therapy had been delayed until cord clamping or postdelivery.

## Treatment

Various studies have compared the outcomes in women with chorioamnionitis who did not receive antibiotic therapy before parturition with the outcomes of such patients who received ampicillin and gentamicin therapy for at least three hours. In one study, 5 of the 26 neonates whose mothers had not received antibiotic therapy were documented to have perinatal septicemia caused by GBS, *E. coli*, *K. pneumoniae*, *H. influenzae*, and *Gardnerella vaginalis*. In the case of perinatal septicemia due to *E. coli*, the mother developed chorioamnionitis while she was in the hospital with premature and prolonged rupture of the fetal membranes. A maternal urine culture demonstrated more than 100,000 colony-forming units of *E. coli* with sensitivities identical to those of the septicemic isolate. Of the 17 premature and 23 term infants born to mothers with chorioamnionitis who received ampicillin and gentamicin therapy at least three hours prior to parturition, none exhibited infectious morbidity in the immediate neonatal period.

Many of the studies of perinatal septicemia have focused on the effect of antibiotic therapy. The outcome of perinatal septicemia with onset in the immediate postpartum period, but not *in utero*, is closely tied to how quickly the patient receives appropriate antibiotic therapy. If appropriate therapy is implemented within three hours of the onset of signs or symptoms, then the probability that the baby will survive and remain free of long-term sequelae is very good. If more than three hours have elapsed, that probability falls dramatically—into the neighborhood of 35%.

## Prevention

### Prolonged Rupture of Membranes

The prospective risk criteria developed for GBS antibiotic prophylaxis are applicable to the Enterobacteriaceae. For maximum effectiveness in treating perinatal septicemia, the broadest spectrum of coverage achievable is advocated. Aggressive use of a broad-spectrum antibiotic effective against *E. coli*, *Salmonella* species, *L. monocytogenes*, and *H. influenzae* will markedly reduce the incidence of perinatal septicemia. The cephalosporins are not effective against *L. monocytogenes*.

Preterm premature rupture of the fetal membranes should be an indication for antibiotic prophylaxis (10–13). In the author's experience, the single greatest risk factor for perinatal septicemia is prolonged rupture of the membranes, and antibiotic prophylaxis should be used in this clinical situation as well (9). Drug administration should be continued until the results of admission cultures become available.

## Asymptomatic Bacteriuria

All pregnant women should be screened for asymptomatic bacteriuria using appropriate culture techniques. When asymptomatic bacteriuria is documented, a test of cure is imperative. Women with a history of multiple episodes of urinary tract infection should be rescreened at 36 weeks' gestation, irrespective of the initial culture results. Women with a history of multiple episodes of pyelonephritis should be serially monitored throughout their pregnancies.

## Chorioamnionitis

A major issue for perinatologists and neonatologists has been the point at which to institute antibiotic therapy for a woman with chorioamnionitis. In many institutions, when delivery is imminent, maternal therapy is delayed until the umbilical cord is clamped, so as to avoid influencing the neonatal cultures. Other facilities advocate delaying maternal therapy until the cord is clamped to preclude sending a child into the intensive care nursery with suboptimal serum/tissue concentration of an antibiotic, which might induce resistance among the Enterobacteriaceae.

Once the diagnosis of chorioamnionitis is made, regardless of the possibility of early delivery, women with chorioamnionitis should receive prompt antibiotic therapy. The selection of antibiotic therapy for maternal disease should be consistent with the preferences of newborn intensive care personnel. The pharmacokinetics should be such that not only fetal blood levels, but also amniotic fluid levels are rapidly achieved.

## References


1. St. Geme JW III, Polin RA. Neonatal sepsis: progress in diagnosis and management. Drugs 1988;36:784–800.
2. Polin RA, St. Geme JW III. Neonatal sepsis. Adv Pediatr Infect Dis J 1992;7:25–61.
3. Bada HS, Alojipan LC, Andrews BF. Premature rupture of membranes and its effects on the newborn. Pediatr Clin North Am 1977;24:491–500.
4. Bergqvist G, Eriksson M, Zelterstrom R. Neonatal septicemia and perinatal risk factors. Acta Pediatr Scand 1979;68:337–339.
5. Eriksson M. Neonatal septicemia. Acta Pediatr Scand 1983;72:1–8.
6. Hurley R. Neonatal septicaemia and meningitis. J Hosp Infect 1982;3:323–328.
7. Klein JO. Bacteriology of neonatal sepsis. Pediatr Infect Dis J 1990;9:778.
8. Monif GRG. Intrapartum bacteriuria and postpartum endometritis. Obstet Gynecol 1991;78:245–248.
9. Monif GR, Hume H Jr, Goodlin RC. Neonatal considerations in the management of premature rupture of the fetal membranes. Obstet Gynecol Surv 1986;41:531–537.
10. Mercer BM, Miodovnik M, Thurnau GR, et al. Antibiotic therapy for reduction of infant morbidity after preterm premature rupture of membranes. JAMA 1997;278:989–995.
11. Lovett SM, Weiss JD, Diogo MJ, et al. A prospective, double-blind, randomized, controlled clinical trial of ampicillin-sulbactam for preterm premature rupture of membranes in women receiving antenatal corticosteroid therapy. Am J Obstet Gynecol 1997;176:1030–1038.
12. Mercer BM, Arheart KL. Antimicrobial therapy in expectant management of preterm premature rupture of the membranes. Lancet 1995;346:1271–1279.
13. Egarter C, Leitich H, Karas H, et al. Antibiotic treatment in preterm premature rupture of membranes and neonatal morbidity: a meta-analysis. Am J Obstet Gynecol 1996;174:589–597.

CHAPTER

7

# Postpartum Endometritis

*J. M. Ernest*
*Philip B. Mead*

## Background and Incidence

Postpartum infection of the uterus, a condition that is the most common reason for puerperal fever, indicates the presence of endometritis, endomyometritis, or endoparametritis, depending on its severity. Cesarean section delivery causes most of these infections, especially when the procedure is performed after labor or when membranes have been ruptured and nonelective cesarean section is undertaken. Other possible predeterminants of postcesarean endometritis include bacterial vaginosis, numerous vaginal examinations, use of internal fetal monitoring, and low neonatal birthweight.

The reported incidence of these conditions occurring after vaginal delivery ranges from 0.9% to 3.9%; after cesarean section, it increases dramatically—from 10% in the private-care sector to 50% or higher in large teaching services that care for indigent patients. Although prolonged membrane rupture, anemia, midforceps delivery, and maternal soft-tissue trauma are known to predispose patients who deliver vaginally to postpartum endometritis, these factors are not identified in most patients who develop this infection. In addition, indigent patients have a substantially higher risk of developing endometritis after vaginal or cesarean section delivery, though the reasons for this increase have never been clearly delineated.

## Etiology

Endometritis is a polymicrobial infection caused by a wide variety of bacteria commonly found in the vagina, including group B streptococci, enterococci, other aerobic streptococci, *Gardnerella vaginalis*, *Escherichia coli*, *Prevotella bivius*, *Bacteroides* species, and peptostreptococci. Group B streptococci and *G. vaginalis* are the most common pathogens isolated from infected patients' blood.

It appears that *Ureaplasma urealyticum* and *Mycoplasma hominis* cause the infection as well, as these organisms have been isolated from the endometrium and blood of patients with endometritis. Favorable clinical responses, however, have been achieved in women who have had mycoplasmas cultured from their blood but who received antibiotics that did not affect these organisms.

*Chlamydia trachomatis* is associated with a late form of endometritis that appears between two days to five weeks postpartum in women who deliver vaginally. Group A ß-hemolytic streptococcal endometritis is rare and epidemiologically unique—it is caused by exogenous infection, most often transmitted by caregivers, and is characterized by early onset and rapid progression with poor localization.

## Diagnosis

A fever of 38.5 °C (101.3 °F) or higher anytime during the first 24 hours postpartum or one of 38.0 °C (100.4 °F) or higher that occurs more than 24 hours after delivery and lasts for at least 4 consecutive hours suggests endometritis. Other signs include uterine tenderness, lower abdominal pain, and leukocytosis.

When you suspect endometritis, the following diagnostic techniques and management plan are recommended:

1. Rule out other causes of fever before treating the patient for endometritis; this infection is rare after uncomplicated vaginal delivery. Carefully determine whether the fever is caused by retained placental fragments and, if so, perform uterine curettage.

2. If the patient has postpartum fever, consider other possible causes. The differential diagnosis can include urinary tract infection, appendicitis, viral syndrome, pneumonia (particularly common in women who are smokers and were given general anesthesia), and noninfectious fever caused by a drug reaction or breast engorgement, which rarely exceeds 38 °C (100.4 °F).

3. Some clinicians do not perform endometrial cultures in the course of selecting therapy for postpartum fever. In fact, because most therapy for postpartum endometritis is empiric, the results of endometrial cultures may not change the antibiotic selected. In addition, vaginal flora could possibly contaminate endometrial specimens.

To increase the likelihood of obtaining an uncontaminated sample, use the following technique when taking cultures. First, perform a pelvic examination after placing the patient on an appropriate examining table. With a speculum, visualize the cervix, wipe it with sponges or cotton balls to remove extraneous secretions, and obtain endocervical swabs for *C. trachomatis* and *Neisseria gonorrhoeae*, if indicated. Next, cleanse the cervix with povidone iodine-soaked gauze and obtain endometrial cultures with a cotton-tipped swab grasped in a sponge forceps. Place the swab directly into an aerobic/anaerobic tube containing transport media and immediately send it to the laboratory.

Alternatively, double- or triple-lumen brush cultures or aspirates of amniotic fluid with a cannula can be used. Obtain cultures or rapid antigen detection tests for *C. trachomatis* from patients with late-onset infection or those at high risk for chlamydial colonization (for example, pregnant teenagers or women with a history of multiple sexual partners). Examine the vagina and perineum to exclude an infected laceration or episiotomy site.

4. Perform a bimanual examination to determine uterine size, consistency, and tenderness as well as to rule out an adnexal mass or pelvic abscess. A rectal exam can eliminate suspicion of an infected episiotomy or cul-de-sac abscess.

5. Obtain a complete blood count and two sets of blood cultures. Blood is an important source for cultures, because 10% to 20% of patients with postpartum endometritis have a documentable bacteremia, which is not predictive of the

severity of clinical illness nor of the length of clinical recovery. If pneumonia is suspected, as it would be with auscultatory findings in a smoker who has received general anesthesia, perform a chest X ray as well.

## Treatment

Patients can be classified as having mild/moderate or severe endometritis based on their clinical course or findings such as general systemic toxicity, increased pulse pattern, and fever.

Treat patients who have severe endometritis but normal renal function with a regimen of clindamycin (900 mg IV every 8 hours) plus gentamicin (loading dose of 2.0 mg/kg IV, followed by a maintenance dose of 1.5 mg/kg IV every 8 hours). Gentamicin also may be given as a single daily dose of 5 mg/kg. Note that gentamicin and clindamycin can be combined in the same intravenous solution. Some clinicians add ampicillin to this regimen to cover enterococci early in the course of treatment. An alternative regimen relies on imipenem (500 mg IV every 6 hours).

For mild to moderate cases, use an extended-spectrum cephalosporin or penicillin, such as one of the following agents:

- Cefoxitin, 2.0 g IV every 6 hours
- Cefotetan, 2.0 g IV every 12 hours
- Piperacillin, 4.0 g IV every 6 hours
- Ampicillin/sulbactam, 3.0 g IV every 6 hours
- Mezlocillin, 4.0 g IV every 6 hours
- Ticarcillin/clavulanic acid, 3.1 g IV every 4 to 6 hours

Theoretically, the same antibiotic that was used as prophylaxis at the time of cord clamping should not be used for therapy.

Continue parenteral therapy until the patient's temperature has remained below 37.5 °C (99.5 °F) for 24 to 48 hours and she is free of pain. It is unnecessary to use oral antibiotics after discharge.

Women whose cultures are positive for *C. trachomatis* and who have been treated with a ß-lactam antibiotic should receive erythromycin or doxycycline therapy for 10 days, even if they show an initial clinical response. (If they have received a clindamycin-containing regimen, which is effective for *C. trachomatis*, they would need to complete 10 days of therapy with clindamycin, doxycycline, or erythromycin.)

For patients who receive aminoglycosides, perform a creatinine determination every other day. After 24 hours of therapy, adjust the gentamicin maintenance doses such that peak dosage (5 to 8 μg/mL) is reached 15 to 30 minutes after the end of a 30-minute infusion and trough level (less than 1 μg/mL) is reached immediately before the next dose. Patients with diminished renal function can receive aztreonam (2 g IV every 6 to 8 hours) as an alternative to gentamicin. Aztreonam is a monocyclic ß-lactam agent with a spectrum of activity similar to that of gentamicin.

## Antimicrobial Failure

Enterococcal superinfection or inadequate coverage of a multiresistant anaerobe is usually the cause of antimicrobial therapy failure. In particular, enterococcal superinfection is suggested when the patient fails to respond to antimicrobials or relapses while taking drugs that are ineffective against enterococci (cephalosporins, clindamycin plus gentamicin), especially if this organism is isolated in pure culture or grows heavily in an endometrial specimen. If you suspect enterococcal superinfection, administer one of the following regimens:

- Clindamycin or metronidazole plus ampicillin plus gentamicin
- Ampicillin/sulbactam
- Cefoxitin or cefotetan plus ampicillin
- Piperacillin
- Mezlocillin
- Ticarcillin/clavulanic acid

Patients who experience antimicrobial failure because of a lack of coverage for a multiresistant anaerobe often respond to a regimen containing metronidazole, clindamycin, or imipenem.

If fever persists despite the administration of appropriate antimicrobial therapy, search for a hidden abscess by evaluating the abdominal wound and performing a bimanual examination.

If the physical examination fails to reveal a suspected wound infection or abscess, use ultrasonography or computed tomography (CT). In the event of either condition, surgical drainage usually is necessary.

Patients in whom an abscess has been ruled out but who remain febrile with hectic fever spikes must be evaluated for possible septic pelvic thrombophlebitis or puerperal ovarian vein thrombosis. Although patients with septic pelvic thrombophlebitis have a plateau tachycardia and often a mild ileus, they otherwise may appear well despite a high fever pattern. Women with puerperal ovarian vein thrombosis typically present with right paramedian pain that develops on the second or third postpartum day. In 50% of these patients, a tender mass is palpable just to the right of the uterine fundus. CT or MRI scans may be necessary to make the diagnosis. Treatment of either condition with full IV heparin anticoagulation usually will relieve fever within 48 hours.

If group A ß-hemolytic streptococci are isolated from more than one patient over a brief timespan, do the following:

- Notify local health authorities.
- Isolate all infected patients for 24 hours after the start of effective therapy.
- Establish a cohort nursery system.
- Culture all involved professional and other hospital staff, and relieve from duty any who have positive results.
- Culture all newborns for group A streptococci.
- Consider stringent reduction of visitors.
- Stress rigid adherence to aseptic technique, especially handwashing.
- Save all positive group A streptococcal isolates for typing.

## Prophylaxis

Antibiotic prophylaxis at the time of cord clamping (to prevent fetal exposure) has been shown to reduce the incidence of postpartum endometritis in both elective and emergent cesarean section. The small risk of allergic reaction is outweighed by the greater benefit of reducing postpartum morbidity due to endometritis. Both lavage and intravenous routes of administration have been reported, and many antibiotics have been used. A first-generation cephalosporin given intravenously usually proves to be an adequate prophylactic regimen. Consider antibiotic prophylaxis for all cesarean section patients.

## Suggested Readings

Currier JS, Tosteson TD, Platt R. Cefozolin compared to cefoxiten for cesarean section prophylaxis: the use of a two-stage study design. J Clin Epidemiol 1993;46:625–630.

Del Priore G, Jackson-Stone M, Shim EK, et al. A comparison of once-daily and 8-hour gentamicin dosing in the treatment of postpartum endometritis. Obstet Gynecol 1996;87:994–1000.

Duff P. Antibiotic selection for infections in obstetric patients. Semin Perinatol 1993;17:367–378.

Hager WD, Pascuzzi M, Vernon M. Efficacy of oral antibiotics following parenteral antibiotics for serious infections in obstetrics and gynecology. Obstet Gynecol 1989;73:326–329.

Hoyme UB, Kiviat N, Eschenbach DA. Microbiology and treatment of late postpartum endometritis. Obstet Gynecol 1986;68:226–232.

Keogh J, MacDonald D, Kelehan P. Septic pelvic thrombophlebitis: an unusual treatable postpartum complication. Aust N Z J Gynaecol 1993;33:204–207.

Lev-Toaff AS, Baka JJ, Toaff ME, et al. Diagnostic imaging in puerperal febrile morbidity. Obstet Gynecol 1991;78:50–55.

Nathan L, Peters MT, Ahmed AM, et al. The return of life-threatening puerperal sepsis caused by group A streptococci. Am J Obstet Gynecol 1993;169:571–572.

Watts DH, Eschenbach DA, Kenny GE. Early postpartum endometritis: the role of bacteria, genital mycoplasmas, and *Chlamydia trachomatis*. Obstet Gynecol 1989;73:52–60.

CHAPTER

# 8

# *Lower Urinary Tract Infections in Pregnancy*

*S. Gene McNeeley, Jr.*
*David C. Kmak*

## Background and Incidence

Urinary tract infection (UTI) is one of the most common medical complications occurring in pregnancy (1). The majority of such infections remain confined to the lower urinary tract and are classified as asymptomatic bacteriuria in asymptomatic cases or cystitis in symptomatic cases. Approximately 5% to 7% of pregnant women have asymptomatic bacteriuria at their first prenatal visit. The prevalence of bacteriuria in pregnancy matches that seen in nonpregnant patients; it also reflects prior colonization rather than acquisition after pregnancy (2). The prevalence of bacteriuria in the general population is approximately 1% in school-aged children, but increases to 2% to 5% by the early teens and is as high as 5% to 7% in women of childbearing age.

Known risk factors for bacteriuria in pregnancy include socioeconomic status, sickle cell disease, and anatomic abnormalities of the urinary system. In addition, women with conditions associated with neurogenic urinary retention, such as spinal cord injuries or multiple sclerosis, diabetes, or a history of UTI, are at increased risk for bacteriuria (3). Some suspect that pregnancy itself is a risk factor for bacteriuria secondary to the urostasis effect of progesterone and the obstructive effect of the gravid uterus.

Asymptomatic bacteriuria in pregnancy predisposes the

pregnant patient to the development of pyelonephritis and potential complications such as sepsis, renal dysfunction, and preterm labor, with its consequent sequelae for the newborn (1–4). Without treatment, as many as 50% of these women will develop symptomatic UTI—that is, pyelonephritis—during their pregnancies. Screening programs for detecting and treating bacteriuria have been shown to reduce the incidence of pyelonephritis in pregnancy to less then 3% and to decrease the incidence of preterm labor (5). Few women whose cultures are negative at the first prenatal visit will subsequently develop bacteriuria during their pregnancies.

Recurrence of bacteriuria affects 10% to 40% of pregnant women treated for bacteriuria. Current recommendations call for patients who are diagnosed as having asymptomatic bacteriuria or cystitis to be screened monthly with urine cultures.

## Pathology and Etiology

More than 90% of the organisms responsible for asymptomatic and symptomatic UTIs are gram-negative rods, such as *Escherichia coli, Klebsiella* sp., *Enterobacter* sp., and *Proteus* sp. *E. coli* is the organism most commonly isolated from the urinary tract during pregnancy. The majority of the remaining infections are caused by group B streptococci and *Staphylococcus saprophyticus* (1).

Bacterial characteristics associated with pathogenicity include an ability to attach to human uroepithelial cells. That is, the virulence of the infecting organism reflects both its ability to attach to these uroepithelial cells and its ability to induce an inflammatory response and, hence, scarring. Nonvirulent strains induce less of an inflammatory response than do the more virulent strains. Other characteristics that affect an organism's pathogenicity include its resistance to the bactericidal effect of serum, serotype identified, and hemolysin production. Isolates recovered from pregnant women with asymptomatic bacteriuria and acute cystitis are less likely to demonstrate these characteristics than isolates recovered from pregnant women with pyelonephritis.

## DIAGNOSIS

Culture and susceptibility testing are the standard means of diagnosing and managing UTI during pregnancy. Bacteriuria is traditionally defined as the presence of more the $10^5$ colony-forming units per milliliter (CFU/mL) of urine from two consecutive first-void, midstream, clean-catch urine specimens. Because most pregnant women cannot provide a first-void specimen at routine prenatal visits, it has been suggested that the presence of more than $10^2$ CFU/mL of a single pathogen from a non–first-void specimen should signify bacteriuria. The recovery of a single uropathogen by suprapubic aspiration or urethral catheterization is indicative of bacteriuria.

Acute cystitis generally requires detecting only $10^2$ CFU/mL or more of a uropathogen on a clean-catch specimen along with associated symptoms such as frequency, dysuria, urgency, and suprapubic tenderness.

Many clinicians believe that nonculture testing is inappropriate as a screening technique for detecting bacteriuria in pregnancy, even though it is an accepted practice for detecting uncomplicated symptomatic UTIs in nonpregnant patients. Reasons for this skepticism about nonculture testing include the lower sensitivity of such testing and the potentially serious maternal and neonatal complications of bacteriuria in pregnancy. On the other hand, testing for leukocyte esterase and microbe-produced nitrites by urine dipstick has been shown to be cost-effective in populations who do not show a high prevalence of asymptomatic bacteriuria (6).

In populations in whom resistant bacteria are frequently encountered, such as women with recurrent bacteriuria or upper-urinary tract abnormalities, collection of urine specimens for culture and susceptibility testing becomes necessary. Women with acute urinary symptoms should be appropriately tested for organisms associated with urethritis. In addition to a urine culture, testing for *Neisseria gonorrhoeae* and *Chlamydia trachomatis* should be performed, with appropriate treatment as recommended for pregnancy if results are positive (see Chapters 11 and 13).

**Table 8-1.** Suggested Treatment Regimens for Lower UTI

| Indication | Regimen |
|---|---|
| Bacteriuria and acute cystitis | Trimethoprim/sulfamethoxazole, 160/800 mg b.i.d. for 7–10 days, except near term<br>Nitrofurantoin, 50–100 mg q 6–8 hours for 7–10 days<br>Amoxicillin, 500 mg q 8 hours for 7–10 days<br>Cephalexin, 250–500 mg q 6 hours for 7–10 days |
| Long-term suppositories | Nitrofurantoin, 50–100 mg at bedtime or 50 mg b.i.d.<br>Cephalexin, 250–500 mg b.i.d. |

## Treatment

Appropriate management of lower UTI during pregnancy will prevent most upper tract infections and their sequelae. A variety of antibiotics can be prescribed to pregnant patients for UTI (Table 8-1).

The sulfonamides should be used with caution when the patient is close to delivery because of their potential for displacing fetal bilirubin and inducing kernicteris. The sulfonamides and nitrofurantoin may also produce a fetal hemolytic anemia in the presence of glucose-6-phosphate dehydrogenase (G6PD) deficiency. Administration of quinolones should be avoided in pregnancy.

Nitrofurantoin is very effective for treating of lower UTIs during pregnancy; this medication becomes highly concentrated in the urinary system but appears in relatively low levels in tissue. Because of the high prevalence of resistance, ampicillin and related penicillins should not be prescribed as first-line therapy on an empiric basis, even though they achieve high concentrations in the urine and often are clinically effective. Many studies have demonstrated the effectiveness of a trimethoprim/sulfamethoxazole regimen in eradicating bacteriuria in pregnancy, but this approach should be used with caution at term in pregnancy.

Several studies have shown that a 7- to 10-day course of therapy is more effective than single-dose therapy for asymptomatic bacteriuria and acute cystitis during pregnancy; 3- and 5-day courses also have proved very effective (1).

Cephalosporins should not be used for single-dose treatment because of their consistently high failure rate (40%).

Regardless of the regimen prescribed, a follow-up test of cure is mandatory, and the pregnant patient should undergo monthly testing for bacteriuria for the remainder of her pregnancy. Treatment of women with recurrent episodes of bacteriuria or cystitis should employ long-term daily suppression with nitrofurantoin or a cephalosporin.

## References

1. Sweet RL, Gibbs R. Infectious diseases of the female genital tract, 3rd ed. Baltimore: Williams and Wilkins, 1995.
2. Andriole VT, Patterson TF. Epidemiology, natural history, and management of urinary tract infections in pregnancy. Med Clin North Am 1991;75:359–373.
3. Guinn DA, Wigton T, Owen J, et al. Prediction of preterm birth in nulliparous patients. Am J Obstet Gynecol 1994;171:1111–1115.
4. Lucas M, Cunningham FG. Urinary infection in pregnancy. Clin Obstet Gynecol 1993;36:855–868.
5. Gratacos E, Torres PJ, Vila J, et al. Screening and treatment of asymptomatic bacteriuria in pregnancy prevent pyelonephritis. J Infect Dis 1994;169:1390–1392.
6. Rouse DJ, Andrews WW, Goldenberg RL, et al. Screening and treatment of asymptomatic bacteriuria of pregnancy to prevent pyelonephritis: a cost-effectiveness and cost-benefit analysis. Obstet Gynecol 1995;86:119–123.

CHAPTER

# 9

# *Pyelonephritis in Pregnancy*

*Penny Clark*
*Patrick Duff*

## Background

Pyelonephritis, a condition that occurs in 1% to 2% of all pregnancies, is the most common severe bacterial infection that causes obstetrical complications. It typically develops when patients have undiagnosed or inadequately treated asymptomatic bacteriuria. Approximately 2% to 10% of expectant mothers have asymptomatic bacteriuria at their initial prenatal visit. As many as one-third of untreated patients will progress from asymptomatic bacteriuria to acute pyelonephritis (1).

Gilstrap and colleagues demonstrated that 67% of mothers with acute pyelonephritis develop symptoms during their second or third trimester (2). Several other studies have shown that 80% to 90% of these infections can be prevented when asymptomatic bacteriuria is recognized and treated (1–4). In particular, Harris and Gilstrap reported a decrease in incidence of pyelonephritis—from 4% to 0.8%—that they attributed to prevention efforts, such as frequent culture follow-up, as well as identification and eradication of bacteriuria (5).

Even with antibiotic treatment, pregnant women who have asymptomatic bacteriuria have a 3% risk (range of 0% to 17%) of developing pyelonephritis during their pregnancies (6). This increased frequency generally is attributed to pregnancy-related anatomic and physiologic alterations: The enlarging uterus can cause ureteral obstruction, incomplete bladder emptying, vesicoureteral reflux, glycosuria, and aminoaciduria.

Other factors that may increase an expectant mother's

predisposition to pyelonephritis are related to the immunosuppressive effects of pregnancy. In a study by Petersson and colleagues, infection in both pregnant and nonpregnant women was accompanied by increased serum and urine levels of IgG-, IgA-, and IgM-specific antibody to *Escherichia coli* antigens (7). The pregnant group showed a less pronounced and significantly lower serum antibody response, however. Similarly, serum and urinary levels of interleukin-6 (IL-6) were elevated in the nonpregnant women who had pyelonephritis, but were low in the pregnant group. These results suggest that pregnancy suppresses the active cytokine and specific antibody responses to gram-negative organisms.

The combination of bacterial virulence and host-tissue ligands also may play a role in increasing the susceptibility of pregnant patients to pyelonephritis. Nowicki and other researchers observed that increased expression of virulence factors such as *E. coli* fimbriae and bacterial adhesins, together with a high density of human chorionic gonadotropin (hCG) hormone receptors, contributes to the pathogenesis of acute pyelonephritis because these hCG hormone receptors are recognized by *E. coli* fimbriae (8).

## Etiology

Uropathogens that are frequently isolated from pregnant women with pyelonephritis include *E. coli* (in more than 70% of all cases), *Klebsiella/Enterobacter* sp. (15%), and *Proteus* sp. (4%) (9,10). *E. coli* is the most common isolate in both acute and chronic pyelonephritis. If *Proteus* strains are identified, the patient may have nephrolithiasis. *Pseudomonas aeruginosa* generally is associated with nosocomial origin, particularly in neutropenic, immunocompromised patients. Staphylococci, group B streptococci, and enterococci also may cause pyelonephritis, usually in association with urinary stones. Anaerobic infections are distinctly uncommon unless patients have chronic obstruction.

The uropathogenic strains of *E. coli* belong to a small group of O:K:H serotypes that usually produce both hemolysin and aerobactin and have specific pili that facilitate their attachment to uroepithelial cells (11). These specific virulence determinants enable the uropathogens to infect the upper urinary tracts of healthy women.

Hart and colleagues collected *E. coli* isolates from 57 pregnant patients who had acute pyelonephritis at different gestational ages. The researchers performed repetitive sequence-based polymerase chain reaction (PCR) tests and assays for plasmid profiles, hemolysin, and O serotypes on the isolate (12). The authors found that *E. coli* strains associated with acute pyelonephritis during different trimesters represent nonrandom, closely related isolates, and some of these strains may be found in pregnant patients only (12).

## Diagnosis

Women who have antepartum pyelonephritis typically develop fever, nausea, chills, vomiting, flank pain, and tenderness. Approximately 75% of cases affect the right kidney, 10% to 15% affect only the left side, and 10% to 15% are bilateral. Nearly 40% of women with this condition also complain of urinary symptoms such as urgency, frequency, and dysuria. Fever may reach 40 °C (104 °F) and frequently shows characteristic spikes.

Confirmation of the diagnosis of acute pyelonephritis typically relies on a positive urine culture, defined as a clean-void, midstream specimen that contains 100,000 or more colonies per milliliter. In a study by Stamm and colleagues, this traditional diagnostic criterion identified only 51% of women whose bladders contained coliforms, however (13). These authors showed that bacterial counts of more than $10^2$ colonies/mL of midstream urine were a more sensitive diagnostic criterion for women with symptomatic coliform infection. Microscopic examination of the urine usually reveals white cell casts, red blood cells (RBCs), and bacteria. The leukocyte esterase and nitrite tests usually give positive results. Blood cultures are positive in nearly 15% of cases.

## Treatment

The pregnant woman with pyelonephritis generally becomes quite ill, particularly when she is in her late second or third trimester. Accordingly, hospitalization is recommended in most cases. Initially, treatment should be directed toward restoring the contracted blood volume. It is essential to administer IV crystalloids—either physiologic saline or lactated Ringer's solution—along with antibiotics. Give fluids rapidly at the start of treatment to establish an hourly urinary output of at least 30 to 50 mL, and carefully monitor the patient's respiratory status for possible pulmonary edema.

Laboratory assessment should include a complete blood cell count and urine culture. Blood cultures should be obtained from women who are at increased risk for bacteremia or endocarditis and from those who show a poor initial response to therapy.

The choice of antimicrobials is empiric. Nevertheless, you must carefully consider the antibiotic susceptibility of the suspected bacterial pathogens when selecting an agent. In pregnancy, the most common antibiotic regimen is a first-generation cephalosporin, such as cefazolin, given as 1 g every 8 hours. Newer and broader-spectrum cephalosporins are not necessarily more effective against the common gram-negative pathogens and usually are considerably more expensive.

Administer combination therapy with gentamicin, 1.5 mg/kg every 8 hours, plus ampicillin, 2 g every 6 hours, or cefazolin, 1 g every 8 hours, to critically ill patients. Women who have a previous history of multiple urinary tract infections (UTIs) should receive the same treatment, as they likely harbor a resistant organism. Currently, there is insufficient evidence that single daily doses of aminoglycosides are safe for pregnant women.

Ampicillin has a long history of use in the treatment of uncomplicated pyelonephritis. In the past decade, however, the prevalence of ampicillin-resistant uropathogens has risen to as high as 20% for *E. coli* and 30% for *Klebsiella pneumoniae* (14). In contrast, significantly fewer of the same uropathogens show resistance to a limited-spectrum, first-generation cephalosporin. In a more recent controlled, randomized trial reported by Millar and co-workers, *E. coli* was the major uropathogen (86%, 95 out of 111 cases) isolated from 120 pregnant women with pyelonephritis (10). Of these isolates, 12% (13 of 111 cases) were resistant to cefazolin. The results of this investigation clearly indicate the need to constantly monitor the antibiotic susceptibilities of uropathogens at each institution and to make periodic adjustments in antibiotic selection as patterns of resistance change.

Continue parenteral antibiotic therapy until the patient has been afebrile and asymptomatic for approximately 24 to 48 hours. At this point, she may be discharged and continued on comparable oral antibiotics for another 7 to 10 days. Possible choices for this therapy include cephalexin (500 mg four times daily), sustained-release nitrofurantoin macrocrystals (100 mg twice daily), or double-strength trimethoprim–sulfamethoxazole (twice daily).

After the treatment is completed, the patient should receive suppressive doses of a drug such as sustained-release nitrofurantoin macrocrystals (100 mg daily) or sulfisoxazole (1 g daily) for the duration of her pregnancy. Recurrent infections develop in 20% to 30% of patients who do not receive prophylaxis. Selection of a specific oral agent for treatment or prophylaxis should be based on efficacy, toxicity, and cost considerations.

## Other Treatment Considerations

When treating a patient with pyelonephritis, you must make several decisions: What type of antibiotic will best suit her? Should it be a single or multiple daily-dose regimen? Is oral or IV administration the best route? Should therapy begin on an inpatient or outpatient basis? The following studies provided some results that may help you determine the best options for your patient.

### Single versus Multiple Daily-Dose Antibiotics

A single daily dose of antibiotics was shown to be effective for treatment of pyelonephritis in a double-blind, randomized clinical trial performed by Sanchez-Ramos and coworkers (15). In this study, the researchers compared the efficacy of a single daily dose of IV ceftriaxone with that of multiple doses of cefazolin in the treatment of pregnant women hospitalized with acute pyelonephritis.

A single daily dose of ceftriaxone was given intravenously to 90 women in the study group; the 88 members of the comparison group received three daily doses of 2 g cefazolin intravenously. Once the patients were afebrile, IV antibiotics were discontinued and patients were discharged on oral antibiotics. Follow-up cultures demonstrated that the single daily IV dose of ceftriaxone was as effective as the multiple-dose regimen of cefazolin.

Despite the slightly higher cost per dose of ceftriaxone, the mean total cost of antibiotic therapy for the ceftriaxone group was $1676, versus $4828 for the cefazolin group. The mean total cost of antibiotic therapy included the total cost per actual antibiotic dose (drug plus administration fee) multiplied by mean number of doses of administered antibiotic. Thus cost savings may be realized with the single dose of ceftriaxone, at least at some institutions.

## Oral versus IV Antibiotics

Angel and colleagues studied the efficacy of oral versus IV antibiotics in women hospitalized with antepartum pyelonephritis (16). In nonbacteremic patients, oral antibiotics appeared to be effective for treating acute pyelonephritis.

Ninety pregnant women with acute pyelonephritis were randomly assigned to oral or IV antibiotics. The oral group received an initial dose of 1 g of cephalexin followed by 500 mg every 6 hours, and the IV group received 1 g of cephalothin every 6 hours. Treatment continued until costovertebral-angle tenderness decreased and temperature remained lower than 38.0 °C for 48 hours. Patients then were discharged with the appropriate oral agent, which was chosen on the basis of sensitivities, to complete a 14-day course. The average hospital stay for both groups was four to five days. Blood cultures taken upon admission showed bacteremia in 14% of patients.

In the authors' protocol, IV therapy was mandatory for patients with bacteremia, who were excluded in the analysis of successful therapy. Of the 77 nonbacteremic patients, 91.4% (32 of 35) and 92.9% (39 of 42) were treated successfully with oral and IV therapy, respectively.

## Inpatient versus Outpatient Therapy

Most patients who develop pyelonephritis during early pregnancy may be candidates for outpatient therapy. In an attempt to reduce health care costs without increasing morbidity and mortality, Millar and colleagues conducted a randomized, controlled trial to determine whether pregnant women whose gestational age was less than 24 weeks could be treated for pyelonephritis as outpatients through a combination of IM and oral antibiotics—a therapeutic regimen that is used successfully in nonpregnant women (10). Sixty patients were randomized to receive cefazolin, 1 g IV every 8 hours until afebrile for 48 hours; another 60 outpatients received a third-generation cephalosporin, ceftriaxone, 1 g IM in the emergency room and another injection 18 to 36 hours after discharge. Both groups completed a 10-day course of oral cephalexin, 500 mg four times per day. All subjects receiving outpatient therapy showed a good initial response to treatment, with resolution of fever and flank pain.

The authors concluded that most patients with pyelonephritis in early pregnancy are candidates for outpatient therapy with IM ceftriaxone and oral cephalexin. They recommended that outpatient therapy follow an initial period of observation in the hospital and that close follow-up be undertaken to document clinical response and patient compliance. The safety and efficacy of this regimen have not been investigated in women in later stages of pregnancy.

# Complications

Failure to improve within two or three days after therapy begins suggests a complication, such as urinary tract obstruction or a resistant microorganism. Use susceptibility testing to determine whether the patient's antibiotic therapy should be modified. The use of a ureteral stent normally will relieve ureteral obstruction caused by the mother's enlarged uterus. Obstruction from a ureteral or renal calculus may require surgery to remove the stones and clear the infection. If you suspect the presence of an obstruction, perform renal ultrasonography. Intravenous pyelography should be obtained only if sonography proves nondiagnostic.

## SEQUELAE

As noted previously, 20% to 30% of obstetric patients with acute pyelonephritis develop a recurrent UTI later in their pregnancies. The administration of a daily dose of prophylactic antibiotic such as sulfisoxazole (1 g) or sustained-release nitrofurantoin macrocrystals (100 mg) can reduce the frequency of recurrence in a cost-effective manner. At each subsequent prenatal appointment, the urine of patients receiving prophylaxis should be screened for leukocyte esterase and nitrites. If either of the screening tests gives positive results, or if the patient shows new symptoms, obtain a urine culture to determine whether reinfection has occurred.

Among pregnant women with severe pyelonephritis, approximately 5% to 10% will develop potentially life-threatening maternal complications, such as bacteremia, septic shock, and adult respiratory distress syndrome (17,18). Pyelonephritis also may precipitate preterm labor.

### Respiratory Insufficiency

An estimated 2% of severe cases of pyelonephritis lead to some form of respiratory compromise. Towers and colleagues attempted to identify clinical risk factors for acute respiratory distress in pregnant women with pyelonephritis (19). Their study compared 11 patients with pyelonephritis and pulmonary injury with 119 patients with pyelonephritis only. In gestations longer than 20 weeks, maternal heart rate greater than 110 beats/minute and fever of 103 °F 12 to 24 hours before respiratory symptoms were highly predictive of pulmonary injury. The best predictors of pulmonary injury were, in fact, factors related to treatment, such as fluid overload, use of tocolytic agents, and, perhaps to a lesser extent, choice of antibiotic. Although the researchers' results were inconclusive, initial treatment with ampicillin alone was implicated as a risk factor in the development of pulmonary injury.

### Hematologic and Vascular Changes

Anemia appears in approximately 25% of women whose pregnancies are complicated by pyelonephritis (20). Antepartum infection does not alter erythropoietin production, either acutely or subacutely, indicating that hemolysis is the contributing factor to anemia associated with renal infection. With a scanning electron microscope, Cox and colleagues observed a high frequency of morphologically aberrant red blood cells (RBCs) in pregnant women with pyelonephritis (21). Moreover, these RBC aberrations could be induced in vitro by lipopolysaccharides, which are known to cause premature RBC destruction in vivo. Therefore, the anemia in pregnant women with pyelonephritis most likely derives from lipopolysaccharide-induced RBC membrane damage.

Uncomplicated antepartum pyelonephritis is associated with measurable depression of systemic vascular resistance. Ultrasonographic evaluation of central and end-organ hemodynamics in patients with antepartum pyelonephritis has demonstrated that, during acute infection, total peripheral resistance was significantly decreased and cardiac output was increased (22). In women with unilateral signs and symptoms, an increased resistive index was observed in the symptomatic kidney compared with the nonsymptomatic side; this difference disappeared after treatment. The increased resistive index of the symptomatic kidney may be attributed to local effects of infection—perhaps representing the effects of infection that, in the extreme, would constitute septic shock syndrome.

## Septic Shock

Although as many as 10% of women with severe antepartum pyelonephritis have bacteremia, septic shock remains rare. You should differentiate hypotension and diminished perfusion as a consequence of endotoxemia from that caused by dehydration from nausea, vomiting, and fever. Aggressive IV fluid resuscitation usually restores cardiac output. Vasopressor drugs rarely are required.

## Preterm Labor

Although preterm labor occurs in pregnancies complicated by pyelonephritis, its pathogenesis remains unclear. Graham and colleagues noted that the number of uterine contractions occurring in pregnant patients with pyelonephritis significantly increased one to two hours after antibiotic administration (23). This increase in contraction frequency was observed primarily in women infected with gram-negative bacteria; no such increase was seen in women infected with gram-positive bacteria. In this study, *E. coli* was the most common isolate, being found in 87% of urine cultures and 100% of blood cultures. Thus, uterine contractions may begin because of the endotoxins released by lysis of gram-negative bacteria following antibiotic therapy. The released endotoxins may stimulate production of inflammatory mediators, such as cytokines and prostaglandins associated with uterine contractions, and subsequently lead to preterm labor.

## References


1. Whalley PJ. Bacteriuria in pregnancy. Am J Obstet Gynecol 1967;97:723–728.
2. Gilstrap LC, Cunningham FG, Whalley PJ. Acute pyelonephritis in pregnancy: an anterospective study. *Obstet Gynecol* 1981; 57:409–413.
3. Norden CW, Kass EH. Bacteruria in pregnancy. A critical appraisal. Annu Rev Med 1968;19:431–470.
4. Harris RE. The significance of eradication of bacteriuria during pregnancy. Obstet Gynecol 1979;53:71–73.
5. Harris RE, Gilstrap LG. Prevention of recurrent pyelonephritis during pregnancy. Obstet Gynecol 1974;44:637–641.
6. Rouse DJ, Andrews WW, Goldberg RL, et al. Screening and treatment of asymptomatic bacteriuria in pregnancy to prevent pyelonephritis: a cost-effectiveness and cost-benefit analysis. Obstet Gynecol 1995;86:119–123.
7. Petersson C, Hedges S, Stenqvist K, et al. Suppressed antibody and interleukin-6 responses to acute pyelonephritis in pregnancy. Int Soc Nephrol 1994;45:571–577.
8. Nowicki B, Martens M, Hart A, et al. Gestational age-dependent distribution of *Escherichia coli* fimbriae in pregnant patients with pyelonephritis. Ann NY Acad Sci 1994;730:290–291.
9. Duff P. Pyelonephritis in pregnancy. Clin Obstet Gynecol 1984;27:17–31.
10. Millar LK, Wing DA, Paul RH, et al. Outpatient treatment of pyelonephritis in pregnancy: a randomized controlled trial. Obstet Gynecol 1995;86:560–564.

11. Stamm WE, Hooton TM. Management of the urinary tract infection in adults. N Engl J Med 1993;329:1328–1334.
12. Hart A, Pham T, Nowicki S, et al. Gestational pyelonephritis-associated *Escherichia coli* isolates represent a nonrandom, closely related population. Am J Obstet Gynecol 1996;174: 983–989.
13. Stamm WE, Counts GW, Running KR, et al. Diagnosis of coliform infection in acutely dysuric women. N Engl J Med 1982;307:463–468.
14. Dunlow S, Duff P. Prevalence of antibiotic resistant uropathogens in obstetric patients with acute pyelonephritis. Obstet Gynecol 1990;76:241–244.
15. Sanchez-Ramos L, McAlpine KJ, Adair CD, et al. Pyelonephritis in pregnancy: once-a-day ceftriazone versus multiple dose of cefazolin. A randomized double-blind trial. Am J Obstet Gynecol 1995;172:129–133.
16. Angel JL, O'Brien WF, Finan MA, et al. Acute pyelonephritis in pregnancy: a prospective study of oral versus intravenous antibiotic therapy. Obstet Gynecol 1990;76:28–32.
17. Cunningham FG, Morris GB, Mickal A. Acute pyelonephritis of pregnancy: a clinical review. Obstet Gynecol 1973;43:112–117.
18. Cunningham FG, Lucas MJ, Hankins GDV. Pulmonary injury complicating antepartum pyelonephritis. Am J Obstet Gynecol 1987;156:797–807.
19. Towers CV, Kaminskas CM, Garite TJ, et al. Pulmonary injury associated with antepartum pyelonephritis: can patients at risk be identified? Am J Obstet Gynecol 1991;164:974–978.
20. Cox SM, Cunningham FG. Ureidopenicillin therapy for acute antepartum pyelonephritis. Curr Ther Res 1988;44:1029.
21. Cox SM, Shelburne P, Mason R, et al. Mechanisms of hemolysis and anemia associated with acute antepartum pyelonephritis. Am J Obstet Gynecol 1991;164:587–590.
22. Twickler DM, Lucal MJ, McIntire DD, et al. Ultrasonographic evaluation of central and end-organ hemodynamics in antepartum pyelonephritis. Am J Obstet Gynecol 1994;170:814–818.
23. Graham JM, Oshiro BT, Blanco JD, et al. Uterine contractions after antibiotic for pyelonephritis in pregnancy. Am J Obstet Gynecol 1993;168:577–580.

CHAPTER

# 10

# *Mastitis*

*W. David Hager*

## Puerperal Mastitis

### Background

Inflammatory disorders of the breast have caused problems among mothers for as long as they have nursed their infants. In 1953, Gibberd categorized these inflammatory disorders as being either epidemic or nonepidemic (sporadic) (1).

Epidemic mastitis is an acute adenitis and cellulitis that primarily involves the lactiferous apparatus of the breast and often includes nonadjacent lobes. Epidemic outbreaks frequently result from *Staphylococcus aureus* infections in the hospital nursery.

Nonepidemic mastitis is an acute puerperal cellulitis that extends to the periglandular connective tissue. A V-shaped area between the lobes results from the connective tissue infection. Thomsen and coworkers classified nonepidemic mastitis into three categories based on the progression of the disease: milk stasis, noninfectious inflammation, and acute mastitis (2). Milk stasis results from incomplete emptying of the breast and causes engorgement and pain. When stasis is persistent and severe, noninfectious inflammation may follow with edema, erythema, pain, and tenderness. Each condition may last for a few days and, if unresolved, lead to acute mastitis, which is characterized by edema, erythema, pain, myalgias, chills, fever, and tenderness.

In the past, acute mastitis often was epidemic and associated with longer postpartum hospital stays and outbreaks of *S. aureus* infection in nurseries. Few antibiotics were available to treat the infection. Today, mastitis is more likely to be of the nonepidemic variety.

Studies show that 7% to 11% of nursing mothers will develop inflammation or acute mastitis. Nursery outbreaks of *S. aureus* infections may be avoided, however, when infants share a hospital room with their mothers. A study from Finland supports this notion: A 30-fold decrease in acute mastitis was achieved when infants were allowed to share a hospital room with their mothers (3).

## Etiology

The onset of symptoms and signs of acute puerperal mastitis often results from a vicious cycle of events. Bacteria from the infant's mouth or from the mother's skin may enter the breast through a cracked nipple (Table 10-1). Infection may occur after these bacteria encounter milk that remains in the breast when the organ fails to empty completely. Infection, in turn, causes pain and tenderness that further impede emptying and promote engorgement; the latter condition prevents the infant from drawing the nipple and areola into its mouth completely. The result is nibbling and further cracking, which allows more bacteria to enter and infect the breast.

Relatively few well-designed studies have focused on the bacterial etiology of mastitis. Niebyl and coworkers isolated pathogenic bacteria from 53% of their patients who had nonepidemic mastitis. Of those women with bacteria isolated, 37% had *S. aureus* alone or in combination with other bacteria (4). Marshall and co-workers recovered *S. aureus* from more than 50% of their patients with puerperal mastitis (5). In the only prospective, randomized, blinded study of acute puerperal

**Table 10-1.** Bacteriology (Principal Isolates) of Sporadic Acute Puerperal Mastitis

| |
|---|
| *Staphylococcus aureus* (PCN-R, Ceph-S) |
| Staphylococcal species (PCN-R, Ceph-S) |
| Alpha streptococci |
| Group B streptococci |
| *Propionibacterium acnes* |

mastitis, the authors isolated staphylococci from 60% of patients (coagulase-positive *S. aureus*, 28%; coagulase-negative *S. aureus*, 32%) (6). Bacteria isolated in other reports include coagulase-negative *S. aureus*, group A and group B ß-hemolytic streptococci, *Escherichia coli*, and *Bacteroides* species.

Several factors predispose the nursing mother to mastitis. Failure to empty the breast adequately is undoubtedly the most important consideration. Nipple fissures and bacterial inoculum from the infant's mouth or mother's skin also have been noted. Incorrect preparation and care of the nipples and improper positioning of the infant for nursing may foster nipple fissuring. In addition, lowered maternal immune defenses must be considered; they may result from fatigue, stress, or improper nutrition.

## Diagnosis

Clinical symptoms and signs are used to confirm the diagnosis of acute puerperal mastitis. The most frequent symptoms are malaise, myalgias, fever, chills, and pain. Signs of disease include edema, erythema, temperature higher than 37.8 °C (100 °F), and breast tenderness. The erythema frequently occurs in a V-shaped distribution. Engorgement of the breast from milk stasis often takes a bilateral form and is not associated with fever or erythema; in contrast, noninfectious inflammation and mastitis are more frequently unilateral.

Diagnosis rarely is based on culture results alone. When performing a culture, obtain the specimen from expressed milk after discarding the first 2 to 3 mL. Differentiating milk stasis from noninfectious inflammation and infectious mastitis by quantitative evaluation of the mother's milk has been described by Thomsen and coworkers (Table 10-2) (2). This classification relies on quantitative leukocyte counts and quantitative bacterial cultures (per milliliter of milk).

## Treatment

The key to managing mastitis is recognizing a potential problem early. To prevent infection, treat milk stasis with adequate breast emptying. Among patients with noninfectious inflammation, 79% had a poor outcome when their breasts were

**Table 10-2.** Stages of Breast Inflammation

| Stage | Fever | Breast Appearance | Leukocytes per mL Milk | Bacteria per mL Milk | Treatment |
|---|---|---|---|---|---|
| Milk stasis | Low grade | Engorged, nodular | $<10^6$ | $<10^3$ | Empty breasts, acetaminophen, moist heat |
| Noninfectious inflammation | Low grade | Tender, swollen, red, hot | $>10^6$ | $<10^3$ | Empty breasts, acetaminophen, moist heat |
| Infectious mastitis | High grade | Tender, swollen, red, hot | $>10^6$ | $>10^3$ | Empty breasts, acetaminophen, moist heat, antibiotics |

SOURCE: Adapted from Thomsen AC, Espersen T, Maigaard S. Course and treatment of milk stasis, noninfectious inflammation of the breast, and infectious mastitis in nursing women. Am J Obstet Gynecol 1984;149:492–495.

not emptied regularly and adequately. Because the infection site in acute puerperal mastitis is extraductal, continued nursing is not detrimental to the baby and no data indicate adverse effects on the infant. Furthermore, weaning the infant from the breast during an acute infection has been shown to increase the risk of prolonged infection and of developing an abscess.

In addition to emptying the breasts, the following supportive measures may help:

- Application of moist heat to the infected breast
- Adequate hydration of the mother
- Use of anti-inflammatory agents such as acetaminophen

If the pain is so severe that the mother cannot nurse, she may use a breast pump or express milk while lying in a tub of warm water, where the breast can float comfortably.

The selection of an antibiotic is made empirically. Devereux has shown that the best response to treatment occurs when antibiotics are initially administered in the first 24 hours of infection (7). Thomsen's data indicate a good response in 15% of women with no treatment, in 51% of those who only emptied their breasts regularly, and in 96% of those who emptied their breasts regularly and received oral antibiotics (2).

Effective antibiotic regimens include the following: penicillin, 500 mg orally every 6 hours; ampicillin, 500 mg orally every

6 hours; oxacillin, 500 mg orally every 6 hours; dicloxacillin, 500 mg orally every 6 hours; erythromycin base, 500 mg every 6 hours; and cephalosporins such as cephalexin, 500 mg orally every 6 hours, or cephradine, 500 mg orally every 6 hours. Recent data indicate that amoxicillin and cephradine are equally effective in treating mastitis (6).

## Sequelae

The most frequent consequences of mastitis are persistent infection and development of an abscess. Devereux diagnosed an abscess in 11.1% of women treated for puerperal mastitis, while Marshall and coworkers found this condition in 4.6% of their patients (5,7).

Discourage cessation of nursing, because this tactic increases the risk of prolonged infection and abscess. Alert the mother that, because milk from the infected breast has increased sodium, the infant may reject it. In addition, milk from mastitis patients has been reported to be lower in lactose, fat, and total protein. If the infant continues to reject the mother's breast, investigate the possibility of carcinoma of the breast.

If a breast abscess is diagnosed, instruct the patient to stop nursing from that breast. Treat her with parenteral antibiotics such as cefazolin (1 g IV every 6 to 8 hours), ampicillin (1 g IV every 6 hours), or methicillin (1 to 2 g every 6 to 8 hours). Provide anaerobic coverage with clindamycin (900 mg every 8 hours) or metronidazole (500 mg every 6 hours). If the response is not favorable within 48 to 72 hours, incise and drain the abscess and administer appropriate wound care. Careful follow-up must be performed to evaluate for recurrent abscess formation.

Acute nonepidemic puerperal mastitis is a frequent cause of morbidity among recently pregnant women. Most patients, however, will have a successful outcome when they stay alert to the possibility of infection, have an early diagnosis, and receive appropriate therapy.

## Prevention

Any program for avoiding acute mastitis must stress regular emptying of the breasts, proper positioning of the infant for nursing, and appropriate nipple care. Although good data are lacking to confirm the protective benefit of nipple care, we have found UPS-modified lanolin applied directly onto the nipple and areola to be the best preparatory agent available.

## Nonpuerperal Mastitis

### Background

Infection of the breast in nonpregnant women is an uncommon clinical problem. Nevertheless, it is important to understand the presentation of this disease and its etiology because, if left untreated, it can lead to chronic sinus tract infection and severe abscesses.

Nonpuerperal mastitis is characterized as a partial blockage of the lactiferous ducts by keratotic debris and squamous metaplasia of the epithelium lining the milk sinus.

### Etiology

The etiology of nonpuerperal mastitis has been uncertain because the literature disagrees about which bacteria cause the infection. Most case reports have identified *S. aureus* as the predominant microbial isolate. Recent data indicate that anaerobic cocci and bacilli often are isolated from breast secretions and from abscesses. Edmiston and coworkers have reported that peptostreptococci are the most common isolates among women with nonpuerperal mastitis (8). Thus the literature would seem to confirm that the etiology frequently involves mixed aerobes and anaerobes in chronic disease.

Unlike puerperal mastitis, in which bacteria that are introduced into the cracked nipples and ascend to areas of milk stasis are an obvious predisposing factor, the factors that lead to nonpuerperal disease are less certain. Some authors have suggested that manipulative breast procedures or oral stimulation of the breast are possible inciting factors. In addition, cutaneous infections may invade nearby breast tissue.

## Diagnosis

Nonpuerperal mastitis can present as acute, subacute, or chronic disease. Patients with acute disease usually complain of pain, fever, and edema and erythema of the involved breast and have a firm, tender mass in the subareolar region. Patients with subacute disease present similarly to those with acute disease but have a tender, fluctuant mass. Chronic disease may occur after multiple, recurrent infections, leading to sinus tract formation, suppuration, and possibly a fluctuant mass, along with pain and edema.

## Treatment

Women who have nonpuerperal mastitis usually respond to antibiotic therapy that combines a penicillinase-resistant penicillin with an agent, such as metronidazole (500 mg orally, every 6 to 8 hours), that provides anaerobic coverage (see the "Treatment" section for puerperal mastitis). Another option is to administer a broad-spectrum antibiotic, such as one of the fluoroquinolones, in doses of 300 to 400 mg orally every 12 hours.

Subacute disease usually necessitates surgical drainage, along with broad-spectrum antimicrobial therapy. In contrast, chronic disease requires aggressive surgical excision and debridement, followed by extended antibiotic treatment. Preventive measures, such as treating skin lesions aggressively and encouraging avoidance of oral breast stimulation, may help decrease the prevalence of disease.

### References

1. Gibberd CF. Sporadic and epidemic puerperal breast infections. Am J Obstet Gynecol 1953;65:1038–1041.
2. Thomsen AC, Espersen T, Maigaard S. Course and treatment of milk stasis, noninfectious inflammation of the breast, and infectious mastitis in nursing women. Am J Obstet Gynecol 1984;149:492–495.
3. Jonsson S, Pulkkinen MO. Mastitis today: incidence, prevention, and treatment. Ann Chir Gynaecol 1994;208(suppl):84–87.
4. Niebyl JR, Spence MR, Parmley TH. Sporadic (nonepidemic) puerperal mastitis. J Reprod Med 1978;20:97–100.

5. Marshall BR, Hepper JK, Zirbel CC. Sporadic puerperal mastitis—an infection that need not interrupt lactation. JAMA 1975;233:1377–1379.
6. Hager WD, Barton JR. Treatment of sporadic acute puerperal mastitis. Infect Dis Obstet Gynecol 1996;4:97–101.
7. Devereux WP. Acute puerperal mastitis: evaluation of its management. Am J Obstet Gynecol 1970;108:78–81.
8. Edmiston CE, Walker AP, Krepel CJ, et al. The nonpuerperal breast infection: aerobic and anaerobic microbial recovery from acute and chronic disease. J Infect Dis 1990;162:695–699.

## Suggested Readings

Goldsmith HS. Milk rejection sign of breast cancer. Am J Surg 1974;127:280–281.

Leach RD, Eykyn SJ, Phillips I, et al. Anaerobic subareolar breast abscess. Lancet 1979;1:35–37.

Puerperal mastitis. Editorial. Br Med J 1976;1:920.

CHAPTER

# 11

# Chlamydia Trachomatis *Infections in Pregnancy*

*Abner P. Korn*

## BACKGROUND

During recent decades, genital *Chlamydia trachomatis* infection has become the most prevalent sexually transmitted bacterial pathogen in the United States. In 1993, approximately 4 million cases occurred in the United States. The estimated direct and indirect costs for care of illness following from *C. trachomatis* infections exceed $3.4 billion annually.

Serious consequences of *C. trachomatis* infections in non-pregnant women include salpingitis, acute urethral syndrome, bartholinitis, proctitis, tubal factor infertility, ectopic pregnancy, and chronic pelvic pain. During pregnancy, endometritis (post-partum and postabortal) and transmission to the neonate create concern. The neonatal risks of exposure to *C. trachomatis* include conjunctivitis (18% to 50%) and pneumonia (11% to 18%). Other conditions possibly associated with *C. trachomatis* infection include spontaneous abortion, poor prognosis of in vitro fertilization, premature rupture of membranes (PROM), preterm labor, and low birthweight.

Risk factors for *C. trachomatis* infection include young age, single marital status, young age at onset of coitus, multiple sex contacts, mucopurulent cervicitis, and oral contraceptive use.

## Pathophysiology

*C. trachomatis* is an obligate intracellular bacterium that depends on host cells for nutrients and energy. Infection occurs when the metabolically inactive elementary body attaches to host cells, which ingest it by phagocytosis. The elementary body then becomes transformed into the metabolically active and dividing reticulate body. Reticulate bodies divide for 8 to 24 hours, but then revert to elementary bodies. After 48 to 72 hours, the host cell bursts or releases the phagosome, thereby spreading the infection. A latent state has been documented in vitro.

Most genital *C. trachomatis* infections remain asymptomatic. Women with symptomatic cases complain of nonspecific symptoms such as vaginal discharge, intermenstrual bleeding, dysuria, and pelvic pain. *C. trachomatis* is transmitted to the glandular epithelium of the endocervix, where it can persist for many months. Ascent to the endometrium, the fallopian tubes, and peritoneal cavity can occur in the absence of symptoms. Risk factors for development of upper tract disease are poorly defined. This type of disease might result from repeated exposure to sexually transmitted organisms as a result of high-risk sexual behavior. Also, vaginal douching could force organisms mechanically from the lower to the upper genital tract.

The majority of women with tubal factor infertility show serologic evidence of *C. trachomatis* infection but do not have histories of recognized pelvic inflammatory disease. A negative endocervical *C. trachomatis* culture does not exclude *C. trachomatis* infection of the urethra or fallopian tubes, however.

Tubal obstruction after infection with *C. trachomatis* appears to be caused by a delayed hypersensitivity reaction, which occurs (in animal models) only after repeated exposure to *C. trachomatis*. Perinatal *C. trachomatis* infection has been reported even after cesarean section delivery with intact membranes.

## Diagnosis

In most family planning and prenatal care clinics, routine screening for *C. trachomatis* is a cost-effective strategy. In other settings, if the overall prevalence of *C. trachomatis* infection is less than 2% to 6%, screening may be limited to women with mucopurulent cervicitis, women younger than 20 years of age, and older women who do not consistently use barrier contraception or who have a new sex partner or multiple sex partners.

The "gold standard" for diagnosing *C. trachomatis* infection has traditionally been cell culture. The validity of this method depends on the viability of the organisms in transport media; false-negative results can occur if cells die during transport from the office to the laboratory. The sensitivity of culture for detection of *C. trachomatis* infection is estimated to be 70% to 80%, but it may be improved by use of a blind second passage for initially negative specimens and by use of an endocervical brush to obtain specimens.

Other detection methods include direct fluorescent antigen (DFA) testing, enzyme immunoassay (EIA), rapid enzyme tests, and DNA detection. In the DFA test, monoclonal antibody is applied to a fixed slide that is then examined microscopically. This test offers a sensitivity of 90% and specificity of 98% as compared with culture. The EIA test is performed with a spectrophotometer; it has a sensitivity of 92% to 97% but a specificity of only 67% to 91%. Its low specificity means that positive results must be confirmed with another test (usually the DFA test). Rapid enzyme tests have lower sensitivity than DFA or EIA tests but can be performed in the physician's office. DNA probe assays provide a high sensitivity (98% compared with culture) and specificity (99%). DNA detection by polymerase chain reaction (PCR) or ligase chain reaction (LCR) has been used to detect *C. trachomatis* from cervical swabs, but it can also be applied to urine or vaginal introitus swabs. DNA amplification tests offer greater sensitivity than tissue culture.

## TREATMENT

Several nonrandomized studies have shown that treatment of *C. trachomatis* infection is associated with improved outcome of pregnancy (reduction in preterm PROM, preterm labor, small-for-gestational-age infants, and low-birthweight infants, as well as improved neonatal survival). In pregnant women, erythromycin base, 500 mg four times daily for 7 days, has been considered the treatment of choice for *C. trachomatis* infection. (Erythromycin estolate is contraindicated during pregnancy because it carries a risk of drug-related hepatotoxicity.) Unfortunately, erythromycin often causes gastrointestinal side effects, which may lead to discontinuation of therapy in approximately 15% to 20% of women using this drug. Alternative medications include amoxicillin and azithromycin.

Several clinical trials have compared amoxicillin, 500 mg three times daily for 7 days, with erythromycin. A meta-analysis of these trials suggests that amoxicillin is superior to erythromycin, mostly because it produces less gastrointestinal morbidity.

Use of azithromycin, 1 g orally in one dose, has been reported in relatively few pregnant women. This single-dose regimen, made possible by azithromycin's three-day half-life in tissue, could be advantageous in patient populations who are at high risk for treatment noncompliance. The entire course of medication can be administered (and consumption observed) in the office. A disadvantage of this drug is its relatively high cost.

In a recent randomized trial, azithromycin-treated pregnant women with *C. trachomatis* infection were significantly less likely to discontinue treatment because of an adverse reaction to the medication than were those treated with erythromycin. In this study, eythromycin and azithromycin provided similar efficacy (93% and 88%, respectively).

Antichlamydial medications such as doxycycline or fluoroquinolones (ofloxacin) should be avoided in pregnancy. Doxycycline can affect fetal tooth and bone development, and fluoroquinolones have been associated with fetal cartilage defects in animal studies.

Two first-line treatment approaches seem logical at this time:

1. Use erythromycin as a first-line agent. If gastrointestinal disturbance results, decrease the dose from 500 mg to 250 mg and continue for two weeks or switch to amoxicillin.
2. Use amoxicillin as a first-line agent.

Alternatively, single-dose azithromycin may be prescribed, especially for patients who would be unlikely to comply with a one-week course of therapy.

Treatment of sex contacts of infected women is important

to reduce further transmission or reinfection. Many treatment failures in pregnancy reflect reinfection by an untreated sex contact. A routine test of cure after treatment of *C. trachomatis* infection is recommended by the Centers for Disease Control and Prevention. Preferably, a culture test should be performed three weeks after completion of therapy.

## Suggested Readings

Adair CD, Gunter M, Stovall TD, et al. Chlamydia in pregnancy: a randomized trial of azithromycin and erythromycin. Obstet Gynecol 1998;91:165–168.

Bell TA, Stamm WE, Kuo CC, et al. Risk of perinatal transmission of *Chlamydia trachomatis* by mode of delivery. J Infect 1994;29:165–169.

Bush MR, Rosa C. Azithromycin and erythromycin in the treatment of cervical chlamydial infection during pregnancy. Obstet Gynecol 1994;84:61–63.

Centers for Disease Control and Prevention. Recommendations for the prevention and management of *Chlamydia trachomatis* infections. MMWR 1998;47(RR-1):53–56.

Friede A, O'Carroll PW, Nicola RM, et al. Centers for Disease Control and Prevention guidelines: a guide for action. Baltimore: Williams and Wilkins, 1997.

Gibbs RS, Eschenbach DA. Use of antibiotics to prevent preterm birth. Am J Obstet Gynecol 1997;177:375–380.

Turrentine MA, Newton ER. Amoxicillin or erythromycin for the treatment of antenatal chlamydial infection: a meta-analysis. Obstet Gynecol 1995;86:1021–1025.

Weber JT, Johnson RE. New treatments for *Chlamydia trachomatis* genital infection. Clin Infect Dis 1995;20(suppl 1):S66–S71.

CHAPTER 12

# *Neonatal Chlamydial Infections*

*William R. Crombleholme*

## Background

At present, the most common sexually transmitted organism in the United States is *Chlamydia trachomatis*. This organism is responsible for several distinct infectious illnesses in adults, including urethritis and epididymitis in men and cervicitis and salpingitis in women. Moreover, endocervical infection in women during pregnancy *may* lead to vertical transmission of the infection to their infants during the course of vaginal delivery (see Chapter 14).

## Incidence

The prevalence of cervical infections with *C. trachomatis* among pregnant women differs according to the population studied. Women who are younger, unmarried, nonwhite, and of lower socioeconomic status tend to have higher rates of infection. In reported series, prevalence has ranged from 2% to 26%, with an overall estimate of 6% to 8% of all pregnant women harboring the organism. More importantly, most of these women were asymptomatic.

## Pathophysiology

Perinatally acquired *C. trachomatis* causes two major infectious complications among infants: inclusion conjunctivitis and pneumonitis.

Inclusion conjunctivitis affects 35% to 50% of infants born to untreated mothers with cervical *C. trachomatis* infection. Clinical findings usually emerge between the fifth and twelfth day of life. Symptoms include a mucoid discharge that becomes more purulent, followed by edema of the eyelids with erythema of both the palpebral and bulbar conjunctivas.

Chlamydial pneumonia is seen in 11% to 20% of infants born to untreated mothers. Onset of symptoms often occurs as early as two to three weeks of age, gradually worsening and prompting the diagnosis by four to six weeks of age. Symptoms include tachypnea with a staccato cough and rales; the chest X ray shows hyperexpansion with diffuse interstitial and patchy alveolar infiltrates.

Treatment for both infections involves a two-week course of oral erythromycin, which offers the advantage of clearing all colonization sites, including the nasopharynx. Such clearance is not accomplished when only topical antibiotic therapy is administered to treat conjunctivitis.

## Diagnosis

Chlamydiae have a unique growth cycle and therefore are quite different from the other common agent causing endocervical infection, *Neisseria gonorrhoeae*. With *C. trachomatis*, the infectious particle is called the elementary body and is the extracellular form. It is not metabolically active and appears quite resistant to environmental influences. This elementary body attaches to the host cell and appears to induce phagocytosis so as to gain access to the host. In the host, it remains within the phagocytic vesicle but changes to a metabolically active and dividing form called the reticulate body.

*C. trachomatis* thus is an obligate intracellular parasite. It cannot synthesize high-energy compounds itself; instead, it must use host cell substrates to synthesize its proteins, including RNA and DNA. For this reason, for purposes of identification, *C. trachomatis* can be grown only in tissue culture, not in artificial media. Alternatively, it can be identified by immunofluorescence staining of smears with monoclonal antibody or by detection of chlamydial antigen by enzyme-linked immunoassay (ELISA).

The introduction of these two techniques made the screening of pregnant women for *C. trachomatis* more practical.

More recently, DNA amplification techniques have been employed to improve screening and diagnosis of *C. trachomatis* even more. Ligase chain reaction (LCR) testing for cervical infection has yielded a sensitivity of 94% and a specificity of 99.9% compared with 65% and 100%, respectively, for cell culture. Similarly, polymerase chain reaction (PCR) testing offers equally high sensitivity (91.7%) and specificity (100%). Use of PCR has permitted accurate screening in pregnancy, even in low-prevalence populations.

## Treatment

### Neonatal Prophylaxis

Although oral antibiotics can be prescribed to treat chlamydial infection, the more preferable course is to prevent the development of infection at the outset. Initial strategies for preventing inclusion conjunctivitis due to *C. trachomatis* infection have focused on newborn ocular prophylaxis. Prevention of gonococcal ophthalmia neonatorum by prophylactic instillation of silver nitrate drops had long been standard practice in almost all newborn nurseries.

With the recognition that *C. trachomatis* is the most common organism causing neonatal conjunctivitis in more currently studied populations, attention has turned to ocular antibiotic preparations that would cover both *N. gonorrhoeae* and *C. trachomatis*. In 1980, Hammerschlag and coworkers suggested that 0.5% erythromycin ophthalmic ointment could prevent chlamydial conjunctivitis as well as gonococcal ophthalmia. In 1988, Laga and coworkers reported that 1% tetracycline ointment was also effective in preventing conjunctivitis caused by either *N. gonorrhoeae* or *C. trachomatis*.

Hammerschlag and colleagues later prospectively evaluated use of silver nitrate drops, erythromycin ointment, and tetracycline ointment for preventing neonatal conjunctivitis among infants born in a large urban hospital. The total incidence of gonococcal ophthalmia was low in this group of newborns

(0.06%), and the failure rate for prophylaxis with each regimen was roughly the same. The frequency of prophylaxis failure for each regimen was also comparable with respect to chlamydial conjunctivitis. On the other hand, the rate of failure was disturbingly high and not significantly different: 20% in the silver nitrate group, 14% in the erythromycin group, and 11% in the tetracycline group. The investigators concluded that ocular prophylaxis with any of the regimens was effective for gonococcal conjunctivitis but that chlamydial conjunctivitis would be prevented most effectively by the screening and treatment of pregnant women before delivery.

## Maternal Therapy

Two studies initially addressed the issue of preventing vertical transmission of *C. trachomatis* by screening and treating women during pregnancy. In 1986, Schachter and coworkers reported their experience using erythromycin ethylsuccinate, 400 mg four times daily for 7 days at 36 weeks' gestation. The infants of treated mothers were followed for one year or until maternal antichlamydial antibody disappeared. Overall, 92% (98 of 107) of women who completed a course of therapy and had tests of cure were successfully cleared of their chlamydial infection. Vertical transmission was prevented in 93% (55 of 59) of their infants, with no evidence of chlamydial infection by culture and/or antichlamydial serology. On the down side, 6.6% of treated women experienced gastrointestinal side effects so severe that half of them stopped their therapy.

Occurrence of gastrointestinal side effects led the same investigators to seek an alternative regimen for women intolerant of, or allergic to, erythromycin. They compared amoxicillin, 500 mg three times daily for 7 days, with erythromycin base, 500 mg four times daily for 7 days. Chlamydial infection was eradicated in 98% (63 of 64) of women treated with amoxicillin and in 95% (55 of 58) of women treated with erythromycin base. Similarly, vertical transmission was prevented in 95% (37 of 39) of infants whose mothers received amoxicillin compared with 89% (32 of 36) of infants whose mothers were in the

**Table 12-1.** Azithromycin versus Erythromycin Therapy for Chlamydial Infection

| | **Total Patients Treated** | | **Failure of Therapy** | | **Frequency of Side Effects** | |
|---|---|---|---|---|---|---|
| **Study** | **Azithromycin** | **Erythromycin** | **Azithromycin** | **Erythromycin** | **Azithromycin** | **Erythromycin** |
| Bush and Rose | 15 | 15 | 0 | 1 | 0 | 15 |
| Rosenn et al. | 23 | 22 | 2 | 5 | 4 | 10 |
| Edwards et al. | 62 | 64 | 4 | 18 | 12 | 42 |
| Adair et al. | 42 | 43 | 5 | 3 | 5 | 25 |
| **Total** | 142 | 144 | 11 (7.8%) | 27 (18.8%) | 21 (14.8%) | 92 (63.8%) |

erythromycin base group. Of eight patients (8.6%) in the amoxicillin group who experienced side effects, only two stopped their therapy. In contrast, of 15 patients (15%) in the erythromycin group who experienced side effects, 13 discontinued their therapy.

Subsequently, at least four other studies have compared the efficacy and side effects of therapy with amoxicillin and erythromycin for the treatment of cervical infection with *C. trachomatis.* As noted in the meta-analysis by Turrentine and Newton, infection was eradicated in 92.6% (225 of 249) of amoxicillin-treated patients and in 94.9% (206 of 217) of patients treated with erythromycin. More importantly, these investigators demonstrated that discontinuation of therapy because of gastrointestinal side effects could be reduced by 86% with use of amoxicillin for therapy.

In its 1998 guidelines, the Centers for Disease Control and Prevention recommends either of two regimens as first-line therapy for *C. trachomatis* infection in pregnancy:

- Erythromycin base, 500 mg four times daily for 7 days
- Amoxicillin, 500 mg three times daily for 7 days

Azithromycin, 1 g orally in a single dose, is listed as an alternative regimen.

To date, the number of well-studied pregnant patients treated with azithromycin remains small, but the outcomes are striking (Table 12-1). In one study, chlamydial infection was eradicated in 92.2% (131 of 142) of women treated with azithromycin compared with 81.2% (117 of 144) of women treated with erythromycin. One obvious contributor to the lower success rate with erythromycin was the 63.8% frequency of side effects with this drug; the comparable rate for azithromycin was only 14.8%.

In addition to a relatively small patient experience with azithromycin, the higher cost of therapy with this drug also must be taken into account. Nevertheless, given the high frequency of side effects with erythromycin—which can lead to noncompliance and the need to reculture and retreat—azithromycin may ultimately prove to be the better choice for first-line therapy.

## Suggested Readings

Adair CD, Gunter M, Stovall TG, et al. *Chlamydia* in pregnancy: a randomized trial of azithromycin and erythromycin. Obstet Gynecol 1998;91:165–168.

Bush MR, Rosa C. Azithromycin and erythromycin in the treatment of cervical chlamydial infection during pregnancy. Obstet Gynecol 1994;84:61–63.

Catry MA, Borrego MJ, Cardoso J, et al. Comparison of the Amplicor *Chlamydia trachomatis* test and cell culture for the detection of urogenital chlamydial infections. Genitourin Med 1995;71:247–250.

Centers for Disease Control and Prevention. 1998 guidelines for treatment of sexually transmitted diseases. MMWR 1998;47 (RR-1):53–56.

Crombleholme WR, Schachter J, Grossman M, et al. Amoxicillin therapy for *Chlamydia trachomatis* in pregnancy. Obstet Gynecol 1990;75:752–756.

Edwards M, Newman R, Carter S, et al. Randomized clinical trial of azithromycin versus erythromycin for the treatment of chlamydial cervicitis in pregnancy. Infect Dis Obstet Gynecol 1996;4:333–337.

Hammerschlag MR, Chandler JW, Alexander ER, et al. Erythromycin ointment for ocular prophylaxis of neonatal chlamydial infection. JAMA 1980;244:2291–2293.

Hammerschlag MR, Cummings C, Roblin PM, et al. Efficacy of neonatal ocular prophylaxis for the prevention of chlamydial and gonococcal conjunctivitis. N Engl J Med 1989;320:769–772.

Harrison HR, Alexander ER. *Chlamydia trachomatis* infections of the infant. In: Holmes KK, Mårdh PA, Sparling PF, et al., eds. Sexually transmitted diseases. New York: McGraw-Hill, 1990:811–820.

Laga M, Plummer FA, Piot P, et al. Prophylaxis of gonococcal and chlamydial ophthalmia neonatorum: a comparison of silver nitrate and tetracycline. N Engl J Med 1988;318:653–657.

Rosenn MF, Macones GA, Silverman NS. Randomized trial of erythromycin and azithromycin for treatment of chlamydial infection in pregnancy. Infect Dis Obstet Gynecol 1995;3:241–244.

Schachter J, Stamm WE, Quinn T, et al. Ligase chain reaction to detect *Chlamydia trachomatis* infection of the cervix. J Clin Microbiol 1994;32:2540–2543.

Schachter J, Sweet RL, Grossman M, et al. Experience with the routine use of erythromycin for chlamydial infections in pregnancy. N Engl J Med 1986;314:276–279.

Turrentine MA, Newton ER. Amoxicillin or erythromycin for the treatment of antenatal chlamydial infection: a meta-analysis. Obstet Gynecol 1995;86:1021–1025.

CHAPTER 13

# *Gonococcal Infections in Pregnancy*

*Walter J. Morales*

## Background and Incidence

*Neisseria gonorrhoeae* infection is the most common sexually transmitted disease (STD) in the United States, with slightly less than 1 million new cases reported annually and another 1 million unreported new cases estimated to occur each year. The causative organism, a gram-negative diplococcus, may infect the epithelium of the genitourinary tract as well as the rectum, pharynx, or eye. A localized acute infection may give rise to bacteremia and disseminated disease. In men, *N. gonorrhoeae* can infect the urethra after an incubation period of five to seven days. The risk of transmission from an infected male to an unprotected female partner is about 70%.

Depending on the socioeconomic status of the population studied, the incidence of gonococcal infection in pregnancy ranges from 0.5% to 10%. This condition results in a broad spectrum of maternal and neonatal disease. In some studies, colonized pregnant patients have been reported to have an increased risk of preterm birth and premature rupture of membranes, underscoring the need to diagnose gonococcal disease in pregnancy properly and to provide effective therapy promptly.

## Diagnosis

Culture for *N. gonorrhoeae* and tests for chlamydial infection and syphilis should be performed at the first prenatal visit. For women at high risk of STDs, culture and testing should be repeated late in the third trimester.

## Clinical Diagnosis

Gonococcal infection in women is frequently asymptomatic. In some patients, genitourinary infection may result in dysuria and purulent discharge after a one- to three-week incubation period. On examination, the cervix may be erythematous and friable, with a mucopurulent discharge. Frequently, the findings are minimal. Pus may be expressed from the urethra, Skene's ducts, or Bartholin's gland. Ascending infection occurs only very rarely in pregnancy; when it does occur, it tends to appear in the first trimester.

Untreated gonococcal infection may progress to disseminated disease. This serious complication follows an initial bacteremic phase characterized by a pustular dermatitis. During this first stage of disseminated disease, blood cultures are positive for *N. gonorrhoeae* in half of the patients. In contrast, cultures from the pustules are positive in only one-fifth of cases. Lesions are frequently located in the periphery of the arms and eventually resolve without residual scarring. Typically, lesions have necrotic centers and hemorrhagic bases caused by gonococcal emboli. In addition to bacteremia, patients with disseminated gonococcal infection (DGI) often experience a low-grade fever, myalgias, and migratory polyarthralgia. The bacteremia may lead to endocarditis, pericarditis, and meningitis.

Disseminated gonococcal infection can also take the form of an acute febrile illness associated with a severe arthritis (see Chapter 45). In these cases, purulent synovial effusion may cause significant pain and limit the patient's range of motion. The skin overlying the joint—usually the knees, ankles, or wrists—is warm to the touch and erythematous. Aspiration of the purulent effusion permits identification of the organism, although blood cultures usually give negative results.

## Laboratory Diagnosis

A Gram's stain of the purulent material from the genitourinary tract exudate can provide rapid identification of *N. gonorrhoeae.*

Smears are positive on microscopic examination in 90% of infected men but in only 60% of infected women. Detection of the gonococcal antigen by an enzyme immunoassay (Gonozyme, Abbott Laboratories, North Chicago, Illinois) has been described. This test is highly specific (97%) but not especially sensitive (60%). Although its sensitivity improves with increasing numbers of colony-forming units/plate, this enzyme immunoassay should not be employed for diagnostic confirmation of clinical infection or for widespread screening of a low-prevalence asymptomatic population.

The laboratory diagnosis of *N. gonorrhoeae* is best accomplished by isolating the organism on a selective medium such as Thayer–Martin broth. Some colonies may appear as early as 24 hours after incubation; most become evident by 48 hours.

## Perinatal Implications

In their first trimester, pregnant patients with untreated endocervical gonococcal infection are at increased risk for endometritis after elective abortion or chorionic villus sampling. As a result, proper documentation of a negative culture is required before carrying out either procedure.

Acute salpingitis in pregnancy is extremely rare and very difficult to diagnose; when it does occur, it appears most frequently during the first trimester and is associated with substantial fetal wastage. Acute salpingitis should be considered in the differential diagnosis of appendicitis in the febrile patient with abdominal or pelvic tenderness, particularly in those who are at risk for STDs and who have a mucopurulent discharge. Correct diagnosis will permit proper antibiotic therapy, sparing the patient the risk of unnecessary abdominal surgery.

Although subclinical lower genital tract infection has been strongly correlated with prematurity, the specific role played by gonococcal infection in preterm birth remains uncertain. Earlier reports failed to correct for the potentially detrimental contributions of chlamydial, group B streptococcal, trichomonal, and bacterial vaginosis infection to preterm birth and may have overestimated the importance of gonococcal infection. Nevertheless, studies by Elliot and coworkers and Alger and coworkers have associated *N. gonorrhoeae* with preterm delivery. In addition, women with gonococcal endocervical infection are at high risk for concomitant cervical chlamydial infection, which is itself associated with preterm birth. *N. gonorrhoeae* also has been isolated in the amniotic fluid of patients who had intact membranes and ultimately developed clinical amnionitis.

A recent study by McGregor and coworkers, however, failed to confirm a direct relationship between gonococcal infection and preterm birth. Nevertheless, all patients in idiopathic preterm labor—and most certainly those with rupture of membranes—should be cultured for *N. gonorrhoeae* and other STDs and treated if the culture gives positive results. Endocervical infection with *N. gonorrhoeae* has been identified in several studies as a risk factor for postpartum endomyometritis. Therefore, the practice of routine antenatal culture for this organism should continue in all at-risk patients.

Finally, maternal endocervical colonization with *N. gonorrhoeae* can lead to vertical transmission to the newborn, with a risk of conjunctivitis of 30% to 40% (see Chapter 14). Although the detection of penicillinase-producing *N. gonorrhoeae* (PPNG) has increased, no evidence exists (other than requirements for alternative neonatal therapy) that the emergence of this strain has affected the risk of vertical transmission. While neonatal sepsis caused by this organism is a rare event, it has been reported by Hammerschlag and coworkers.

## Treatment

The recommended treatment regimen for pregnant women with gonococcal infection is a single dose of ceftriaxone (125 mg IM) or cefixime (400 mg orally), plus erythromycin base (500 mg orally four times daily for 7 days). Women who are allergic to penicillin should be given a single dose of spectinomycin (2 g IM), followed by erythromycin. Cervical and rectal cultures for *N. gonorrhoeae* should be performed four to seven days after treatment ends.

Pregnant women with gonorrhea should also receive therapy for chlamydial infection if tests for *Chlamydia trachomatis* are positive. They should be treated for chlamydial infection presumptively if the results of such tests are not available. Treatment with tetracyclines, including doxycycline, or fluoroquinolones is contraindicated in pregnancy because of the possibility of adverse effects on the fetus.

Patients with DGI should be hospitalized and examined for clinical signs of endocarditis or meningitis. The recommended regimen for DGI is ceftriaxone, 1 g IM or IV every 24 hours; ceftizoxime, 1 g IV every 8 hours; or cefotaxime, 1 g IV every 8 hours. DGI patients allergic to penicillin should be treated with spectinomycin, 2 g IM every 12 hours. All regimens should be continued for 48 hours after improvement begins; treatment then may be switched to cefixime, 400 mg orally twice a day, to complete seven days of therapy. If the infecting organism is penicillin-sensitive, the patient may be switched to ampicillin, 1 g IV every 6 hours, followed by oral amoxicillin with clavulanic acid, 500 mg three times a day, to complete the seven days of therapy. Women receiving therapy for DGI should be tested for genital chlamydial infection or treated empirically for such infection if the results of such testing are not available.

Gonococcal meningitis and endocarditis require high-dose therapy with ceftriaxone, 1 to 2 g IV every 12 hours, or an antibiotic effective against the strain causing the disease. Although the optimal duration of therapy remains unknown, most authorities advise treating gonococcal meningitis for 10 to 14 days and gonococcal endocarditis for at least 4 weeks.

Women with gonococcal meningitis, endocarditis, or nephritis and those with recurrent DGI should be evaluated for complement deficiencies. Complicated DGI should be managed in consultation with an infectious diseases expert.

Prophylaxis for the newborn against ophthalmia neonatorum has been changed from the use of silver nitrate to use of either erythromycin or tetracycline (see Chapter 14).

## Suggested Readings

Alexander ER. Gonorrhea in the newborn. Ann NY Acad Sci 1988;549:180–186.

Alger LS, Lovchik JC, Hebel JR, et al. The association of *Chlamydia trachomatis, Neisseria gonorrhoeae*, and group B streptococci with preterm rupture of the membranes and pregnancy outcome. Am J Obstet Gynecol 1988;159:397–404.

Amstey MS, Steadman KT. Asymptomatic gonorrhea and pregnancy. J Am Vener Dis Assoc 1976;3:14–16.

Blanchard AC, Pastorek JG II, Weeks T. Pelvic inflammatory disease during pregnancy. South Med J 1987;80:1363–1365.

Christmas JT, Wendel GD, Bawdon RE, et al. Concomitant infection with *Neisseria gonorrhoeae* and *Chlamydia trachomatis* in pregnancy. Obstet Gynecol 1989;74:295–298.

Elliott B, Brunham RC, Laga M, et al. Maternal gonococcal infection as a preventable risk factor for low birth weight. J Infect Dis 1990;161:531–536.

Hammerschlag MR, Cummings C, Roblin PM, et al. Efficacy of neonatal ocular prophylaxis for the prevention of chlamydial and gonococcal conjunctivitis. N Engl J Med 1989;320:769–772.

Lieberman RW, Wheelock JB. The diagnosis of gonorrhea in a low-prevalence female population: enzyme immunoassay versus culture. Obstet Gynecol 1987;69:743–746.

Mason PR, Katzenstein DA, Chimbira TH, et al. Vaginal flora of women admitted to hospital with signs of sepsis following normal delivery, cesarean section, or abortion. The Puerperal Sepsis Study Group. Cent Afr J Med 1989;35:344–351.

McGregor JA, French JI, Parker R, et al. Prevention of premature birth by screening and treatment for common genital tract infections: results of a prospective controlled evaluation. Am J Obstet Gynecol 1995;173:157–167.

Smith LG Jr, Summers PR, Miles RW, et al. Gonococcal chorio-amnionitis associated with sepsis: a case report. Am J Obstet Gynecol 1989;160:573–574.

Thomason JL, Gelbart SM, Sobieski VJ, et al. Effectiveness of Gonozyme for detection of gonorrhea in low-risk pregnant and gynecologic populations. Sex Trans Dis 1989;16:28–31.

CHAPTER

# 14

# *Ophthalmia Neonatorum*

*Mara J. Dinsmoor*

## Background and Incidence

Ophthalmia neonatorum (ON)—conjunctivitis that occurs within an infant's first month of life—was first discovered during the mid-1700s, when the association between maternal vaginal discharge and neonatal conjunctivitis was identified. By 1881, as many as 10% of infants developed ON (1). Since the advent of silver nitrate prophylaxis and the subsequent discovery of antibiotics, however, blindness from ON has become increasingly rare. In this century alone, the incidence has dropped 100-fold.

The incidence of ON parallels that of maternal gonorrhea and chlamydial infections. Overall, approximately 3 to 10 cases of ON occur for every 1000 live births. Some prospective studies, however, report incidences of chlamydial conjunctivitis alone of as many as 63 cases for every 1000 births.

Chemical conjunctivitis, which is characterized by conjunctival edema, hyperemia, and watery discharge, affects as many as 90% of infants following prophylaxis with topical 1% silver nitrate prophylaxis. It typically occurs within a few hours of administration and always is sterile.

Although the proportion of ON caused by infectious agents is fairly constant, the relative proportion of specific pathogens associated with this infection varies among institutions. This variation may be attributed to the fluctuating prevalence of maternal infection and differences in prenatal surveillance and treatment for sexually transmitted diseases. Microbiological differences also may arise because of variations in ocular prophylactic regimens and diagnostic techniques.

## Etiology

*Chlamydia trachomatis* is a common cause of ON that often manifests itself after administration of silver nitrate prophylaxis, which is not effective against *C. trachomatis*. Approximately 20% to 40% of newborns exposed intrapartum to *C. trachomatis* will develop ON, usually within 5 to 10 days after delivery. The overall incidence of ON from this source has been estimated to be eight in every 1000 births. Characteristically, a large amount of mucopurulent exudate is present; likewise, pseudomembrane formation is common. The lower portion of the eye is more often affected than is the upper portion.

*Staphylococcus aureus* and other bacteria cause a milder conjunctivitis that rarely affects the cornea. Other organisms frequently implicated in ON are *Streptococcus pneumoniae*, *Haemophilus influenzae*, *Escherichia coli*, and α-hemolytic streptococci. Mixed infections also can occur.

Approximately 30% to 50% of newborns born to women who have gonococcal cervicitis will develop gonococcal conjunctivitis. The incidence appears to be higher in premature infants and in cases involving premature rupture of membranes. Gonococcal ophthalmia, which typically emerges as bilateral, purulent conjunctivitis within the first week of life, occurs in approximately one of every 2000 live births.

Although viruses rarely cause ON, 15% to 20% of newborns infected with herpes simplex virus (HSV) will develop ocular complications. The eye is the only affected organ in approximately 4% of infected newborns. Ocular herpes infection usually appears within the first two weeks of life.

## Diagnosis

When conjunctivitis develops after the first day of life, persists for more than three days, or progresses, it is unlikely to be chemical. A diagnostic evaluation should therefore be performed. Although the type and timing of symptoms can be useful, such information is not diagnostic.

Gram's stain of the exudate may reveal gram-negative intracellular diplococci (suggesting gonococcal infection), gram-positive cocci (*S. aureus*), or gram-negative bacilli (*H. influenzae*). Evidence of multinucleated giant cells on Papanicolaou staining is characteristic of a herpes infection. It is also useful to perform cultures of the exudate, including specific tests for *Neisseria gonorrhoeae* using chocolate or Thayer–Martin agar. If you suspect *N. gonorrhoeae*, culture the oropharynx and anus as well.

If possible, perform cultures for *C. trachomatis* and HSV. Because of their low sensitivity, do not rely solely on Giemsa stains of conjunctival scrapings to eliminate chlamydial infection as a possible cause of ON. Positive findings can be used, however, to guide early treatment. Acceptable alternatives to culture for detecting *Chlamydia* include direct fluorescent antibody tests, enzyme immunoassays, and DNA probes. Early studies of polymerase chain reaction (PCR) for detection of *Chlamydia* also show promise.

## Treatment

Chlamydial conjunctivitis requires systemic treatment with erythromycin for two weeks. Although topical erythromycin ointment will effectively cure the conjunctivitis, nasopharyngeal carriage may persist and place the infant at risk for chlamydial pneumonia. If oral erythromycin regimens fail, as happens in approximately 20% of cases, IV treatment is recommended.

All infants born to women who have cervical gonorrhea should receive prophylaxis of a single dose of ceftriaxone. Treatment for gonococcal ON consists of IV or IM ceftriaxone or cefotaxime for seven days combined with eye irrigation with saline or ophthalmic solutions. It has been suggested that a single dose of ceftriaxone may prove effective if no evidence of disseminated infection is found. Because of the high prevalence of penicillin-resistant *N. gonorrhoeae*, most experts discourage treatment with penicillin. Isolate infants with gonococcal ophthalmia for the first 24 hours of treatment, as this condition is very contagious. Examine and treat the mother and her sex partner(s) when a diagnosis of chlamydial or gonococcal conjunctivitis is made.

Treatment of ON caused by HSV infection relies on isolation and use of topical antiviral agents such as trifluorothymidine or adenine arabinoside. Consider evaluating the patient for systemic involvement and initiating systemic antiviral therapy, as ocular involvement may precede manifestations of systemic disease.

ON caused by gram-negative bacilli may be treated with gentamicin ophthalmic ointment given four times daily for one week. When you suspect pseudomonal infections, administer parenteral antibiotics as well. Treat infections caused by gram-positive cocci or "nonspecific" inflammation with erythromycin ophthalmic ointment four times daily for one week.

## SEQUELAE

Undertreated or untreated bacterial conjunctivitis may result in septicemia, nasolacrimal duct obstruction, corneal ulceration, or blindness. ON caused by *S. aureus* may be complicated by corneal ulcers or infiltrates, hypopyon (puslike fluid in the anterior chamber), endophthalmitis, and exfoliative dermatitis. Although untreated ON caused by *C. trachomatis* usually will resolve spontaneously and rarely results in visual loss, it can lead to conjunctival scarring and pannus formation (neovascularization of the cornea). Furthermore, it may precede colonization of the upper respiratory tract and chlamydial pneumonia. Early treatment, however, can prevent such ocular sequelae. ON that results from herpes infection also may lead to keratitis, cataracts, chorioretinitis, or optic neuritis.

## PREVENTION

Introduced as prophylaxis against gonococcal ON in 1881, silver nitrate drops remained the "gold standard" in the United States until the 1970s, when concerns arose about their effectiveness in preventing chlamydial conjunctivitis. Recent studies have found that both 0.5% erythromycin and 1% tetracycline ointment effectively prevent gonococcal conjunctivitis, the most serious pathogen in terms of long-term sequelae (2,3).

Studies have produced conflicting results, however, as to whether these ointments can effectively prevent chlamydial disease. A recent trial of povidone-iodine as prophylaxis revealed that, overall, this regimen was more effective in preventing infectious conjunctivitis (including cases caused by *Chlamydia*) than were both silver nitrate and erythromycin (4). In addition, the incidence of noninfectious conjunctivitis (most likely a local reaction to the treatment) was significantly lower in the infants treated with povidone-iodine.

The relative costs of the different prophylactic regimens and the local disease prevalence are important factors when selecting a prophylactic regimen. The American Academy of Pediatrics currently recommends prophylaxis with a 1% silver nitrate solution in single-dose ampules, or a single-use tube of an ophthalmic ointment containing 0.5% erythromycin or 1% tetracycline.

The effectiveness of erythromycin or tetracycline in preventing ON caused by penicillinase-producing *N. gonorrhoeae* has not been established as yet. In addition, no topical regimen has proven efficacy in preventing chlamydial conjunctivitis. As noted by Hammerschlag and coworkers, most cases of gonococcal ON occur in infants born to women who received no prenatal care (2). Consequently, diagnosis and treatment of maternal genital infections with *C. trachomatis* and *N. gonorrhoeae* before delivery remain of utmost importance.

## References


1. Rothenberg R. Ophthalmia neonatorum due to *Neisseria gonorrhoeae*: prevention and treatment. Sex Trans Dis 1979;6(suppl):187–191.
2. Hammerschlag MR, Cummings C, Roblin PM, et al. Efficacy of neonatal ocular prophylaxis for the prevention of chlamydial and gonococcal conjunctivitis. N Engl J Med 1989;320:769–772.
3. Laga M, Plummer FA, Piot P, et al. Prophylaxis of gonococcal and chlamydial ophthalmia neonatorum: a comparison of silver nitrate and tetracycline. N Engl J Med 1988;318:653–657.
4. Isenberg SJ, Apt L, Wood M. A controlled trial of povidone-iodine as prophylaxis against ophthalmia neonatorum. N Engl J Med 1995;332:562–566.

## Suggested Readings

American Academy of Pediatrics. Prevention of neonatal ophthalmia. In: 1994 red book: report of the Committee on Infectious Diseases, 23rd ed. Elk Grove Village, IL: American Academy of Pediatrics, 1994:533.

Jarvin VN, Levine R, Asbell PA. Ophthalmia neonatorum: study of a decade of experience at the Mount Sinai Hospital. Br J Ophthalmol 1987;71:295–300.

Prentice MJ, Hutchinson GR, Taylor-Robinson D. A microbiological study of neonatal conjunctivae and conjunctivitis. Br J Ophthalmol 1977;61:601–607.

Sandstrom KI, Bell TA, Chandler JW, et al. Diagnosis of neonatal purulent conjunctivitis caused by *Chlamydia trachomatis* and other organisms. In: Mårdh PA, Holmes KK, Oriel JD, et al., eds. Chlamydial infections. New York: Elsevier Biomedical Press, 1982.

CHAPTER

# 15

# *Syphilis in Pregnancy*

*Larry C. Gilstrap III*
*George D. Wendel, Jr.*

## Background and Incidence

The number of cases of syphilis in the United States began to rise in the latter part of the 1980s, peaked in 1990, and then began to decrease. According to the Centers for Disease Control and Prevention (CDC), the rate of primary and secondary syphilis in 1997 was 3.2 per 100,000. In the same year, more than 1000 cases of congenital syphilis were reported.

Klass and associates at Boston City Hospital found that congenital syphilis was associated with substance abuse, HIV infection, lack of prenatal care, treatment failures, and reinfection. Although pregnancy itself does not affect the course of syphilis, this infection may cause premature birth, stillbirth, and neonatal morbidity and mortality.

## Pathophysiology

Infection is accomplished when *Treponema pallidum*, the etiologic agent, gains entrance to the host through a break in a mucous membrane. A lesion, chancre, or ulcer develops at the site of inoculation. This chancre is the hallmark of primary syphilis. If the patient is not treated, spirochetemia will likely occur.

Spirochetes readily cross the placenta to produce chronic infection in the fetus, although clinical disease does not generally become evident before 18 weeks' gestation. The most common

**Table 15-1.** Findings in Newborns with Congenital Syphilis

| |
|---|
| **Clinical** |
| Hepatosplenomegaly |
| Osteochondritis/periostitis |
| Lymphadenopathy |
| Jaundice |
| Ascites/edema/hydrops |
| Petechiae/purpura |
| **Laboratory** |
| Reactive serologic test in blood/cerebrospinal fluid |
| Anemia/thrombocytopenia |
| Hyperbilirubinemia |
| Abnormal liver function tests |
| Elevated cerebrospinal fluid cell count/protein |

clinical findings in newborns with congenital syphilis are hepatosplenomegaly, osteochondritis or periostitis, jaundice or hyperbilirubinemia, petechiae, purpura, lymphadenopathy, and ascites or hydrops (Table 15-1).

Newborns also may manifest with rhinitis ("snuffles"), pneumonia alba, myocarditis, or nephrosis. The placenta may be affected as well, characteristically being very large and "waxy" in appearance. Microscopic examination of the placenta frequently will reveal focal villitis, immature villi, and endarteritis. The umbilical cord may show necrotizing funisitis.

## Diagnosis

Primary syphilis in pregnant and nonpregnant women can be diagnosed either by the identification of *Treponema pallidum* through dark-field examination of material taken from a chancre or via serologic testing. As the majority of pregnant women with syphilis do not have lesions when they present for prenatal care, the diagnosis of antepartum syphilis frequently is made by serologic testing. Nonspecific, nontreponemal tests used to screen patients include the Venereal Disease Research Laboratory (VDRL) and rapid plasma reagin (RPR) tests.

Serum samples of individuals with positive screening results should undergo confirmatory tests, such as the microhemagglutination assay for antibodies specific for *T. pallidum* (MHA-TP) or the fluorescent treponemal antibody absorption test (FTA-ABS). All pregnant women with syphilis should be carefully examined for the presence of other sexually transmitted diseases (STDs), such as gonorrhea, trichomoniasis, chlamydial infection, hepatitis B, or HIV infection.

It is important to remember that the chancre of primary syphilis is asymptomatic and that individuals with secondary syphilis may not exhibit any obvious lesions. The clinician may therefore miss the diagnosis of syphilis unless the patient's history indicates that she is at risk. The presence of trichomoniasis, gonorrhea, chlamydial infection, herpes, recently acquired hepatitis B infection, or HIV infection should immediately suggest testing for syphilis.

Serologic testing is important not only in establishing the presence of syphilis, but also for determining the success of the treatment. In most cases, the VDRL or RPR test will revert to negative or become fixed at a low titer. The specific treponemal test, such as MHA-TP or FTA-ABS, will remain positive for life in more than 95% of the cases. Such specific tests are therefore not useful in evaluating individuals who have contracted syphilis in the past.

The diagnosis of congenital syphilis is based primarily on clinical findings, suspicious history, and positive serologic tests (see Table 15-1). For the asymptomatic baby without clinical signs of syphilis, diagnosis can prove much more difficult. Maternal IgG antibody readily crosses the placenta and may cause the newborn's serologic test to be positive. All newborns with suspected syphilis should receive a lumbar puncture for cerebrospinal fluid analysis and radiographic studies of the bones; in approximately 95% of infected infants, these studies will reveal significant changes in metaphyseal bone.

Confirmation of congenital syphilis in a stillborn infant may prove extremely difficult, especially in the severely macerated infant. Staining the fetal tissue to identify spirochetes, performing X-ray studies to look for osteochondritis, and evaluating the placenta may prove helpful in such cases.

**Table 15-2.** Penicillin Regimens for the Treatment of Syphilis

| |
|---|
| **Primary, Secondary, and Early (< 1 year) Latent Syphilis** |
| Benzathine penicillin G, 2.4 million U administered IM in a single dose |
| **Late (> 1 year or unknown duration) Latent Syphilis or Tertiary (gumma or cardiovascular) Syphilis** |
| Benzathine penicillin G, 2.4 million U administered IM weekly for 3 weeks |
| **Neurosyphilis** |
| Aqueous penicillin G, 3 to 4 million U administered IV every 4 hours for 10 to 14 days |
| or |
| Procaine penicillin, 2.4 million U administered IM daily, plus probenecid, 500 mg orally four times daily, for 10 to 14 days. |

SOURCE: Centers for Disease Control and Prevention. 1998 guidelines for treatment of sexually transmitted diseases. MMWR 1998;47:1.

## TREATMENT

Treatment, which is the same for both pregnant and non-pregnant women, consists primarily of the administration of long-acting benzathine penicillin G in doses appropriate for the stage of infection (Table 15-2). Some experts recommend that pregnant women receive benzathine penicillin twice, with doses being administered one week apart. This approach is especially pertinent to women diagnosed with syphilis in the third trimester or those with secondary syphilis.

After receiving treatment for early-stage disease, more than 60% of women will exhibit the Jarisch–Herxheimer reaction, an acute febrile reaction that occurs within the first 12 to 24 hours after administration of penicillin. The Jarisch–Herxheimer reaction may induce premature labor or cause fetal distress. Pregnant patients should be warned to watch for decreases in fetal activity and for signs of preterm labor.

The efficacy of the treatment regimens overall is about 98%, but is lower (95%) with secondary syphilis. All treated pregnant women should receive monitoring in the form of monthly serologic tests and clinical examinations to detect both therapeutic failures and recurrent disease. The patient's RPR or VDRL titer may not rise after treatment, but should fall at least 4-fold or become negative (see chapter 46).

Treatment prior to 20 weeks' gestation can effectively prevent congenital syphilis. Treatment fails in 1% to 2% of patients because of advanced, irreversible fetal infection. These failures are seen more frequently with maternal secondary syphilis or treatment in the late second or third trimester. Ultrasonography prior to treatment may identify fetuses with severe infection (hepatomegaly, ascites, hydrops, or hydramnios). Unfortunately, treatment of the severely affected fetus may lead to preterm labor or fetal death.

The pregnant woman with syphilis who is allergic to penicillin presents a therapeutic challenge. Although erythromycin offers a high cure rate for adults with early syphilis, it may not treat the fetus adequately and therefore is not recommended by the CDC. Tetracycline and doxycycline are contraindicated in the pregnant patient because they may discolor fetal deciduous teeth. No acceptable, proven alternatives to penicillin have been identified.

In 1998, the CDC recommended that pregnant patients with documented syphilis who are known or suspected to be allergic to penicillin undergo skin testing and desensitization. Desensitization can be accomplished either orally or intravenously. Patients who undergo successful desensitization and treatment with penicillin will again require desensitization if they need to receive penicillin again in the future.

Treatment of the newborn who has congenital syphilis should consist of 100,000 to 150,000 U/kg of aqueous crystalline penicillin G, administered intravenously at a dosage of 50,000 U/kg every 8 to 12 hours, or 50,000 U/kg of procaine penicillin G, given IM once daily for 10 days.

## Prevention

Congenital syphilis may be prevented only by early detection, appropriate treatment, and assiduous follow-up. All pregnant women should have serologic testing for syphilis at their first prenatal visit, and again in the third trimester of pregnancy, if they are at high risk for syphilis. The CDC currently recommends that all seropositive pregnant women should be considered infected and treated unless a history of adequate treatment is obtained and confirmed with serologic antibody titers. Finally, all syphilis patients should be counseled about the risks of HIV infection and be encouraged to receive testing for HIV antibody.

## Suggested Readings

Alexander JM, Sheffield JS, Sanchez PJ, et al. Efficacy of treatment for syphilis in pregnancy. Obstet Gynecol 1999;93:5–8.

Centers for Disease Control and Prevention. 1998 guidelines for treatment of sexually transmitted diseases. MMWR;47:1.

Centers for Disease Control and Prevention. Primary and secondary syphilis—United states, 1997. MMWR 1998;47:493–497.

Hira SK, Bhat GJ, Patel JB, et al. Early congenital syphilis: clinico-radiologic features in 202 patients. Sex Trans Dis 1985;12: 177–183.

Klass PE, Brown ER, Pelton SI. The incidence of prenatal syphilis at the Boston City Hospital: a comparison across four decades. Pediatrics 1994;94:24–28.

Rolfs RT. Treatment of syphilis, 1993. Clin Infect Dis 1995; 20(suppl 1):S23–S38.

Sanchez PJ, Wendel GD Jr. Syphilis in pregnancy. Clin Perinatol 1997;24:71–90.

Sheffield JS, Wendel GD Jr. Syphilis in pregnancy. Clin Obstet Gynecol 1999;42:97–106.

Wendel GD, Stark BJ, Jamison RR, et al. Penicillin allergy and desensitization in serious infection during pregnancy. N Engl J Med 1985:312;1229–1232.

CHAPTER

# 16

# *Lyme Disease in Pregnancy*

*Marvin S. Amstey*

## BACKGROUND

Lyme disease is caused by the spirochete *Borrelia burgdorferi*. This organism is transmitted to humans by the bite of a tick. The tick bite produces an early-stage disease, erythema chronicum migrans (ECM), that is a characteristic dermatologic condition. If the infection is treated at this stage, later stages do not occur. If it goes untreated, the systemic manifestations of this spirochetal disease develop: a flu-like syndrome with headache, photophobia, and dysesthesias, followed by acute and chronic neurologic, arthritic, and cardiac diseases.

The tick most commonly found to transmit *B. burgdorferi* is the *Ixodes dammini* (deer tick). At least three other *Ixodes* ticks and the *Amblyomma america* tick, however, also may be vectors for this organism. Most of these ticks are found not on deer but on small rodents, such as field mice.

Since first described in 1975, total Lyme disease cases—in all their manifestations—have increased from approximately 8000 cases in 1989 to more than 16,000 cases in 1996, as reported by the Centers for Disease Control and Prevention (CDC). Ninety percent of these cases were reported from the Northeastern United States, with a peak incidence of rash from ECM occurring in the summer months. The incidence of the disease in pregnant women remains unknown, but estimates based on serologic surveys indicate that 1% of pregnant women in the United States have been infected.

## Maternal Lyme Disease

All reported cases of Lyme disease in pregnancy have demonstrated the same manifestations of the disease that appear in nonpregnant women. This finding suggests that pregnancy itself does not change the disease presentation or progression. The effect of the disease on the pregnancy relates to two problems:

- Illness in the mother severe enough to jeopardize the pregnancy (for example, AV heart block or myopericarditis)
- Placental transmission of the spirochete

## Fetal/Neonatal Disease

Given that *Borrelia* is a spirochete, it is reasonable to assume that this organism crosses the placenta in the same way as does the spirochete that causes syphilis. Such transmission was first demonstrated by Schlesinger and coworkers in 1985. In that case, the infant died 39 hours after birth from complications related to a complex congenital heart problem. Although spirochetes were not found in the heart, they did appear in the infant's kidney, spleen, and bone marrow. Although no cultures were done for this organism, the mother's serum had antibodies to *B. burgdorferi.*

The following year, Markowitz and colleagues at the CDC collected 19 cases of Lyme disease in pregnancy retrospectively. Of these 19 cases, 5 had adverse outcomes, including syndactyly, cortical blindness, intrauterine fetal death, prematurity, and rash. These adverse outcomes occurred regardless of trimester or administration of appropriate therapy. No cardiac lesions were found, no spirochetes were cultured, and no IgM antibody was detected in the five cord-blood samples studied.

A collection of 58 cases of ECM was reported from Slovenia—13 first-trimester cases, 27 second-trimester cases, and 18 third-trimester cases. Outcomes included one missed abortion and five preterm infants, one of which had a cardiac anomaly. These authors concluded that no causal relationship existed between *Borrelia* infection in pregnancy and adverse fetal outcome.

Williams and colleagues conducted a study of 463 infants after birth, dividing them into groups that were serologically positive or negative to *B. burgdorferi.* They found no differences in incidence of malformations based on the infants' serology or geographic location (that is, based on whether they were born in an area endemic for Lyme disease or a county with no cases).

## DIAGNOSIS

The ideal diagnostic approach is to save the tick found on the patient's body and have it tested for the spirochete. Usually, however, this tactic is not possible. The next best approach is to be aware of and recognize ECM. This characteristic skin rash with a target macule or plaque surrounded by a clear zone and circumscribed by an erythematous macular rash lasts three to four weeks. It is associated with pruritus and burning and often appears in multiple sites.

The ELISA and indirect fluorescent antibody (IFA) serologic tests are insensitive with such early-stage infection, and only 50% of patients have positive results on these tests even when the disease has progressed to flu-like symptoms. Only during the late stages, when neurologic, cardiac, or arthritic problems appear, do the serologic tests become sensitive enough to be used with confidence. More importantly, variability of serologic test results among laboratories is great and standards are not available. Although Western blot testing has been used for confirmation of ELISA and IFA tests, its results also vary considerably from laboratory to laboratory. Therefore, the decision to treat relies more heavily on geography, index of suspicion, and whether ticks were seen and removed. When treatment is begun early for any of these reasons, destruction of the spirochete may alter the serologic response, resulting in no laboratory confirmation of the diagnosis.

Serologic tests for syphilis also should be performed because of cross-reactivity. Be aware, however, that a patient with Lyme disease is more likely to have a negative result from a nonspecific test, such as the rapid plasma reagin (RPR) or Venereal Disease Research Laboratory (VDRL) test, but also is more likely to have a positive result from a specific one, such as the fluorescent treponemal antibody (FTA) test. Patients with rheumatoid factor may give false-positive IgM and IgG serological results for *Borrelia*, as they do for syphilis.

## Treatment

The best treatment for Lyme disease is removing the tick before it can transmit the spirochete by inoculation. Individuals should examine their skin completely after venturing into woodlands or meadows known to harbor rodents and deer and remove all ticks. Usually, if this step is taken less than 24 hours after tick attachment, infection from *B. burgdorferi* may be aborted. Even more useful is dressing appropriately to prevent ticks from getting onto the skin. Tick repellents can be helpful, but their use is problematic in pregnancy because of the potential toxicity of the agents. The risk-benefit equation for using such repellents must be weighed. In addition, overuse of repellents in children has produced convulsive symptoms.

Prophylactic treatment of tick bites is common, at least for pregnant women, when protective strategies fail or are not practiced—even though the risk of Lyme disease is estimated to be less than 5% after a tick bite. For early-stage disease and ECM, a three-week course of amoxicillin, 500 mg orally four times daily, or penicillin V, 500 mg four times daily, is commonly recommended. The alternative is erythromycin, 250 mg orally four times daily for three weeks. Later-stage disease (and, according to some, any-stage disease in pregnancy) should be treated with IV antibiotics such as penicillin G, 5 million U every 6 hours for three to four weeks (every 4 hours also is acceptable). An alternative is ceftriaxone, 2 g IM daily for three to four weeks. As with syphilis, consider desensitizing any patient who is allergic to penicillin instead of using erythromycin, which seems to be less effective.

The decision to treat the baby further if the mother has just started therapy or has not completed therapy depends on many factors and should be made with the help of a pediatric infectious disease specialist.

## Suggested Readings

Centers for Disease Control and Prevention. Lyme disease surveillance—United States, 1996. MMWR 1997;46:531–535.

Maraspin V, Cimperman S, Lotric-Furlan S, et al. Treatment of erythema migrans in pregnancy. Clin Infect Dis 1996;22:788–793.

Markowitz LE, Steere AC, Benach JL, et al. Lyme disease during pregnancy. JAMA 1987;255:3394–3396.

Schlesinger PA, Duray PH, Burke BA, et al. Maternal-fetal transmission of the Lyme disease spirochete, *Borrelia burgdorferi.* Ann Intern Med 1985;103:67–68.

Weber K, Pfister HW. Clinical management of Lyme borreliosis. Lancet 1994;343:1017–1020.

Williams CL, Strobino BA. Lyme disease transmission during pregnancy. Contemp Ob/Gyn 1990;35:48–64.

CHAPTER

# 17

# Listeria *Infections in Pregnancy*

*M. Lynn Yonekura*
*Philip B. Mead*

## Background and Incidence

*Listeria monocytogenes* has been recognized as a cause of human disease since 1929. Today, it causes 1700 cases of meningitis and sepsis in the United States each year, with a mortality rate of 33%. Listeriosis primarily affects pregnant women, neonates, the elderly, and individuals with immune system dysfunction. Neonatal disease was first described in 1936, and maternal and fetal infections account for about 50% of reported cases. Although most maternal infections are mild, *Listeria* infection in pregnancy may result in abortion, preterm labor, and fetal infection, with reported rates of neonatal mortality ranging from 7% to more than 50%.

## Pathophysiology

Several epidemics of listeriosis in the 1980s, as well as a substantial proportion of sporadic cases, were caused by foodborne organisms. Thus, while listeriosis is less common than infections due to other foodborne pathogens, *L. monocytogenes* causes more deaths in the United States than any other foodborne pathogen. The median incubation period is 31 days (range 11 to 70 days). Prodromal symptoms include fever, myalgias, headache, diarrhea, nausea, and vomiting.

The pathogenesis of fetal *Listeria* infection starts with maternal hematogenous infection, which leads to placental infection and results in fetal septicemia and multiorgan involvement. Amniotic fluid becomes infected as the agent is excreted in fetal urine. Aspiration and swallowing of infected amniotic fluid then engenders respiratory and gastrointestinal tract involvement.

Variend and Blumenthal have reported two cases that lend support to this proposed transplacental route of infection—one involving early-onset neonatal listeriosis after elective cesarean section at term and the other involving vaginal birth of twins (twin A was uninfected but twin B was seropositive for *Listeria*). Alternatively, an ascending route of infection associated with rectovaginal colonization by *L. monocytogenes* may account for some fetal infections.

Nosocomial transmission of listeriosis between newborns has been reported on two occasions.

## ETIOLOGY

*L. monocytogenes* is a small, aerobic, non–spore-forming, gram-positive rod that is ß-hemolytic on blood agar. Major serotypes causing infection are 1a, 1b, 2a, 2b, and 4b. *L. monocytogenes* is widely distributed in the environment and in animals. Foodborne outbreaks have been traced to consumption of soft cheeses, milk, raw vegetables, and paté. Sporadic cases have been caused by the ingestion of undercooked chicken, unheated hot dogs, and foods purchased from store delicatessen counters. Asymptomatic fecal and vaginal carriage occurs in humans; this source may account for a few sporadic cases.

Both early- and late-onset forms of neonatal listeriosis occur, much as in group B streptococcal infection. The early type presents within two days of birth, with signs of septicemia and pneumonia, and probably derives from transplacental infection. Early-onset disease is most commonly associated with serotypes 1a and 4b. The late form of the disease appears after the fifth day of life and usually presents as meningitis. Late-onset neonatal listeriosis, which is associated with serotype 4b, probably results from infection acquired during or after delivery.

## Diagnosis

Maternal infection with *L. monocytogenes* is often asymptomatic, though patients may experience a flu-like syndrome characterized by chills, fever, and back pain, occasionally mimicking the symptoms of pyelonephritis. Although diarrhea is commonly believed to be a symptom of listeriosis, it was not reported by any pregnant patients in a recent outbreak. Most infected gravidas present with fever, active preterm labor, and brown-stained amniotic fluid that is frequently mistaken for meconium. Intrapartum fetal monitoring commonly shows nonspecific abnormalities consistent with intrauterine infection —for example, fetal tachycardia, decreased variability, and absence of accelerations.

Infants with early-onset disease characteristically are delivered preterm but of appropriate weight for gestational age. Typically, they will experience respiratory distress at birth and evidence of congenital pneumonia. Some will exhibit a fleeting, salmon-colored maculopapular rash.

## Treatment

Maternal listeriosis should be suspected in a pregnant woman with a flu-like syndrome, especially if she has back pain and premature labor. Blood culture, which is often positive, and rectovaginal culture and Gram's stain should be performed as part of the evaluation of such a patient. Amniocentesis specimens for Gram's stain and culture have also been employed for diagnosis. Antimicrobial therapy with intravenous ampicillin plus gentamicin is essential for infection diagnosed during pregnancy, as it may prevent fetal infection and its consequences. In penicillin-allergic patients, trimethoprim/sulfamethoxazole or erythromycin has been used successfully.

Congenital listeriosis should be considered in the differential diagnosis of a depressed preterm infant who is delivered after a labor complicated by fetal distress with meconium- or brown-stained amniotic fluid. The clinician should perform Gram's stain of amniotic fluid and of the newborn's gastric aspirate, cerebrospinal fluid, or skin lesions. Gram's stain of a fecal smear from an infected newborn may show the organism in profusion. The findings of gram-positive rods or coccobacillary forms should prompt a presumptive diagnosis of listeriosis. Inform the microbiologist that *Listeria* infection is a concern, as *L. monocytogenes* can easily be mistaken for diphtheroids and ignored.

Presumptive diagnosis of *Listeria* infection by Gram's stain demands immediate institution of therapy; awaiting confirmation by culture may result in fatal delay. The optimal therapeutic regimen for the infected newborn remains unknown, but initial therapy with ampicillin plus gentamicin is recommended because this combination has proved highly effective in animal models of *Listeria* infection.

## Sequelae

In a recent report of listeriosis identified at perinatal autopsy, gross pathologic lesions were encountered in only one of seven cases; these lesions consisted of a skin rash and small hepatic abscesses. In six cases, the microscopic lesions consisted of rare, localized microabscesses and granuloma-like lesions. One patient had no gross or microscopic findings. Placental lesions, consisting of chorioamnionitis and villitis, appeared in all cases, while three of five examined cords showed acute funisitis.

Although fetal or neonatal infection with *L. monocytogenes* is known to have high fatality, long-term morbidity has not been ascertained. Some studies have found an increased incidence of developmental delays among *Listeria*-infected infants who weighed less than 1250 g and who required assisted ventilation. Others have reported neurodevelopmental handicaps, hydrocephalus, ptosis, and strabismus. In contrast, one author found no evidence of neurodevelopmental sequelae in six of eight survivors and concluded that sequelae for neonatal early-onset listeriosis were uncommon if meningitis was not present. Because meningitis is not characteristic for early-onset disease, the outcome may be generally good. The prognosis for infants with late-onset neonatal sepsis and meningitis has not been extensively studied.

## Prevention

The Centers for Disease Control and Prevention offer the following recommendations for preventing foodborne listeriosis.

### *For All Persons*

1. Thoroughly cook raw food from animal sources.
2. Thoroughly wash raw vegetables before eating.
3. Keep uncooked meats separate from vegetables, cooked foods, and ready-to-eat foods.
4. Avoid consumption of raw (unpasteurized) milk or foods made from raw milk.
5. Wash hands, knives, and cutting boards after handling uncooked foods.

### *Additional Recommendations for Persons at High Risk**

1. Avoid soft cheeses (for example, Mexican-style, feta, Brie, Camembert, and blue-veined cheese). (There is no need to avoid hard cheeses, cream cheese, cottage cheese, or yogurt.)
2. Reheat leftover food or ready-to-eat foods (such as hot dogs) until steaming hot before eating.
3. Although the risk for listeriosis associated with food from delicatessen counters is relatively low, pregnant women and immunosuppressed persons may choose to avoid these foods or to reheat cold cuts thoroughly before eating.

The risk for developing listeria infection after eating a contaminated product is low. Persons who have eaten a contaminated product and do not have any symptoms do not need any special medical evaluation or treatment, even if they are in high-risk groups. However, persons in high-risk groups who become ill with fever or influenza-like illness within 2 months of eating a contaminated product should inform their physicians about this exposure.

* Persons immunocompromised by illness or medications, pregnant women, and the elderly.

## Suggested Readings

Bortolussi R, Seelinger HPR. Listeriosis. In: Remington JS, Klein JO, eds. Infectious diseases of the fetus and newborn infant, 3rd ed. Philadelphia: WB Saunders, 1990:812.

Centers for Disease Control and Prevention. Update: multistate outbreak of listeriosis—United States 1998–1999. MMWR 1999;47:1117–1118.

Cruikshank DP, Warenski JC. First-trimester maternal *Listeria moncytogenes* sepsis and chorioamnionitis with normal neonatal outcome. Obstet Gynecol 1989;73:469–471.

Farber JM, Peterkin PI, Carter AO, et al. Neonatal listeriosis due to cross-infection confirmed by isoenzyme typing and DNA fingerprinting. J Infect Dis 1991;163:927–928.

Kalstone C. Successful antepartum treatment of listeriosis. Am J Obstet Gynecol 1991;164:57–59.

Liner RI. Intrauterine *Listeria* infection: prenatal diagnosis by biophysical assessment and amniocentesis. Am J Obstet Gynecol 1990; 163:1596–1597.

Linnan MJ, Mascola L, Lou XD, et al. Epidemic listeriosis associated with Mexican-style cheese. N Engl J Med 1988;319:823–828.

Lorber B. Listeriosis. Clin Infect Dis 1997;24:1–9.

Schuchat A, Swaminathan B, Broome CV. Epidemiology of human listeriosis. Clin Microbiol Rev 1991;4:169–183.

Teberg AJ, Yonekura ML, Salminen C, et al. Clinical manifestations of epidemic neonatal listeriosis. Pediatr Infect Dis J 1987; 6:817–820.

Variend S, Blumenthal I. Neonatal listeriosis. Postgrad Med J 1975;51:96–99.

CHAPTER

# 18

# *Tuberculosis in Pregnancy*

*Charles V. Sanders*
*Michael K. Hill*

## Background and Incidence

Congenital and neonatally acquired tuberculosis are frequently underdiagnosed, resulting in delayed treatment and a mortality rate approaching 50%. Most fatal cases are diagnosed at autopsy. In contrast, if the diagnosis is suspected early and appropriate treatment initiated promptly, prospects for recovery are excellent.

Although tuberculosis in pregnancy and neonatal and congenital tuberculosis are rare, recent statistics suggest that their incidence will increase in coming years. Higher birth rates in women at risk, coupled with the AIDS epidemic, are the chief factors underlying this trend (Table 18-1).

## Pathophysiology

Opinions about the influence of pregnancy on the prognosis for tuberculosis have varied widely. Good data are now available

**Table 18-1.** Risk Factors for Acquiring Tuberculosis

| |
|---|
| Lower socioeconomic class |
| Poor living conditions |
| Crowded housing conditions |
| Poor nutrition |
| Drug abuse |
| Exposure to infected individuals |
| Lack of prenatal care |

that suggest pregnant women or postpartum women do not face any increased risk of progression as compared with nonpregnant women of the same age.

The most common manifestation of disease in pregnancy includes asymptomatic purified protein derivative (PPD) skin test conversions and pulmonary tuberculosis. Less common entities are peritonitis, meningitis, mastitis, and paraplegia secondary to spinal osteomyelitis (Pott's disease).

Fetal ingestion or aspiration of infected amniotic fluid (AF) and hematogenous infection have been proposed as modes of congenital infection. The liver or regional lymph nodes represent the most frequent sites of involvement, owing to direct seeding from the umbilical vein. Disease may spread to the lungs by direct transplacental transport of organisms through the ductus venosus branch of the umbilical vein or aspiration of infected AF. Although the liver and lungs are the primary organs affected, diffuse hematogenous seeding usually takes place, involving the bone marrow, bone, gastrointestinal tract, adrenal glands, spleen, kidneys, abdominal lymph nodes, and skin.

Lymphohematogenous spread or smoldering endometritis during pregnancy often causes the transmission of infection to the newborn at delivery. Untreated mothers with active pulmonary tuberculosis may infect their infants through close postpartum physical contact.

## Diagnosis

Pregnant women considered to be at high risk for tuberculosis should receive a skin test. These patients include any women with signs or symptoms suggesting either tuberculosis or a history of exposure to it, as well as all HIV-positive patients. In addition, pregnant women who have had a gastrectomy or who work in a hospital, nursing home, or prison should be considered candidates for screening. Women from high-risk ethnic groups, such as Asian refugees and recent Haitian immigrants, should also be tested routinely.

Although some controversy has emerged regarding the validity of PPD testing during pregnancy, overwhelming evidence now shows that such testing is valid at all times. A positive reaction requires further investigation for active disease. Obtain a chest X ray with abdominal shielding. In addition, submit sputum specimens for smear and culture, along with appropriate biopsy specimens if evidence of extrapulmonary disease is found.

Identification of *Mycobacterium tuberculosis* by traditional culture techniques, followed by biochemical testing, requires four to eight weeks; in contrast, radiometric culture methods combined with a DNA probe for *M. tuberculosis*-specific ribosomal RNA sequence can permit identification in one to three weeks. Newer methods based on the polymerase chain reaction (PCR)—though not yet widely in use—have the potential to provide a specific diagnosis within one day.

In all respects, clinical manifestations of active tuberculosis in pregnant women resemble those seen in nonpregnant patients. No substantial evidence suggests that extrapulmonary disease occurs more often in the former patients.

Infants with congenital tuberculosis usually do not manifest signs of disease for several days to weeks after delivery. In most cases, signs and symptoms are nonspecific, including respiratory distress, fever, poor feeding, lethargy, failure to thrive, lymphadenopathy, abdominal distention, hepatomegaly, and splenomegaly. Eventually, extensive progressive infiltrates will appear on the chest X ray, and approximately half will show a miliary pattern.

Diagnosis of congenital or neonatal tuberculosis is difficult. The PPD skin test is almost always initially negative, although it frequently becomes positive six weeks to four months later. Positive smear and culture results can frequently be obtained from liver biopsy specimens, spinal fluid, urine, bone marrow, middle ear fluid, tracheal aspirates, and biopsies of skin lesions or peripheral lymph nodes. Although direct smears from gastric aspirates are unreliable, culture of early morning aspirates may prove highly productive.

## Treatment

Therapy in pregnant women does not differ from that employed in nonpregnant women. Two drugs in standard

**Table 18-2.** Treatment of Tuberculosis in Pregnancy

| Condition | Regimen |
|---|---|
| Active disease | Isoniazid, 300 mg daily, plus rifampin, 600 mg daily, or ethambutol, 2.5 g daily, for minimum of 9 months |
| Positive purified protein derivative (PPD) skin test (recent seroconversion, no evidence of active disease) | Isoniazid, 300 mg after first trimester for 6 to 9 months |
| Positive PPD (no evidence of active disease) | Isoniazid, 300 mg after delivery for 6 to 9 months |
| Neonatal prophylaxis | Isoniazid, 10 mg/kg daily for 3 months; recheck PPD skin test at 3 months; continue treatment |

doses should be administered for nine months (Table 18-2). Extensive experience has been accumulated with isoniazid in pregnancy. Although isoniazid crosses the placenta, it does not appear to be associated with teratogenic effects. Likewise, ethambutol appears to be safe, as no relationship has been identified between its use during pregnancy and fetal abnormalities, including optic deformities. Although rifampin crosses the placenta and theoretically could cause fetal damage because of its ability to inhibit DNA-dependent RNA polymerase production, no such damage has been proven.

In some cases, streptomycin has been associated with severe, irreversible bilateral hearing loss and marked vestibular abnormalities in infants exposed to it in utero. Its use is therefore contraindicated in pregnancy. Capreomycin and kanamycin, which could have the same potential toxicity as streptomycin, are contraindicated as well. Teratogenic effects also have been linked to ethionamide, and cycloserine is known to cause central nervous system side effects; both should be avoided in pregnant patients. As the potential adverse effects of pyrazinamide in pregnancy have not been delineated, it is wise to avoid this agent's use as well.

Pregnant women with active tuberculosis should receive isoniazid and rifampin daily. Always give 50 mg of pyridoxine daily with isoniazid. Ethambutol should be added if isoniazid resistance is a threat. If sensitivities prove all drugs to be effective, treatment may be administered twice weekly after the first one to two months of therapy.

Duration of therapy must last nine months. In most cases, this time is needed because usually the patient receives only two active drugs. It may be necessary to consider therapeutic abortion if the mother is infected with a multidrug-resistant organism and requires treatment with potentially teratogenic medications.

The consensus is that unless the infant is receiving antituberculous therapy, a mother undergoing therapy can safely breast-feed her child. Infants receive less than 20% of the mother's isoniazid dose and less than 11% of other antituberculous drugs in breast milk.

Treatment of congenital or neonatally acquired tuberculosis should begin as soon as a presumptive diagnosis has been made and appropriate smears and cultures obtained. Start with daily isoniazid and rifampin. If a drug-resistant organism is suspected, treatment with four drugs is recommended. Isoniazid, rifampin, streptomycin, and pyrazinamide are recommended for cases involving potentially drug-resistant organisms. Streptomycin appears to be safe in young children. If possible, avoid giving ethambutol to young children and infants because of the potential for retrobulbar neuritis and the inability to check visual acuity in these cases.

When drug susceptibility results are available, treatment can continue with two bactericidal drugs administered twice weekly. A total of six months of treatment is adequate if pyrazinamide, isoniazid, and rifampin are given daily for the first two months. Otherwise, treatment should last for nine months.

Pregnant women younger than age 35 who are PPD-positive but without evidence of active tuberculosis should receive six months of isoniazid prophylaxis starting immediately postpartum. If PPD conversion has occurred within the past one to two years, start isoniazid prophylaxis during the second trimester of pregnancy, regardless of the woman's age.

Infants born to mothers on antituberculous therapy and having negative sputum cultures at the time of delivery are unlikely to develop tuberculosis. One should skin-test the infant at birth and after three months. When the mother has positive sputum cultures, examine the infant thoroughly for tuberculosis. If no evidence of this infection is found, initiate isoniazid prophylaxis (assuming the mother's isolate was not isoniazid-resistant). Bacille Calmette-Guérin vaccination may be an effective alternative to isoniazid prophylaxis in situations where compliance might pose a problem.

## Prevention

Give preventive therapy to pregnant women who have recently converted their PPD skin test and are at high risk of developing progressive disease. Initiating treatment after the first trimester of pregnancy is preferable. On the other hand, treatment of active disease should be started as soon as tuberculosis is diagnosed. Isoniazid, rifampin, and ethambutol—the preferred agents—are considered safe. Mothers taking antituberculous drugs can nurse safely, provided the infant is not also receiving antituberculous therapy.

### Suggested Readings

Barnes PF, Barrows S. Tuberculosis in the 1990s. Arch Intern Med 1993;119:400–410.

Bate TW, Sinclair RE, Robinson MJ. Neonatal tuberculosis. Arch Dis Child 1986;61:512–514.

de March AP. Tuberculosis and pregnancy. Five- to ten-year review of 215 patients in their fertile age. Chest 1975;68:800–804.

Hamadeh MA, Glassroth J. Tuberculosis and pregnancy. Chest 1992;101:1114–1120.

Henderson CE. Management of tuberculosis in pregnancy. J Assoc Acad Minor Phys 1995;6:38–42.

Jacobs RF, Abernathy RS. Management of tuberculosis in pregnancy and the newborn. Clin Perinatol 1988;15:305–319.

Kendig EL Jr. The place of BCG vaccine in the management of infants born of tuberculous mothers. N Engl J Med 1969;281:520–523.

Mofenson LM, Rodriguez EM, Hershow R, et al. *Mycobacterium tuberculosis* infection in pregnant and nonpregnant women infected with HIV in the Women and Infants Transmission Study. Arch Intern Med 1995;155:1066–1072.

Nemir RL, O'Hare D. Congenital tuberculosis. Review and diagnostic guidelines. Am J Dis Child 1985;139:284–287.

Nitta AT, Mulligan D. Management of four pregnant women with multidrug-resistant tuberculosis. Clin Infect Dis 1999;28:1298–1304.

Peterson EM, Lu R, Floyd C, et al. Direct identification of *Mycobacterium tuberculosis*, *Mycobacterium avium*, and *Mycobacterium intracellulare* from amplified primary cultures in BACTEC media using DNA probes. J Clin Microbiol 1989;27:1542–1547.

Robinson CA, Rose NC. Tuberculosis: current implications and management in obstetrics. Obstet Gynecol Surv 1996;51:115–124.

CHAPTER

# 19

# *Postabortal Infections*

*A. Karen Kreutner*

## Background and Incidence

Postabortal infection encompasses a wide range of conditions, from simple febrile morbidity associated with uterine tenderness to pelvic inflammatory disease (PID) with abscess. Septic pelvic thrombophlebitis, bacteremia, and septic shock are possible sequelae.

Although these adverse events have occurred at a low rate after suction procedures, the frequency of complications after the newer medical techniques remains unknown. Both mifepristone (RU-486, an antiprogestin) and methotrexate (an antimetabolite) combined with misoprostol (a prostaglandin given days later) rely on patient compliance for their effectiveness. In the small number of cases where failed or incomplete evacuation occurs, infection becomes a possibility if the patient does not return for follow-up care.

## Etiology

Postabortal infections are polymicrobial in nature. *Chlamydia trachomatis* and bacterial vaginosis (BV) are associated with serious postabortal infections. Identification of these organisms and appropriate therapy are essential before any termination procedure is performed. Other causative organisms include *Neisseria gonorrhoeae*, group B ß-hemolytic streptococci, *Escherichia coli*, and *Staphylococcus aureus*, as well as anaerobes such as *Bacteroides* sp. and peptostreptococci.

## Pathophysiology

Infection after abortion is an ascending process, occurring more commonly in the presence of retained products of conception or operative trauma. Perforation of the uterus, with or without bowel injury, may be followed by severe infection. Risk factors include greater duration of pregnancy, technical difficulties, and the presence of unsuspected sexually transmitted diseases. Short-term prophylaxis with agents such as doxycycline reduces the rate of infection in both high- and low-risk individuals; its use is now recommended.

## Diagnosis

Symptoms of postabortal infection include fever, chills, abdominal pain, and vaginal bleeding, often with the passage of placental tissue. This type of infection generally emerges within four days of the procedure. BV is frequently associated with early symptoms with uterine tenderness, whereas *C. trachomatis* causes the later, more serious, pelvic infections.

Physical findings include an elevated temperature, tachycardia, and tachypnea. In the presence of bacteremia, low blood pressure or frank shock may occur, and the patient may become agitated or disoriented. Pelvic examination will reveal a sanguinopurulent discharge and uterine tenderness, with or without adnexal and parametrial tenderness or fluctuance. It is important to look for cervical and vaginal lacerations, especially in a suspected illegal abortion.

Septic abortion due to *Clostridium perfringens* infection follows a characteristic clinical picture. In the severe case, massive intravascular hemolysis very rapidly produces jaundice, mahogany-colored urine, and severe anemia. This hemolysis frequently leads to acute renal failure secondary to lower-nephron nephrosis. Although critically ill, these patients may appear composed and unconcerned about their illness. The pulse is often disproportionately higher than the fever.

Laboratory diagnostic evaluation for patients with more than early endometritis should include a complete blood count, urinalysis, blood cultures, anteroposterior X ray or ultrasound of the abdomen or pelvis, and upright chest X ray. Endometrial aspiration is the preferred way to obtain material for Gram's stain and culture of the pathogens involved.

## TREATMENT

Because of the polymicrobial etiology of postabortal infections, therapy of even simple endometritis should involve an oral regimen of doxycycline (100 mg twice daily for 14 days), preceded by cefoxitin (2 g IM with probenecid). The alternative outpatient PID regimen of ofloxacin (400 mg twice daily for 14 days) combined with clindamycin or metronidazole is also appropriate. Clinical follow-up within 48 hours must be arranged to evaluate therapeutic response and change the patient's medication if necessary. Persistent bleeding or residual signs of infection require curettage to empty the uterus.

Patients with more serious infection should be admitted to the hospital for surgical removal of infected tissue and appropriate parenteral antibiotic therapy. After the completion of diagnostic procedures, including pelvic ultrasound scans to confirm the presence of retained tissue, broad-spectrum antibiotic therapy with cefoxitin, cefotetan, or clindamycin plus gentamicin should be initiated. For the patient with septic shock, administering clindamycin plus ampicillin, plus either gentamicin or aztreonam, is advisable. In the rare case of clostridial postabortal sepsis, the regimen should include high-dose penicillin.

Surgical drainage is essential. In most cases, the infection can be controlled by prompt curettage of the retained products of conception shortly after admission. When the uterus is too large to permit suction curettage under ultrasound guidance, oxytocin administration may prove successful. Use of prostaglandin suppositories is contraindicated in the presence of acute pelvic infection, but 15-methyl prostaglandin $F_{2\alpha}$ IM injections may be employed (except in asthmatics). Concurrent laparoscopy may be required when curetting a uterus that became perforated at the time of the abortion.

Indications for laparotomy and hysterectomy include failure to respond to curettage and appropriate medical therapy, perforation and infection with suspected bowel injury, pelvic and adnexal abscess, and gas gangrene (clostridial necrotizing myometritis). Isolation of *C. perfringens* does not always mandate hysterectomy. Initial treatment should rely on high-dose parenteral penicillin, curettage, and supportive therapy with intensive cardiovascular monitoring. Laparotomy is indicated if deterioration occurs or the patient does not show any response.

## Sequelae

Prognosis for even severe postabortal sepsis is good. The Centers for Disease Control and Prevention reports that, since 1980, the death-to-case ratio for all abortions has been less than 1 to 100,000. From 1978 to 1985, only five reported deaths from illegal abortion occurred in the United States.

Reproductive potential after a postabortal infection may be compromised by Asherman's syndrome, pelvic adhesions, or incompetent cervix. Tubal infertility is a concern after postabortal infections caused by *N. gonorrhoeae* or *C. trachomatis*.

## Prevention

Avoiding unwanted pregnancies by making contraceptives available is the most important preventive measure. Screening for sexually transmitted diseases before performing elective abortion is optimal but often impractical.

The literature suggests that administration of prophylactic antibiotics reduces infectious morbidity by half when it is used routinely for first-trimester elective suction curettage abortion. Data are not available to support designation of any optimal regimen, but both oral tetracyclines and the nitroimidazoles have been used equally successfully. In some regimens, antibiotic prophylaxis is instituted after the procedure to minimize the common side effects of nausea and vomiting.

## Suggested Readings

Murray S, Muse K. Mifepristone and first trimester abortion. Clin Obstet Gynecol 1996;39:474–485.

Sawaya GF, Grady D, Kerlikowske K, et al. Antibiotics at the time of induced abortion: the case for universal prophylaxis based on meta-analysis. Obstet Gynecol 1996;87:884–890.

Stevenson MM, Radcliffe KW. Preventing pelvic infection after abortion. Int J STD AIDS 1995;6:305–312.

Stubblefield PG, Grimes DA. Septic abortion. N Engl J Med 1994;331:310–314.

CHAPTER

# 20

# *Immunization in Pregnancy*

*Marvin S. Amstey*

## Background

Vaccination of pregnant women is an uncommon preventive therapy. Few physicians perform these procedures enough to understand the agents, doses, responses, or risks involved (Tables 20-1 and 20-2). Therefore, it would not be helpful to discuss the use of all possible immunizing agents in pregnancy. For those interested in this topic, summaries are available elsewhere.

On the other hand, the need for active and passive immunization in pregnancy is growing as people travel more often and more widely, leading to more rapid dissemination of infectious agents. The following discussion will focus on a few generalizations, with specifics limited to those products that are likely to be used more frequently.

## Active Immunization

The accepted criteria dictating a need for active immunization are susceptibility to the infection and absence of antibodies. Because antibody testing is not performed routinely, except for rubella and hepatitis B infections, susceptibility information often is unknown. Therefore, the patient's history and record of previous vaccinations are important. Most women of childbearing age in the United States should be immune to measles, mumps, polio, rubella, tetanus, pertussis, and diphtheria because of state requirements for school admissions. Nevertheless,

**Table 20-1.** Vaccines Available for Active Immunization

| |
|---|
| **Live Bacteria** |
| *Bacillus Calmette-Guérin* |
| Tularemia |
| **Killed Bacteria or Product** |
| Cholera |
| *Haemophilus influenzae* |
| *Meningococcus* |
| Pertussis |
| Plague |
| *Pneumococcus* |
| Rocky Mountain spotted fever (*Rickettsia*) |
| Typhoid |
| Typhus |
| **Live Virus** |
| Mumps |
| Polio |
| Rabies |
| Rota |
| Rubella |
| Rubeola (measles) |
| Varicella-zoster |
| **Killed Virus** |
| Hepatitis A |
| Hepatitis B |
| Influenza |
| Polio |
| **Toxoid** |
| Anthrax |
| Diphtheria |
| Tetanus |

one should assume immunity to tetanus and diphtheria only if the last booster injection of vaccine was given fewer than 10 years ago.

In general, the most conservative statement on the subject—"avoid vaccination in pregnancy with any live bacterial or viral product"—is a safe guideline. In the past, this interdiction was applied to all immunizing products; today, however, it should not include nonviable bacteria, bacterial products, inactivated viruses, and toxoids. In fact, proper management calls for

**Table 20-2.** Passive Immunization Materials

| Condition | Immunoglobulin or Serum |
|---|---|
| Botulism | Antitoxin (horse serum) |
| Diphtheria | Antitoxin (horse serum) |
| Hepatitis A and measles | Pooled human IgG |
| Hepatitis B infection | Human hepatitis B hyperimmune IgG |
| Rabies | Human antirabies hyperimmune IgG |
| Snake bite (coral and crotalid snakes) | Antivenin (horse serum) |
| Tetanus | Human antitetanus hyperimmune IgG |
| Varicella-zoster | Human anti-varicella-zoster hyperimmune IgG |

updating a pregnant patient's tetanus immunization, which should be boosted every 10 years with adult formulations of tetanus and diphtheria toxoids.

Some physicians fear that introducing an antigen such as a vaccine product into the mother will make the fetus tolerant, and therefore unable to form antibody. Although this kind of tolerance can be found in some animals, it has never been seen in humans. In fact, a trial of maternal vaccination with *Haemophilus influenzae* type B provided newborns with high antibody levels. Vaccination of these infants at 18 months of age led to the expected boost in antibodies noted for infants of nonvaccinated mothers.

## Tetanus

The most commonly used vaccine for active immunization—whether a patient is pregnant or not—is tetanus. If someone has never been vaccinated, or more than 10 years has elapsed since the last vaccination, the adult formulation of tetanus–diphtheria, consisting of the adsorbed toxoids of these bacteria, is the product of choice. Primary vaccination is given as two doses, one month apart, followed by a third dose 6 to 12 months after the second one. The booster dose consists of a single 0.5 mL injection given every 10 years.

Vaccination should be part of good prenatal care. This therapy clearly prevents neonatal tetanus, which, although very rare in the United States, is an important cause of neonatal mortality in the developing world. A 90% reduction in mortality from neonatal tetanus in Sri Lanka was achieved from 1978 to 1983 by immunizing all pregnant women with tetanus toxoid.

## Hepatitis B Infection

Perhaps the second most common reason for vaccination in pregnancy is the need either for administering primary immunization against hepatitis B virus (HBV) infection because of family, sexual, or work exposure to this virus or for continuing a series of HBV injections begun before conception. Although this vaccine—or, for that matter, any vaccine—is not approved by the U.S. Food and Drug Administration for use in pregnancy, its benefits outweigh any potential risk. Good medical practice is to offer it or continue its use in women at high risk of contracting the disease.

No reports of harm from HBV vaccine in pregnancy have emerged. The vaccine is administered as two 1-mL intramuscular injections given two months apart, with a third dose given six months after the second one.

## Influenza

In the past, influenza vaccine was given to pregnant women at high risk for serious illness. Women who have chronic cardiac or pulmonary disease or chronic metabolic disease, such as diabetes, should receive the most current formulation of influenza vaccine that is available for the "flu" season (that is, November through March).

The Centers for Disease Control and Prevention (CDC) now recommends that the current influenza vaccine be given to any pregnant woman who will be in her third trimester or early puerperium during the "flu" season.

Physicians should consult with local public health officials to learn which variety of influenza vaccine is recommended. Although the type B influenza virus always is the same strain, the type A influenza virus changes its antigenic makeup frequently, making last year's strain (and vaccine) less effective than the current one.

## Poliomyelitis

Although no adverse effects of oral or intravenous poliomyelitis vaccine have been documented among pregnant women or their fetuses, the CDC recommends avoiding vaccination of pregnant women. If a pregnant woman requires immediate protection against poliomyelitis, she may receive either the oral or IV vaccine in accordance with the recommended schedules for adults.

## Typhoid and Other Vaccines

Typhoid vaccine is rarely administered, particularly in pregnancy, unless the woman is traveling to an endemic area or is involved in a natural disaster affecting the water supply. In such situations, the typhoid vaccine may be given either as a primary series of two injections, four weeks apart, or as a single booster dose if primary vaccination was performed within the past five years. The new oral formulation of typhoid vaccine is better tolerated than previous versions.

All other available vaccines are used so infrequently in pregnancy that one should contact public health officials for the proper product and dose if the need for one of these regimens arises. It is self-evident that exposure to a life-threatening disease, even in pregnancy, warrants making an exception and even using live vaccines, such as those for rabies or yellow fever.

The CDC maintains a registry of women who receive live virus vaccines three months before or after conception. Physicians are urged to report such cases to the CDC (404-329-3091) so that pregnancy can be followed prospectively. This registry has allowed the CDC to inform the medical community about such things as inadvertent rubella vaccination during pregnancy. It has enabled us to learn, for example, that administering live but attenuated rubella virus vaccine—which was once thought to be a potential tragedy—actually poses very little or no risk to the developing fetus.

# Passive Immunization

There is no contraindication to using any immunoglobulin or serum in pregnancy. The danger of serum sickness from using horse serum in a pregnant woman is the same as for a non-pregnant woman and calls for the same precautions. Passive immunity is accomplished with heterologous antibody, which is metabolized with a finite half-life. Protection is therefore limited to 30 days.

Passive immunization becomes necessary when a woman is exposed to an infectious agent or toxin and time doesn't allow her to develop her own antibodies by active immunization. For example, splashing HBV-contaminated blood in an eye requires passive immunization for antibodies to be available immediately. This measure must be followed by active immunization to provide long-lasting protection.

## Future Developments

In addition to protecting the mother, immunization in pregnancy may protect the newborn against infectious agents likely to cause serious harm soon after birth or in the first few months of life. Examples of such agents include group B streptococcal infection and invasive *H. influenzae* infection. In these instances, maternal vaccination may confer passive immunity on the fetus and newborn because immunoglobulin G antibodies produced by the mother will cross the placenta.

The Vaccine Act passed by Congress in 1986 requires physicians to maintain accurate records, including lot numbers, of any vaccinations with diphtheria-pertussis-tetanus, oral polio, measles-mumps-rubella, and *H. influenzae* type B vaccines. The Vaccine Act also requires reporting to public health officials any untoward reactions. Although these four vaccines currently have no place in obstetrics (with the possible exception of *H. influenzae* type B), this requirement should apply to all immunizing agents. Other recommendations regarding adult immunization are available from the CDC and the American College of Physicians.

## Suggested Readings

Advisory Committee on Immunization Practices (ACIP). General recommendations on immunization. MMWR 1989;38:205–214.

Advisory Committee on Immunization Practices (ACIP). Poliomyelitis prevention in the United States: introduction of a sequential vaccination schedule of inactivated poliovirus vaccine followed by oral poliovirus vaccine. MMWR 1996;46(RR-3):18.

Advisory Committee on Immunization Practices (ACIP). Update: vaccine side effects, adverse reactions, contraindications, and precautions. MMWR 1996;45(RR-12):1–35.

American College of Obstetrics and Gynecology. Immunization during pregnancy. ACOG Technical Bulletin Number 160—October 1991. Int J Gynaecol Obstet 1993;40:69–79.

American College of Physicians. Guide for adult immunization, 3rd ed. Philadelphia, 1994.

Amstey MS. Vaccination in pregnancy. Clin Obstet Gynecol 1983;10:13–22.

Amstey MS, Insel R, Munoz J, et al. Fetal-neonatal passive immunization against *Hemophilus influenzae*, type b. Am J Obstet Gynecol 1985;153:607–611.

Amstey MS, Insel RA, Pichichero ME. Neonatal passive immunization by maternal vaccination. Obstet Gynecol 1984;63:105–109.

Baker C, Rench M, Edwards M, et al. Immunization of pregnant women with a polysaccharide vaccine of group B streptococcus. N Engl J Med 1988;319:1180–1185.

Centers for Disease Control and Prevention. Prevention and control of influenza. MMWR 1996;45(RR-5):5–6.

Ramalingaswami V. Importance of vaccines in child survival. Rev Infect Dis 1989;11(suppl 3):S498–S502.

CHAPTER 21

# *HIV Infection in Pregnancy*

*Howard L. Minkoff*

## Background

The percentage of human immunodeficiency virus (HIV)-infected persons in the United States who are women has risen steadily, from less than 5% in the mid-1980s to almost 20% by the mid-1990s. National newborn heelstick serosurveys of HIV infection suggest that approximately 7000 women with HIV infection give birth annually. As the Centers for Disease Control and Prevention (CDC) and the American College of Obstetricians and Gynecologists (ACOG) are urging prenatal care providers to offer HIV tests routinely as part of the management of asymptomatic women, these physicians must be prepared to give ongoing care to patients identified as being infected. This care should include post-test counseling as well as antepartum, intrapartum, and postpartum care. It should also take advantage of the newest diagnostic tests (for example, viral loads) and therapies (for example, protease inhibitors), with the dual goals of optimizing the mother's health and minimizing the chances of HIV transmission to the child.

## Pre- and Post-Test Counseling

Given the tremendous recent advances in the care of HIV-infected individuals and dramatic improvements in our ability to prevent mother-to-child transmission of HIV, it is critical that all women be encouraged to learn their HIV status. To assure maximum utilization of HIV tests, protocols for pretest counseling must be simplified while continuing to provide women with the essential information they need to make an informed decision. Optimally, the counseling also should provide an opportunity to reinforce messages about safer sexual behaviors. It should convey basic information about the transmission of HIV and stress the advantages of knowing one's HIV status. Possible adverse consequences of testing can be discussed, as well as techniques to minimize those consequences. The process usually can be completed in five minutes.

Post-test counseling of the HIV-positive woman is a more delicate and time-consuming process. First, providers should become familiar with individual and institutional resources that can offer assistance. The counseling must cover the social as well as the medical and obstetric consequences of being HIV-infected. The counselor must ensure that the woman understands the distinction between being diagnosed as having acquired immunodeficiency syndrome (AIDS) and being infected with HIV. Techniques needed to avoid infecting others should be explained and stressed. Also, it is important early in the counseling process to have the woman identify support people in whom she can confide and who can assist her during difficult times. Beyond these individuals and medical personnel having a need to know her serostatus, the patient should be cautioned not to give out her serostatus, as instances of discrimination against HIV-positive individuals still occur.

Recent advances allow the clinician to give a somewhat more encouraging picture of the medical aspects of HIV disease. New treatments for opportunistic infections, new antiviral regimens, and new prophylactic therapies have substantially increased disease-free intervals for those infected with this virus. Combination antiviral therapy has been shown to reduce viral loads to essentially undetectable levels for prolonged periods of time. Counseling should emphasize the need to avoid reexposure to the virus as well as the need to maintain good general health. In addition, it should stress the importance of being under the long-term care of clinicians who are well versed in the special needs of HIV-infected individuals.

## The Effect of HIV on Pregnancy Outcomes

Relevant obstetric information that should be shared with HIV-infected women includes the effects of the virus on their pregnancies and their offspring and the effects of pregnancy on their disease. In Western countries, short-term pregnancy outcomes have not been found to be substantially altered by HIV infection. In these areas, when seropositive women are matched with seronegative women from the same risk groups, factors such as smoking, drinking, and drug use are found to be more important determinants of short-term outcome than HIV infection is. The data from Africa differ in that HIV-infected women may experience poorer pregnancy outcomes. Fertility rates, gestational age, and birthweight may all be adversely affected by HIV infection. The difference between the Western and African experience may reflect the higher percentage of clinically ill women in Africa.

Although concerns have been raised that pregnancy might accelerate the course of HIV disease, empiric data are lacking to prove this relationship. Small studies comparing the natural history of HIV infection in pregnant and nonpregnant women have not shown a substantial difference between the two groups. A slightly greater rate of decline of CD4 cells may occur during pregnancy. A low CD4 cell level has been shown to carry the same ominous prognosis—higher risk of developing an opportunistic infection—in both pregnant and nonpregnant women. In all circumstances, consideration of pro phylactic agents is warranted in the patient who has a low CD4 count.

Prior to the introduction of perinatal zidovudine (ZDV), rates of HIV transmission from mother to child were reported in the 20% to 30% range. With the appropriate use of ZDV (vide infra), that rate can be reduced to approximately 8%. The risk of transmission has been reported to increase with more advanced maternal disease (lower CD4 counts, higher viral loads), prematurity, breast feeding, smoking, and drug use. Currently, no practical tools are available to perform prenatal diagnosis of fetal infection.

## ANTEPARTUM MANAGEMENT

When presented with the aforementioned facts and offered reproductive options, including abortion, the large majority of infected pregnant women choose to maintain their pregnancies. All HIV-infected women want their children to be born uninfected, so the first responsibility of the provider is to inform these women of the tools currently available to minimize rates of transmission and to assure access to those interventions.

The current standard of care for prevention of mother-to-child transmission of HIV involves administration of ZDV. Therefore, at 14 weeks' gestation, or as soon as possible thereafter, the clinician should recommend that HIV-infected women start ZDV therapy to prevent perinatal transmission. Recent data suggests that even when started late (as late as the immediate newborn period) ZDV can still reduce the rate of transmission. Some of the benefits, however, may be attenuated when treatment begins later.

Therefore, if the mother has received no therapy but the opportunity exists to commence fetal therapy within the first 24 hours after birth, consider such a course of action. Therapy should be initiated as soon as possible after delivery. If a women presents with a prior extensive history of antiretroviral exposure (more than six months), consideration of ZDV therapy is reasonable, though specific concerns—such as the existence of resistant strains of virus—may need to be addressed. Consultation with an expert in HIV infection may be appropriate under these circumstances. All women must be informed that the long-term consequences of in utero exposure are unknown.

The dose of ZDV used to prevent perinatal transmission is 100 mg, five times per day until labor, which is the standard therapeutic dose for treatment of HIV disease. The medication can also be given as 200 mg three times a day or 300 mg twice a day. Once the patient arrives in labor, a loading dose of 2 mg/kg should be given during the first hour, followed by a maintenance dose of 1 mg/kg per hour until delivery. In the neonatal period, oral ZDV syrup, given 2 mg/kg four times daily for six weeks, is appropriate. Monitoring for toxic effects is straightforward, including monthly assessment of hematologic and liver chemistry indices. Indications of toxicity that might require interrupting or stopping the dose of ZDV include the following:

- A hemoglobin value less than 8 g/dL
- An absolute neutrophil count less than 750 cells/μL
- AST (SGOT) or ALT (SGPT) values greater than five times the upper limit of normal

In addition to preventing mother-to-child transmission, the provider should place a priority on protecting the mother's health. The cornerstones of medical surveillance are the absolute CD4 cell count and the plasma viral load. Women whose counts remain higher than 500/mm$^3$ have been reported to have no HIV-related complications during pregnancy. Conversely, those whose CD4 levels drop below 200/mm$^3$ are at greater risk of developing opportunistic infections. It is therefore prudent to keep a close eye on patients with low CD4 levels and to give them pentamidine if the absolute count falls below 200/mm$^3$ or the percentage of CD4 cells falls below 20%. Antiretroviral therapy is indicated in any woman whose CD4 drops below 500/mm$^3$ or whose viral load is 5000–10,000 copies. Some providers will treat any woman with any detectable virus.

In addition to allowing providers to tailor pharmacologic interventions to patients' particular risk levels, perhaps the most important role of the CD4 count is to alert the clinician to the patient's susceptibility to opportunistic infections. It signals the need for shortening the interval between visits, educating patients about the potential insidious first signs of infection, and responding quickly to subtle symptoms. If an opportunistic infection is diagnosed, it should be treated aggressively, in consultation with an expert in infectious diseases. In general, the threat to a mother's life in these circumstances is so grave that fetal considerations should not lead to a choice of suboptimal therapies.

Other surveillance steps include obtaining baseline *Toxoplasma* titers and screening for sexually transmitted diseases [syphilis, gonorrhea, chlamydial infection, and hepatitis B virus (HBV) infection]. The availability of many new antiretroviral agents gives clinicians many options that were unavailable just a short time ago. Although no consensus on the optimal regimen has emerged as yet, the general sense is that ZDV monotherapy no longer represents the ideal therapy for HIV infection. As optimal therapeutic strategies become more clearly defined, the clinician must take on the responsibility of ensuring that the pregnant patient has access to them. Many of the newer agents [for example, lamivudine (3TC)] have undergone Phase I trials in pregnancy; others, including protease inhibitors, will do so in the near future.

HIV-infected women should also undergo Mantoux testing to exclude tuberculosis and screening for Hepatitis C. HBV, pneumoccocal, and influenza vaccines are not contraindicated in pregnancy, but the possibility of vaccine-associated HIV viremia should be considered.

## Intrapartum Management

The primary goal of the intrapartum management of HIV-infected women—both pharmacologic and obstetric—is to maintain vigilance against transmission of HIV to the child. The pharmacologic imperative calls for the continuation of antiviral therapy in intravenous form throughout labor. Patients should be informed not to discontinue their anti-retroviral medication when their contractions begin, and hospital staff should approach the institution of intrapartum therapy with requisite urgency. Evidence suggests that the intrapartum period often is the critical interval for mother-to-child transmission.

In addition, obstetric management of a parturient should focus on the prevention of transmission. Membranes should not be artificially ruptured, scalp electrodes should not be applied, and forceps should not be used. The role of cesarean delivery has recently been reassessed. A relationship between duration of ruptured membranes and vertical transmission has been reported, and both meta-analysis and randomized trials have found that cesarean section prior to labor and rupture of membranes is associated with a reduction in HIV transmission. This benefit has not been found among women whose viral load is less than 1000 copies.

## Safety Measures

Assiduous adherence to universal precautions is the obstetrician's best protection against acquiring HIV infection during the intrapartum period. HIV testing for purposes of staff protection is an impractical alternative for the following reasons:

- The need to care for unregistered (and therefore untested) patients
- The existence of a virus-positive antibody-negative period (window phase) beyond the capability of current tests
- The existence of strains (HTLV I, II, IV, and V) for which testing is not routinely available

With universal precautions properly applied, risks should be extremely low. Treat all secretions as though infected, and do not perform mouth suction. Surgeons should utilize goggles, double gloving, and waterproof gowns. Impenetrable needle disposal units should be easily accessible in all patient-care areas. If, despite assiduous enforcement of universal precautions, a contaminated needle-stick injury occurs, rapid initiation of antiviral therapy by the injured provider will provide some protection. At least two agents should be used; if the source patient is known to carry ZDV-resistant virus, a protease inhibitor should be added as well.

## Postpartum Management

The immediate postpartum course is not markedly altered by HIV serostatus. The newborn should receive ZDV syrup four times daily for six weeks. Advise patients not to breast-feed if they live in areas where safe alternatives to breast milk are readily available. Although the data on HIV transmission in breast milk suggest that the risk may be high only at the time of maternal seroconversion, sufficient evidence exists to warrant the advice to bottle-feed. (In Third World countries, continuation of breast feeding may be necessary.) Mother and child may bond, however, with staff observing universal precautions for handling of both.

Finally, it is crucial that HIV-infected women and their children be discharged into the care of physicians who are prepared to provide close follow-up, including provision of antiviral and prophylactic therapies.

## Suggested Readings

Augenbraun A, Minkoff HL. Antiretroviral therapy in pregnant women. Obstet Gynecol Clin North Am 1997;24:833–854.

Burns D, Landesman S, Muenz LR, et al. Cigarette smoking, premature rupture of membranes, and vertical transmission of HIV-1 among women with low CD4+ levels. J Acquir Immune Defic Syndr 1994;7:718–726.

Carpenter CCJ, Fischl MA, Hammer SM, et al. Antiretroviral therapy for HIV infection in 1996: recommendations of an international panel. JAMA 1996;276:146–154.

Centers for Disease Control and Prevention. AIDS in women—United States. MMWR 1990;39:845–846.

Centers for Disease Control and Prevention. Recommendations of the U.S. Public Health Service Task Force on the Use of Zidovidine to Reduce Perinatal Transmission of Human Immunodeficiency Virus. MMWR 1994;43:1–20.

Centers for Disease Control and Prevention. Update: provisional Public Health Service recommendations for chemoprophylaxis after occupational exposure to HIV. MMWR 1996;45:468–472.

Connor EM, Sperling RS, Gelbert R, et al. Reduction of maternal-infant transmission of human immunodeficiency virus type 1 with zidovudine treatment. N Engl J Med 1994;331:1173–1180.

Landesman SH, Kalish LA, Burns DN, et al. Obstetrical factors and the transmission of human immunodeficiency virus type 1 from mother to child. N Engl J Med 1996;334:1617–1623.

Minkoff H, Mofenson M. The role of obstetrical interventions in the prevention of pediatric human immunodeficiency virus infection. Am J Obstet Gynecol 1994;171:1167–1175.

Ryder R, Nsa W, Hassib SE, et al. Perinatal transmission of the human immunodeficiency virus type 1 to infants of seropositive women in Zaire. N Engl J Med 1989;320:1637–1632.

Temmerman M, Chomba EN, Ndinya-Achola J, et al. Maternal human immunodeficiency virus-1 infection and pregnancy outcome. Obstet Gynecol 1994;83:495–501.

The mode of delivery and the risk of vertical transmission of human immunodeficiency virus type 1—a meta-analysis of 15 prospective cohort studies. The International Perinatal HIV Group. N Engl J Med 1999;340:977–987.

Villari P, Spino C, Chalmers TC, et al. Cesarean section to reduce perinatal transmission of human immunodeficiency virus: a meta-analysis. Online J Curr Clin Trials 1993 (July 8): doc no. 74.

CHAPTER

# 22

# *Herpes Simplex Virus Infection in Pregnancy*

*Zane A. Brown*

## Background and Incidence

The seroprevalence of herpes simplex virus type 2 (HSV-2) infections among reproductive-aged women in the the United States is approximately 25% (African Americans, 55%; whites, 19%). Of these infected women, only 25% report localized recurrent genital symptoms such as pain, itching, or a vesiculoulcerative eruption. The remaining 75% are unaware of their infection but probably experience mild, episodic genital symptoms that they do not attribute to genital herpes and for which they either do not seek medical consultation or receive an incorrect diagnosis. Therefore, most of what is generally considered asymptomatic shedding of HSV probably comprises unrecognized, unreported, and mildly symptomatic recurrent genital herpes. With counseling, women can be taught to recognize many of these "asymptomatic" recurrences.

Because of declining immunity, the frequency of both symptomatic recurrences and "asymptomatic" shedding increases with advancing gestation. At the time of labor, 2% of HSV-2 seropositive women report a symptomatic recurrence. Asymptomatic shedding can be detected in 1% to 2% of these women by viral isolation and in 20% by polymerase chain reaction (PCR) testing.

Genital herpes infection is acquired for the first time during pregnancy in approximately 2% of the general obstetric population. Among women who are HSV seronegative in early pregnancy but who have a partner who is HSV-2 seropositive,

13% will acquire genital herpes by the time of labor. Approximately two-thirds of these cases of genital herpes acquired during pregnancy are asymptomatic or at least go unrecognized as symptomatic by the patient and provider. Genital herpes acquired during pregnancy poses little threat to the pregnancy as long as HSV seroconversion is complete by the time of labor.

Neonatal herpes infection is by far the most significant complication of genital herpes occurring during pregnancy. The prevalence of this infection varies considerably on a worldwide basis, with reported rates ranging from 1 of every 2000 to 15,000 live births. At least 95% of these newborns acquire their infections by contact during labor and delivery with HSV that is asymptomatically present in the mother's lower genital tract as a consequence of an unrecognized recurrence or a first episode. First-episode genital herpes acquired late in pregnancy accounts for most infection in newborns.

Herpes simplex virus type 1 (HSV-1) is transmitted significantly more often than HSV-2 is from mother to newborn. This relationship holds true whether HSV-1 is present in a lesion or genital secretions as a consequence of either first-episode or recurrent disease. Neonatal HSV-1 infections are more frequently limited to skin, eye, and mucous membranes than are those due to HSV-2; the latter infections commonly disseminate and invade the central nervous system to cause severe neurodevelopmental sequelae or death.

## Diagnosis

Viral isolation in tissue culture remains the method of viral identification against which all HSV diagnostic procedures are compared. HSV tolerates transport well. Preliminary culture results are available by 72 hours, and a final negative culture report is complete in 10 to14 days. Unfortunately, tissue culture is a relatively insensitive method of viral detection. In contrast, the PCR test for detecting HSV DNA in the genital tract is exquisitely sensitive and type-specific. Specimens do not require a liquid transport medium and can be stored at room temperature indefinitely. At present, however, the PCR test has

**Table 22-1.** Definitions of Maternal HSV Infection Based on Viral Isolation and Type-Specific Serology

| Type of Infection | Genital Isolate | Maternal Sera |
|---|---|---|
| Primary | HSV-1 or HSV-2 | Negative |
| Nonprimary first episode | HSV-2 | HSV-1 |
| Recurrent | HSV-1 or HSV-2 | Same type as isolate |

limited availability and is expensive. In addition, researchers have not determined whether the very low levels of HSV DNA detected by the PCR test represent a risk for transmission to sex partners or newborns. Other indirect means of HSV identification, such as Pap and Tzank smears and the fluorescein-conjugated monoclonal antibody test, have little use during pregnancy.

Because genital herpes is primarily a subclinical infection (for both recurrent and first-episode disease), the identification of already-infected patients as well as those at risk for acquiring the infection must be accomplished by a combination of viral isolation and HSV type-specific serologic testing (Table 22-1). Patient history and the physical appearance of lesions on the genitalia are not reliable in classifying the disease. Until recently, HSV serologic assays available from hospital and commercial laboratories were not type-specific and provided confusing results. In contrast, sensitive and type-specific HSV serologic tests, such as the Western blot, are expensive and available only from research laboratories and one commercial laboratory (Microbiology Reference Laboratory, Cypress, California). Several rapid, type-specific and sensitive, point-of-care-based HSV serologic testing kits are in various stages of testing but as yet are not commercially available.

## Antepartum Management

Prior to labor, neither first-episode disease nor recurrent genital herpes has any adverse effect on pregnancy outcome. Therefore, treatment with antiviral chemotherapeutic agents should be used only to obtain relief of maternal symptoms.

Although the published literature suggests that acyclovir is safe and well tolerated by mother and fetus, prudence would dictate that its use be restricted to highly symptomatic infections, whether they are recurrent or first episodes.

Three antiviral agents currently are available in the United States for treating genital herpes: acyclovir, valacyclovir, and famciclovir. Valacyclovir is the valine ester of acyclovir and exhibits no antiviral activity until it becomes hydrolyzed to acyclovir in the intestinal wall or liver. Using this precursor drug significantly increases the blood levels of acyclovir achievable with oral therapy. Similarly, famciclovir is a precursor molecule that improves the bioavailability of penciclovir, which also is highly active against HSV.

At term, acyclovir transfers readily to the fetal compartment, with a ratio of maternal serum to cord blood of 1.15 to 1. Acyclovir also becomes concentrated in the amniotic fluid, with an amniotic fluid to maternal serum ratio of approximately 5 to 1. Currently, among the drugs available for treating genital herpes, only acyclovir has been studied during pregnancy. An ongoing registry of acyclovir use during pregnancy maintained by the manufacturer and the Centers for Disease Control and Prevention has failed to demonstrate any increase in teratogenicity among more than 700 women who received inadvertent first-trimester exposure to acyclovir. Similar human pharmacokinetic and teratologic data are not available for either valacyclovir or famciclovir. Dosage of acyclovir during pregnancy should be similar to that used in nonpregnant women for similar indications.

## Intrapartum Management

The current standard of care in the United States calls for cesarean section delivery of all women in labor with symptomatic genital herpes infection. In view of the current scientific data, however, this policy does not make sense. Because the vast majority of symptomatic lesions at the time of labor are due to recurrent HSV-2 infection and most neonatal herpes is a consequence of asymptomatic first episodes, cesarean delivery of all women with recurrent genital herpes is not an effective strategy for preventing most cases of neonatal herpes. A recent study of 32,000 laboring women suggested that HSV-2 in the genital tracts of women who were HSV-2 seropositive at the time of labor posed little threat of transmission to the fetus. The same study, however, showed that HSV-1 seropositive women with HSV-1 in the genital tract at the time of labor had a much greater chance of neonatal transmission.

In theory, if recurrences of genital herpes could be prevented via suppressive antiviral chemotherapy beginning severa weeks before term, the number of cesarean sections for symptomatic recurrent genital herpes could be substantially reduced. Suppressive use of acyclovir reduces markedly both symptomatic and asymptomatic shedding in nonpregnant women. Of the three small pilot studies of acyclovir use at term, only two were randomized and placebo controlled, and they have yielded conflicting results. It is as yet unclear whether acyclovir is effective in suppressing viral reactivation in late pregnancy or whether it simply modifies symptoms perceived by the patient, a circumstance that, theoretically, could actually increase fetal exposure. Therefore, until safety and efficacy have been proved, acyclovir should not be routinely administered in late pregnancy for suppression.

As acyclovir would be used to prevent symptomatic recurrences at the time of labor rather than to treat active disease in either mother or fetus, the proof required for efficacy and safety should be stringent. There have been all too many tragic examples in obstetrics of "climbing aboard the bandwagon" with a drug or treatment that then becomes the "standard of care" before adequate clinical trials have been performed.

## Summary and Recommendations

1. Routine HSV cultures of the mother during the last several weeks of pregnancy or on admission in labor have little value in predicting infection in the newborn. Similarly, routine delivery room cultures of the newborn have little predictive value unless lesions suspected of being due to HSV are identified.
2. The use of antiviral chemotherapy in the antepartum period should be reserved for symptomatic maternal disease.

3. At the time of this writing, it appears that antiviral chemotherapy should not be used routinely in late pregnancy for suppression of recurrent genital HSV. (This recommendation may change with the completion of clinical trials in progress.)
4. Given that therapeutic levels of acyclovir can be achieved in the fetal circulation by administering the drug to the mother, symptomatic genital herpes—whether a first episode or recurrent disease—is not an indication for preterm delivery of the fetus.
5. Neonatal HSV-2 transmission occurs in approximately 1 in 4000 HSV-2 seropositive women, whether the source of the virus in the genital tract is secondary to asymptomatic shedding or to a symptomatic recurrence. Because accurate, type-specific HSV-2 serologic testing (for example, by Western blot assay) is not generally available and the typing of the virus is either not accurate or not performed in many parts of the country, most patients presenting in labor at term with genital HSV lesions or symptoms should still be delivered by cesarean section. On the other hand, if the HSV serostatus of the patient has been accurately determined by sensitive, type-specific HSV serologic testing in early pregnancy and the patient has been adequately informed of the risks and has given her consent, then an HSV-2 seropositive woman with HSV-2 in the genital tract at the time of labor could be considered for vaginal delivery. If the lesions are recurrent and remote from the genitalia (for example, on the buttocks or mons) and can be isolated by an occlusive dressing, vaginal delivery can be permitted.
6. During labor and delivery in an HSV-2 seropositive woman, early, artificial rupture of membranes and use of instruments such as spiral electrodes, forceps, and vacuum extractors that might injure the fetal scalp should be avoided. In addition, if a woman who is known to be HSV-2 seropositive delivers vaginally, the pediatrician providing newborn care should be notified and the patient herself informed about the incubation period and signs of neonatal herpes.
7. Mothers with active genital HSV lesions do not require isolation in either the antepartum or postpartum period.

They may be permitted to handle and breast-feed their infants but should be cautioned to wash their hands prior to handling the newborn.

## Suggested Readings

Brocklehurst P, Kinghorn G, Carney O, et al. A randomized placebo controlled trial of suppressive acyclovir in late pregnancy in women with recurrent genital herpes. Br J Obstet Gynaecol 1998;105:275–280.

Brown Z, Hume RF, Selke S, et al. Subclinical shedding of herpes simplex virus at the time of labor. Am J Obstet Gynecol 1998; 178(pt 2):S3. Abstract 6.

Brown ZA, Selke, S, Zeh J, et al.The acquisition of herpes simplex virus during pregnancy. N Engl J Med 1997;337:509–515.

Fleming DT, McQuillan GK, Johnson RE, et al. Herpes simplex virus type 2 in the United States, 1976 to 1994. N Engl J Med 1997; 337:1105–1111.

Scott LL, Sanchez PJ, Jackson GL, et al. Acyclovir suppression to prevent cesarean delivery after first-episode genital herpes. Obstet Gynecol 1996;87:69–73.

Stray-Pedersen B. Acyclovir in late pregnancy to prevent neonatal herpes simplex. Lancet 1990;336:756.

CHAPTER

# 23

# *Herpesvirus 6 Infection (Roseola Subitum)*

*Edward R. Newton*

## BACKGROUND

In 1986, Salahuddin and coworkers described a new herpes virus with physical characteristics similar to those of cytomegalovirus and cytopathic effects for T cells (1). The virion of this agent, subsequently called human herpesvirus 6 (HHV-6), has an envelope covering an icosahedral nucleocapsid. Within the nucleocapsid, the HHV-6 viral genome is a duplex DNA strand consisting of approximately 170 kilobase pairs. It shows a strong homology with cytomegalovirus.

Epithelial cells, megakaryocytes, B cells, and glial cells can be infected by HHV-6 in vitro. Both in vitro and in vivo studies suggest, however, that the target cell line for HHV-6 comprises cells that display mature T-lymphocyte characteristics (CD4+/CD8– and CD3+/CD4+) (2). In particular, monocytes and macrophages appear to be persistently infected with HHV-6 following primary infection and may serve as a reservoir for virus reactivation (3). Tissues rich in T lymphocytes and macrophages appear to serve as sites of replication of the virus; they are also potential sites for persistent HHV-6 shedding. Mucosa-associated lymphoid tissues (MALT) play a major role in permitting the persistence of HHV-6. The tissues of the salivary glands and endocervix are probable sources of infection or reinfection. Leach and colleagues suggest that 10% or more of asymptomatic adult women attending sexually transmitted disease clinics are shedding HHV-6 from their genital tracts (4).

Human herpesvirus 6 warrants interest because of its potential role in the transactivation of other viruses, particularly human immunodeficiency virus (HIV), and neoplastic control and promoter genes. On a practical clinical level, its characteristic presentation—that is, primary infection in small children—exposes many young pregnant women to infection.

## Clinical Manifestations

The clinical syndrome associated with HHV-6 is recognized as exanthem subitum or roseola. The classic presentation involves an abrupt onset of moderate to high fever in a child less than three years of age. The fever lasts approximately 72 hours, followed by defervescence and subsequent appearance of a faint, morbilliform rash. Associated signs are remarkably few: mild oropharyngeal or tympanic membrane erythema and enlarged suboccipital lymph nodes. Febrile seizures are not unusual and represent the most dramatic and serious manifestation of the infection. The severity of clinical symptoms appears to be correlated with the degree of viremia (5). Children whose fever lasts for more than four days have a greater percentage of infected mononuclear cells than children whose fever disappears in less than three days (5).

In a prospective study of 200 children younger than two years of age who were brought to the emergency room with high fever, roseola (HHV-6 infection) was examined as a contributing cause (6). Fourteen percent of these children had HHV-6 isolated from their blood. The children presented at a mean age of less than 10 months with a mean temperature of 39.7 °C. Two-thirds of those who were HHV-6 positive had temperatures exceeding 40 °C, and two-thirds of those who had primary HHV-6 isolated from their blood had viral DNA detected in peripheral blood mononuclear cells; the potential for immortalization within lymphatic tissue was demonstrated. Only 9% of the children had classic fever followed by a rash, and the rash was less obvious than that described in classic roseola. Rash was an uncommon finding in children with culture-proven primary HHV-6 infection.

Adult manifestations of recurrent or new HHV-6 infection

are not well defined. Like other herpes viruses, HHV-6 has been shown to transactivate promoter or growth sequences in cells (7–10). Thus this virus may potentially play a role in the development of lymphoma and perhaps other tumors. The link between HHV-6 and lymphoproliferative disorders remains unproven, however. The virus's relationship to immune diseases and cancer remains an important research question.

The specificity of HHV-6 for CD4+/CD8– and CD3+/CD4+ cells is similar to the tropism demonstrated by HIV. Coupled with the known effects of HHV-6 on promoter or growth sequences in cells, this affinity raises questions about its potential collaboration in HIV infections. Although researchers have shown that HHV-6 transactivates HIV type I promoter sequences, epidemiologic studies have failed to support the theory that HHV-6 alters the course of HIV infection (10–12). This area certainly requires more research.

Chronic fatigue syndrome (CFS) is defined as persistent fatigue associated with neuropathy and adenopathy. It appears to be more prevalent in young women, who often have recurrences or exacerbation under stress. In a 1992 study, patients with CFS had higher HHV-6 antibody levels and higher antibody titers to Epstein-Barr virus capsid antigen than did control patients (13). Immunostaining of infected blood peripheral mononuclear cells revealed a 70% positivity rate for HHV-6 among patients with CFS compared with a 20% rate in patients without symptoms (14). These preliminary associations need confirmation, however.

## Perinatal Effects

Undoubtedly, many young women are exposed to HHV-6 infection during pregnancy, given the occurrence of primary infection in children younger than three years of age. It appears that the perinatal effects of HHV-6 infection are not powerful. Nevertheless, because these effects have not been well studied, we cannot rule out the possibility that this infection may play a role in unexplained adverse pregnancy outcome (15).

Human herpesvirus 6 appears to be shed frequently from the genital tracts of pregnant women, but vertical transmission appears to be rare. Okuno and coworkers performed PCR tests for HHV-6 and HHV-7 on cervical secretions from 72 asymptomatic pregnant women six weeks prior to their delivery dates and compared results with those from age-matched nonpregnant women (16). Detectable genomes for HHV-6 and HHV-7 were found in 19% of the pregnant women but in only 3% of nonpregnant controls. Dunne and Demmler found HHV-6-specific IgM antibody in several cord-blood samples, but did not detect HHV-6 DNA genome with PCR testing (17). On the other hand, HHV-6 does not appear to be transmitted to neonates through breast milk or from contact with their mothers (18).

In a group of 30 women suffering early spontaneous abortion (weeks 6 to 12), HHV-6 antibody titers were higher than those in normal pregnant women (1:160 versus 1:40); three (10%) of the abortions were in women who were positive for HHV-6 IgM, and two of these three patients had HHV-6 antigen in aborted villous tissue (19). In contrast, when 52 electively aborted fetuses were evaluated for documented HHV-6 infection, only one had HHV-6 DNA identified by PCR testing. This fetus had HHV-6 in blood mononuclear cells, liver, spleen, brain, and cerebrospinal fluid but no physical abnormalities (20). The lack of abnormalities suggests a strong association does not exist between HHV-6 infection and other adverse outcomes, such as anatomic defects, psychomotor defects, perinatal infection, preterm birth, or perinatal death. More studies are needed in this area, however.

## Diagnosis

The diagnosis of primary or recurrent HHV-6 infection is made by documenting elevations in serologic titer or seroconversion or a fourfold increase in IgG or IgM titers (21,22). Culture and immunostaining of infected blood peripheral mononuclear cells and PCR methods remain research tools.

The common clinical presentation of many viral infections —upper respiratory symptoms, fever, and rash—obscures many roseola (HHV-6) infections. Virtually all infected children are infected with HHV-6 within the first five years of life (23).

Subsequent reactivation becomes a concern in the presence of immunocompromised states such as lymphoma, human immunodeficiency disease, cancer or transplant chemotherapy, and CFS. The potential for HHV-6 reactivation to enhance the development of lymphoproliferative diseases—a common complication of AIDS—has greatly increased interest in HHV-6.

## MANAGEMENT

Presence of a rash and fever in a young family may raise significant concerns among young mothers. It is apparent that roseola (HHV-6 infection) contributes significantly to the incidence of early childhood fevers, accounting for as many as 15%. At this time, adverse pregnancy does not appear to be frequently associated with perinatal HHV-6 infection. Nevertheless, we know little about the incidence of fetal infection and adverse pregnancy outcome. Thus the patient should be told about the uncertainty of the perinatal effects and informed that adverse pregnancy outcomes are usually a result of coexisting perinatal variables. These variables, which include genetic, environmental, and medical risks, should be assessed by the clinician.

No evidence exists to support abortion as a response to HHV-6 exposure or primary infection. The presence of HHV-6 infection in women with CFS or immunocompromised patients is provocative because of the organism's ability to transactivate promoter genes. Nevertheless, the association with these syndromes in HHV-6 is not well understood. Testing for the organism in these clinical scenarios is not warranted and should be reserved for research purposes. Most laboratories are not equipped to provide accurate serologic, molecular, or culture diagnosis of this infection. As yet, because no treatment exists for HHV-6 infection, diagnosis must be considered to serve academic purposes only.

### REFERENCES

1. Salahuddin SZ, Ablashi DV, Markham PD, et al. Isolation of a new virus, HBLV, in patients with lymphoproliferative disorders. Science 1986;234:596–600.

2. Takahashi K, Sonoda S, Higashi K, et al. Predominant CD4 T-lymphocyte tropism of human herpesvirus 6-related virus. J Virol 1989;63:3161–3163.
3. Kondo K, Kondo T, Okuno T, et al. Latent human herpesvirus 6 infection of human monocytes/macrophages. J Gen Virol 1991;72:1401–1408.
4. Leach CT, Newton ER, McParlin S, et al. Human herpesvirus 6 infection of the female genital tract. J Infect Dis 1994; 169:1281–1283.
5. Asano Y, Nakashima T, Yoshikawa, et al. Severity of human herpesvirus-6 viremia and clinical findings in infants with exanthem subitum. J Pediatr 1991;118:891–895.
6. Pruksananonda P, Hall CB, Insel RA, et al. Primary human herpesvirus 6 infection in young children. N Engl J Med 1992;326:1445–1450.
7. Razzaque A. Oncogenic potential of human herpesvirus-6 DNA. Oncogene 1990;5:1365–1370.
8. Martin ME, Nicholas J, Thomson BJ, et al. Identification of a transactivating function mapping to the putative immediate-early locus of human herpesvirus 6. J Virol 1991;65:5381–5390.
9. Torelli G, Marasca R, Luppi M, et al. Human herpesvirus-6 in human lymphomas: identification of specific sequences in Hodgkin's lymphomas by polymerase chain reaction. Blood 1991;77:2251–2258.
10. Geng YQ, Chandran B, Josephs SF, et al. Identification and characterization of a human herpesvirus 6 gene segment that transactivates the human immunodeficiency virus type 1 promoter. J Virol 1992;66:1564–1570.
11. Fox J, Briggs M, Tedder RS. Antibody to human herpesvirus 6 in HIV-1 positive and negative homosexual men. Lancet 1988;2:396–397.
12. Spira TJ, Bozeman LH, Sanderlin KC, et al. Lack of correlation between human herpesvirus-6 infection and the course of human immunodeficiency virus infection. J Infect Dis 1990; 161:567–570.
13. Buchwald D, Cheney PR, Peterson DL, et al. A chronic illness characterized by fatigue, neurologic and immunologic disorders, and active human herpesvirus type 6 infection. Ann Intern Med 1992;116:103–113.
14. Ablashi DV, Zompetta C, Lease C, et al. Human herpesvirus 6 (HHV6) and chronic fatigue syndrome (CFS). Can Dis Wkly Rep 1991;17(suppl 1E):33–40.
15. Wiersbitzky S, Beyersdorf E, Burtzlaff C, et al. Pre- and perinatal infections due to human herpesvirus-6 and Epstein-Barr virus

with lethal outcome or severe residual encephalopathy. Padiatr Grenzgeb 1993;31:199–201.

16. Okuno T, Oishi H, Hayashi K, et al. Human herpesviruses 6 and 7 in cervixes of pregnant women. J Clin Microbiol 1995; 33:1968–1970.
17. Dunne WM Jr, Demmler GJ. Serological evidence for congenital transmission of human herpesvirus 6. Lancet 1992;340: 121–122.
18. Dunne WM Jr, Jevon M. Examination of human beast milk for evidence of human herpesvirus 6 by polymerase chain reaction. J Infect Dis 1993;168:250.
19. Aubin JT, Poirel L, Agut H, et al. Intrauterine transmission of herpesvirus 6. Lancet 1992;340:482–483.
20. Ando Y, Kakimoto K, Ekuni Y, et al. HHV-6 infection during pregnancy and spontaneous abortion. Lancet 1992;340:1289.
21. Farr TJ, Harnett GB, Pietroboni GR, et al. The distribution of antibodies to HHV-6 compared with other herpesviruses in young children. Epidemiol Infect 1990;105:603–607.
22. Saxinger C, Polesky H, Eby N, et al. Antibody reactivity with BBLV (HHV-6) in U.S. populations. J Virol Methods 1988; 21:199–208.
23. Brown NA, Sumaya CV, Liu CR, et al. Fall in human herpesvirus 6 seropositivity with age. Lancet 1988;2:396.

CHAPTER

# 24

# *Cytomegalovirus Infection in Pregnancy*

*Bryan T. Oshiro*

## Background

Cytomegalovirus (CMV) is a member of the Herpesviridae family of viruses, which was first described in the early 1950s. Like other herpes viruses, CMV shares the properties of latency and reactivation. It is a common viral pathogen and is not restricted to any particular population group or geographical region, although it is more prevalent in indigent populations. CMV represents the most common cause of congenital infection in the United States. The annual cost for treating CMV-related complications in the United States is estimated to approach $2 billion.

## Epidemiology and Pathophysiology

Infection with CMV may be either primary or secondary. Primary infection consists of the patient's first encounter with CMV. Secondary infection may occur upon a reactivation of the same virus or the acquisition of a new infection with a different strain of CMV.

CMV has been isolated from virtually all body fluids. Infection can therefore occur when susceptible individuals come into direct contact with infected bodily secretions. Transmission of the virus may occur through close or intimate physical contact or through the receipt of infected blood products, vital organs, or bone marrow. In addition, congenital infection may be acquired through transplacental viral transmission, and perinatal infection may be acquired intrapartum or through breast feeding.

Approximately 60% to 65% of women in the United States are seropositive to CMV by the time they reach their reproductive years, with the highest rate of seroconversion occurring between the ages of 15 and 35. The seropositive rate in lower socioeconomic groups approaches 85%; in the higher socioeconomic groups, it is approximately 55%. This difference appears to be related to poor hygiene, crowded living conditions, and promiscuity. Risk factors include being African American, having a low level of education, being younger than 30 years old, having a history of sexually transmitted disease (STD), having multiple sexual partners, and coming into close contact with children younger than two years of age.

Primary CMV infection occurs in 0.7% to 4% of pregnant women. Recurrent infection may affect as many as 13.5% of such women. As with nonpregnant women, seropositivity is higher in women in the lower socioeconomic groups (70% to 80%) than in women in the higher socioeconomic groups (50% to 60%).

Congenital CMV infection afflicts 1% to 2% of newborns annually in the United States. Both primary and recurrent maternal CMV infection may lead to congenital infection of the newborn. Primary CMV infection in the mother, however, substantially increases risk of viral transmission, with 30% to 40% of fetuses becoming infected; in contrast, fewer than 1% of fetuses become infected when the mother has recurrent CMV infection. CMV infection also may occur during parturition or with breast feeding. Approximately half of all neonates who are exposed to infected cervicovaginal secretions or breast milk develop CMV infection.

Infants and toddlers not infected at birth may acquire CMV while in a day-care setting. Children in day-care centers have a very high prevalence of CMV shedding, ranging from 23% to 72%. Infected children then become a major source of infection for other family members. The seroconversion rate in families with children in day-care centers approaches 50% in family members who were not previously infected.

## Diagnosis

Most CMV-infected patients remain minimally symptomatic, although an occasional patient will present with a mononucleosis-like syndrome. Symptoms may include fever, sore throat, myalgias, fatigue, and diarrhea. Patients may exhibit a rash, lymphadenopathy, pharyngitis, and hepatosplenomegaly. Elevated liver enzymes, thrombocytopenia, lymphocystosis, or lymphocytopenia may be found as well. A heterophile antibody test will give negative results in a CMV-infected patient, and CMV-specific IgG and CMV-specific IgM antibody levels usually are positive. The virus may be detected by culture or antigen testing of body fluids or secretions.

Although seroconversion represents a reliable method for identifying primary CMV infection, the diagnosis can prove problematic. The rise in CMV-specific antibodies may be delayed for as long as four weeks, and the presence of CMV-specific IgM antibodies can be found in as many as 10% of women with recurrent disease. Persistence of CMV-specific IgM antibodies for as long as 18 months after a primary infection has been documented as well. Therefore, when seroconversion cannot be documented in a patient, detection of CMV antigen or isolation of the virus offers a more reliable method for diagnosing active infection.

Prenatal diagnosis of CMV infection in the fetus may prove problematic as well. Fetal blood culture and detection of IgM antibodies in fetal blood are not reliable indicators. At present, detection of virus in amniotic fluid by either culture or polymerase chain reaction (PCR) testing remains the most accurate means of diagnosis, with sensitivities ranging from 80% to 100%. Infected fetuses may also exhibit abnormal ultrasound findings, including cerebral ventriculomegaly, periventricular calcifications, hepatomegaly, intrauterine growth restriction, ascites or hydrops, and abnormal calcification patterns in the liver or bowel. It should be emphasized, however, that negative studies cannot

**Table 24-1.** Findings in Newborns with Congenital CMV Infection

| |
|---|
| Chorioretinitis |
| Deafness |
| Hemolytic anemia |
| Hepatosplenomegaly |
| Intracranial calcifications |
| Microcephaly |
| Seizures |
| Smallness for gestational age |
| Thrombocytopenia |

exclude a CMV infection and that normal prenatal ultrasound scans do not rule out severe neurologic damage.

## Congenital CMV Infection

In utero viral transmission appears to occur with equal frequency throughout pregnancy. The rate of intrauterine infection is much higher with primary disease than with recurrent disease. Congenital infection occurs in approximately 40% of patients with primary disease. Approximately 10% of infected fetuses will have clinically apparent disease at birth. Of the remaining infected neonates who are asymptomatic at birth, approximately 5% to 15% will go on to develop sequelae from CMV infection. The prognosis is much better for pregnant women with recurrent disease, with their fetuses having only a 1% risk of in utero infection and extremely low risk of developing significant sequelae. Table 24-1 lists common findings in newborns with congenital CMV infection.

## Treatment

Fortunately, most CMV infections are asymptomatic or self-limiting. Ganciclovir, foscarnet, and cidofovir are the only antiviral agents currently approved in the United States for treating severe CMV infection. These agents have not been studied in pregnant patients, and information on the use of these antiviral drugs in pediatric patients remains very limited. Currently, a multicenter trial is assessing the use of ganciclovir in children with symptomatic congenital CMV infection and central nervous system involvement. In addition, CMV-specific monoclonal antibody therapy is being studied in children with congenital CMV infections.

## Prevention

Research on CMV vaccine development is encouraging. Live-attenuated CMV administered to renal transplant patients has been shown to effectively elicit an immune response. Safety studies of recombinant vaccines are currently under way. In addition, vaccine administration in pregnant animals has reduced the incidence of congenital infection by CMV.

Until a CMV vaccine is developed, however, susceptible pregnant women must take precautions to prevent transmission of the virus. Because CMV is transmitted through infected body fluids, at-risk pregnant women should practice good hygiene —that is, frequent hand washing, avoiding kissing on the mouth, and not sharing food and utensils. Women who work in situations with potential exposure to children should ascertain their immune status before attempting to conceive. Those who are CMV-IgG negative should consider avoiding such exposure.

### Suggested Readings

Adler SP. Current prospects for immunization against cytomegaloviral disease. Infect Agent Dis 1996;5:29–35.

Daniel Y, Gull I, Peyser MR, et al. Congenital cytomegalovirus infection. Eur J Obstet Gynecol Reprod Biol 1995;63:7–16.

Demmler GJ. Congenital cytomegalovirus infection and disease. Adv Pediatr Infect Dis 1996;11:135–162.

Hagay ZJ, Biran G, Ornoy A, et al. Congenital cytomegalovirus infection: a long-standing problem still seeking a solution. Am J Obstet Gynecol 1996;174:241–245.

CHAPTER

# 25

# *Varicella-Zoster Infection in Pregnancy*

*James A. McGregor*

## Background and Incidence

Varicella-zoster virus (VZV) is a common and highly infectious herpesvirus that causes two common clinical infections: varicella (chickenpox) and herpes zoster (shingles). Although primary infection (varicella) during pregnancy is rare, this type of infection is associated with significant maternal morbidity and occasional mortality, primarily from pneumonitis. Disease consequences may also be severe for the fetus (infection before 20 weeks' gestation) or neonate (neonatal sepsis, pneumonia, encephalitis). Reactivation of latent VZV manifests itself as herpes zoster, though this form poses little risk to mother or fetus. Herpes zoster can be a source of VZV infection in susceptible individuals, including family members and healthcare providers.

Varicella is a nearly universal disease of children in industrialized countries. In these areas, only 2% of cases occur in the 15-to-49 age group, and incidence among pregnant women is about 5 per 10,000. By contrast, in tropical and subtropical countries, varicella is more frequently a disease of reproductive-age adults. Prenatal serologic surveys have found that 95% of U.S.-born women are immune, compared with only 84% of women born in subtropical countries. Women who spent their childhood in the latter regions and subsequently moved to North America are at increased risk for varicella during pregnancy. (In a North Carolina study, women of African

American origin appeared to be at increased risk of VZV infection during pregnancy.)

As with many other childhood infections, the peak incidence of VZV infection occurs in winter and spring. Attack rates for both pregnant and nonpregnant susceptible women with household contacts approach 90%. Exposures other than household contacts—such as nosocomial, school, or playmate contacts—appear somewhat less likely to result in infection. Pregnancy does not predispose a woman to acquiring the infection, but it may increase risk for both mother and baby.

## PATHOPHYSIOLOGY

Primary infection occurs principally through respiratory inhalation of virus particles by a susceptible host. Direct contact with varicella or zoster lesions can also lead to transference of the virus. An initial transient and asymptomatic viremia ensues, with viral propagation into the reticuloendothelial system. An incubation period of 10 to 21 days (mean 14 days) is followed by a second viremia, with dissemination to skin and viscera. Clinical evidence of infection appears within 24 to 48 hours of the second viremia. Thus virus may be transmitted to unsuspecting close contacts one or two days before the characteristic chickenpox rash becomes visible.

It has generally been accepted that one attack of viremia confers lifelong immunity to reinfection in the nonimmunocompromised patient. Virus-specific antibodies (IgA, IgM, and IgG) rise rapidly during the first five days of clinically apparent infection, peaking at two to three weeks. Thereafter, IgG persists at lower levels. Subclinical reinfection is known to occur, however, as shown by rising antibody titers. Rarely, some patients may experience clinically apparent but mild attacks in the face of demonstrated circulating antibody and cell-mediated immunity (CMI). Circulating antibody does not guarantee immunity, though it will ameliorate symptoms and probably prevent congenital infection. Even more rarely, VZV-immune individuals can manifest an episode of zoster after chickenpox exposure.

Before the onset of the rash, adults experience a prodrome

of fever, malaise, myalgia, and headache. Lesions then appear in crops on the face, scalp, and trunk, with relative sparing of the extremities. Initially, lesions are maculopapular, but they progress rapidly to pruritic vesicles, pustules, and scabs. New crops appear for three to four days, and crusting is generally complete within one week. Characteristically, all stages of lesions will be present simultaneously. Infectivity persists until all of the vesicles become scabs; patients are therefore considered infectious from two days before the onset of rash until all lesions become crusted.

The overall mortality for varicella in normal adults is 50 per 100,000. Comparable data are not available for pregnant women.

Pneumonia is the most common complication of varicella in adults. Hospitalization for pneumonia is required in only 0.25% of cases of adult varicella; in those cases, however, mortality may be as high as 12% in nonpregnant women and 35% in pregnant patients. Varicella pneumonia is a treacherous disease, whose course can range from asymptomatic illness to sudden death. Symptoms develop one to six days after the rash appears and may consist of cough, dyspnea, fever, pleuritic chest pain, and hemoptysis. Chest auscultation often appears unremarkable, even in the face of severe pulmonary involvement. X-ray findings are not specific; they often appear as diffuse bilateral nodular infiltrates but may appear as "white out" or be interpreted as acute respiratory distress syndrome (ARDS).

Although pregnancy may place women at greater risk for varicella pneumonia, case-fatality ratios for pregnant women with this disease remain poorly studied as yet. Claims of rates exceeding 40% based on literature reviews probably represent overreporting of severe cases; 35% is probably a more accurate figure. Nevertheless, severe pneumonia and death are well documented and are probably attributable to altered cell-mediated immunity in pregnancy. As with other potentially severe illnesses during pregnancy, the clinician must take note of the patient's increased risk of preterm labor and delivery. Fetal distress and death during maternal pneumonia have been reported, perhaps as the result of massive cytokine activation and/or hypoxemia. Encephalitis and hepatitis are other serious—albeit rare—complications of varicella in the mother.

The varicella rash is so characteristic that diagnosis usually is based on physical examination alone. Other conditions to consider in the differential diagnosis of a varicella-like exanthem include disseminated zoster, disseminated herpes simplex, eczema vaccinatum, generalized vaccinia (cowpox), hand-foot-and-mouth disease (Coxsackie virus), atypical measles, and rickettsialpox.

## DIAGNOSIS

Varicella-zoster virus may be identified in clinical specimens by means of a Tzanck preparation, although varicella, zoster, and herpes simplex infections are indistinguishable by this method. Culture and nucleic acid, probe, or amplification techniques can be employed for definitive identification. Seroconversion is diagnostic and can be detected by complement fixation (CF) assay, fluorescent-antibody-to-membrane-antigen (FAMA) testing, or enzyme immunoassay (EIA). Such seroconversion assays, however, require acute and convalescent serum samples to be drawn three weeks apart. The presence of varicella-specific IgM, which remains in the blood for four to five weeks, is considered diagnostic.

## TREATMENT

Antiviral agents with activity against VZV include α-interferon, vidarabine, acyclovir, valacyclovir, and famciclovir. None has received FDA approval for use in pregnancy. Only acyclovir has been administered with any frequency to pregnant women, and it does not appear to be teratogenic. The decision to treat a pregnant woman who has active varicella should be made on an individual basis. Previously, treatment was limited to women with visceral VZV involvement, particularly pneumonia or encephalitis, as described by Haake and coworkers. Some providers now prescribe acyclovir to treat extensive varicella without specific evidence of visceral involvement.

High-dose acyclovir therapy (12.4 mg/kg of body weight or 500 mg/m$^2$ IV every eight hours) should be started within

72 hours of the onset of rash. Possible major side effects include local tissue irritation, transient elevation of hepatic transaminases, central nervous system (CNS) toxicity, and renal dysfunction (crystalluria and azotemia).

Transplacental passage of acyclovir is prompt, and therapeutic levels may be reached in both the placenta and fetal blood. Reports of acyclovir use in pregnancy for VZV and other indications have been favorable, with no maternal or fetal side effects noted. Antenatal use of acyclovir in an attempt to prevent or ameliorate congenital varicella syndrome or neonatal infection remains of unproven benefit.

## PREVENTION

The most effective method for preventing the spread of VZV infection is isolation, but infection can occur prior to appearance of lesions with asymptomatic viral shedding. Ideally, pregnant women who are exposed to VZV should have their susceptibility promptly determined by history, serology, or both. If she is susceptible, the exposed and presumably infected person should be isolated from at-risk contacts (other susceptible pregnant women or immunosuppressed individuals) from the eighth to twenty-first day after exposure. Because isolation is often an impractical method of control, passive immunization is more frequently employed for those at risk for varicella-induced morbidity (such as pregnant women and immunocompromised individuals).

Prevention or modification of maternal disease can be accomplished with passive immunization using several available products. The most effective of these agents is varicella-zoster immune globulin (VZIG). Its limited supply and high cost mandate that its use be restricted to susceptible patients with significant exposure to VZV (household contact, close contact indoors for longer than one hour, or hospital contact through roommates or infected personnel).

Determining VZV susceptibility by history can be problematic. As many as half of pregnant patients without detectable antibody may give a history of varicella. Conversely, 80% of patients with a negative or uncertain history are serologically immune. Most investigators agree that expedited serologic screening of an exposed pregnant woman with a negative history of prior infection is an accurate method for determining the need for passive immunization. Although costly, screening of all pregnant women for VZV serostatus regardless of history has been recommended by some authorities.

Routine prenatal testing could facilitate prompt treatment when exposure occurs to susceptible women as well as help avoid "crisis" situations, such as when exposed pregnant women of unknown susceptibility present on weekends. (Rouse has calculated that screening could be cost-effective if seronegative women received VZV vaccinations postpartum.) Serologic tests for detecting antibody against VZV are now widely available and can reliably predict immunity. FAMA (used mainly in research laboratories) and EIA offer comparable sensitivity, specificity, and cost. Complement fixing (CF) antibody is short-lived and not useful for determining immunity.

VZIG's efficacy in preventing or attenuating maternal disease is well established. In a prospective study of pregnant women, 80% of seronegatives receiving VZIG within 96 hours remained symptom-free, whereas 89% of untreated controls developed illness. *Susceptible pregnant women with significant exposure to VZV should be given VZIG, 625 units IM, within 96 hours of exposure.* Laboratory determination of susceptibility will prevent unnecessary administration of this costly preparation.

No evidence suggests that VZIG administration prevents intrauterine infection. VZIG should be used solely to prevent serious complications in the mother; neonates exposed peripartum should be treated with this agent after birth. VZIG does not effectively treat maternal varicella.

## Sequelae

Maternal varicella may lead to several possible adverse outcomes for the fetus. Possible sequelae depend on fetal age at the time of infection. In most cases (up to 97%), the fetus remains healthy without showing any clinical or serologic evidence of illness. When intrauterine infection does occur, it may result in congenital varicella syndrome, neonatal varicella, or asymptomatic seroconversion.

Congenital varicella syndrome comprises abnormalities of the limbs, skin, eyes, and peripheral CNS as well as mental retardation or even death. Specific sequelae include dermatologic scarring, hypoplasia of the extremities, paralysis, Horner's syndrome, intestinal atresia, hydronephrosis, seizures, cortical atrophy, mental retardation, cataracts, and chorioretinitis. Of the cases reported, most were associated with maternal infection occurring before 20 weeks' gestation. Reliable methods for diagnosing this syndrome are being sought. Ultrasound may detect microcephaly, limb deformities, and other abnormalities. Measurement of VZV-specific IgM and detection of virus or VZV nucleic acid in fetal blood obtained by cordocentesis or amniotic fluid at amniocentesis has been used on a research basis. Asymptomatic intrauterine infection has been documented by persistence of antibody in infants. Both intrauterine and peripartum VZV infection predispose the infant to development of childhood zoster. Placental involvement is marked by villitis and lymphohistiocytic or giant cells.

Neonatal or perinatal varicella may result from maternal varicella that occurs in the days preceding or following birth. Exposure around the time of birth leads to newborn infection in the absence of maternal passive immunization. The attack rate ranges from 25% to 50%, with the incubation period averaging 11 days (range 1 to 16 days). The severity of infection is directly proportional to the presence and amount of placentally acquired maternal antibody. As maternal antibody is not transported across the placenta in sufficient quantities until the fifth day of maternal infection, neonates born five days or less from the onset of maternal disease receive no protective maternal antibody. Similarly, women who have onset of disease within two days following delivery were presumably viremic antepartum, so their infants will also be born without antibody.

*If possible, birth should be delayed until at least five days after the onset of the mother's illness.* Administering VZIG to neonates born to mothers with onset of disease five days before to two days after delivery significantly reduces newborn complications, even though it does not entirely prevent mortality or alter the attack rate. Although neonates born to mothers experiencing varicella more than five days before or more than two days after delivery are not at increased risk for complications, some experts recommend VZIG use in this setting. Some pediatric infectious disease experts may give acyclovir preemptively to exposed newborns, especially if preterm birth occurs.

Patients with varicella or zoster should be isolated and receive care only from immune employees. Isolation of the newborn from the varicella-infected mother is commonly recommended. Although excretion of VZV into breast milk has not been demonstrated, breast feeding during the active stage of varicella should be avoided to prevent neonatal exposure from direct maternal contact, unless the neonate is also affected. Some experts allow maternal handling and breast feeding on an individualized basis if the child is passively immunized with VZIG and receives preemptive treatment with acyclovir.

VZV vaccination prior to pregnancy or postpartum is increasingly considered as a way to decrease susceptibility to VZV-induced maternal, fetal, and neonatal morbidity and to mitigate excess costs and liability. Such strategies will likely prove most effective in groups of women who are serosusceptible and at high risk of exposure (child-care providers, health-care providers) and in those who are at higher risk of severe disease (immunosuppressed). The present varicella vaccine employs the live Oka strain and should not be used in pregnancy. All cases should be reported to the Varivax pregnancy registry (800-986-8999).

## Suggested Readings

Centers for Disease Control and Prevention. Prevention of varicella: recommendations of the Advisory Committee on Immunization Practices (ACIP). MMWR 1996;45(RR-11):1–36.

Feder HM Jr. Treatment of adult chickenpox with oral acyclovir. Arch Intern Med 1990;150:2061–2065.

Haake DA, Zakowski PC, Haake DL, et al. Early treatment with acyclovir for varicella pneumonia in otherwise healthy adults: retrospective controlled study and review. Rev Infect Dis 1990; 12:788–789.

Landsberger EJ, Hager WD, Grossman JH 3d. Successful management of varicella pneumonia complicating pregnancy. A report of three cases. J Reprod Med 1986;31:311–314.

McGregor JA, Mark S, Crawford GP, et al. Varicella-zoster antibody testing in the care of pregnant women exposed to varicella. Am J Obstet Gynecol 1987;157:281–284.

Miller E, Cradock-Watson JE, Ridehalgh MK. Outcome in newborn babies given anti-varicella-zoster immunoglobin after perinatal infection with varicella-zoster virus. Lancet 1989;2:371–373.

Paryani SG, Arvin AM. Intrauterine infection with varicella-zoster virus after maternal varicella. N Engl J Med 1986;314:1542–1546.

CHAPTER

# 26

# *Parvovirus B19 Infection*

*Philip B. Mead*

## Background and Incidence

Parvovirus B19, a single-stranded DNA virus, was discovered in 1975. It was first linked to human disease in 1981, when it was found in the blood of a child with sickle cell anemia in hypoplastic crisis. B19 can cause asymptomatic infection and has been associated with five distinct clinical syndromes:

- Erythema infectiosum, or fifth disease
- Acute arthritis in adults
- Transient aplastic crisis in patients with sickle cell disease or other chronic hemolytic states
- Chronic anemia in immunodeficient patients
- Fetal hydrops

## Pathophysiology

The rash of erythema infectiosum and clinical manifestations of B19 arthritis are considered immune phenomena. The more serious hematologic manifestations of B19 infection result from selective infection and lysis of erythroid precursor cells with interruption of normal red cell production. In people with normal hematopoiesis, B19 infection produces a clinically inapparent, self-limited red cell aplasia. In patients who have increased rates of red cell destruction or loss and who depend on compensatory increases in red cell production to maintain stable red cell indices, B19 infection may precipitate aplastic crisis.

B19 fetal hydrops involves hematologic, hepatic, and cardiac factors. B19 infection of erythroid precursor cells induces an arrest of red cell production, which renders the fetus particularly vulnerable because its red cell survival is short and its red cell volume is rapidly expanding. The resulting severe anemia causes high-output cardiac failure followed by generalized edema. Extramedullary erythropoiesis leads to hypoproteinemia and portal hypertension. B19 infection of myocardial cells has been observed, suggesting that direct damage to myocardial tissue may also contribute to heart failure in the fetus.

## Epidemiology

The principal mode of B19 transmission is presumed to be person-to-person, through direct contact with respiratory secretions. In addition, the virus can be transmitted parenterally by transfusion of blood or blood products and vertically from mother to fetus. Transplacental transmission of B19 to the fetus occurs in an estimated one-third of pregnancies involving an infected mother.

Patients with erythema infectiosum are likely to be most contagious before the onset of rash but rarely remain contagious for more than a few days after the rash appears. Patients with transient aplastic crisis are infectious prior to the onset of clinical symptoms through the subsequent week.

Cases of erythema infectiosum occur sporadically and, as part of community outbreaks, are often associated with elementary or junior high schools. Community outbreaks are common from midwinter to early summer, often lasting for several months or until school recesses. The incubation period usually spans 4 to 14 days, but can be as long as 20 days.

The secondary attack rate for infection among susceptible household contacts of patients with erythema infectiosum is 50% to 90%. In school outbreaks, 10% to 60% of students may develop erythema infectiosum and 16% to 54% of susceptible teachers and other staff may develop serologic evidence of B19 infection. In one large school outbreak, the minimal rate of B19 infection in susceptible personnel during the outbreak was 19%. In two studies, approximately 37% of susceptible health care workers became infected with B19 after exposure to children with transient aplastic crisis; a recent study, however, showed that nosocomial exposure to adults with transient aplastic crisis contributed only a small additional risk of acquiring B19 infection as compared with the background community risk.

## Diagnosis

The reported seroprevalence ranges from 2% to 15% in children 1 to 5 years old, 15% to 60% in children 5 to 19 years old, and 30% to 60% in adults. For pregnant women and women of reproductive age, the reported seroprevalence varies between 16% and 72%, with the majority of estimates placing this rate between 35% and 55%. In one study of school personnel, previous B19 infection rates ranged from a low of 43% in nonteaching high school staff to a high of 68% in day-care providers. Overall, 58% of school personnel exhibited evidence of previous B19 infection.

The most sensitive test for detecting recent infection is the immunoglobulin M (IgM) antibody assay. B19 IgM antibody can be detected by enzyme-linked immunosorbent assay (ELISA) or radioimmunoassay in approximately 90% of cases by the third day of symptoms. The IgM antibody titer begins to fall 30 to 60 days after the onset of illness, although the antibody may persist at a low level for four months or longer. B19 IgG antibody appears around the seventh day of illness and persists for years. Serologic assays for this infection are available in commercial laboratories and state health department and research laboratories. Their sensitivity and specificity—especially for IgM antibody—may vary at different laboratories.

To summarize the diagnostic serology, the absence of B19 IgM and IgG indicates no previous infection and a susceptible individual. The presence of only B19 IgG indicates previous infection and an immune individual, although the infection may have occurred as recently as four months earlier. The presence of only B19 IgM indicates a very recent infection, probably within the preceding seven days, whereas the presence of both B19 IgM and IgG suggests recent exposure, from seven days to six months previously. Physicians should be aware that the laboratory will report results of both B19 IgM and IgG antibody determinations. Therefore, only a single specimen taken between four days and four weeks after onset of symptoms is necessary for the serologic diagnosis of acute infection.

## Fifth Disease

Erythema infectiosum is often called fifth disease after an otherwise short-lived numerical classification system of childhood rashes devised around 1900. In children, this mild exanthematous disease is associated with few constitutional symptoms. After a brief prodrome of low-grade fever, facial erythema ("slapped cheek") develops, followed by a lacy reticular rash on the trunk and extremities.

Adults may have a rash on their extremities, but rarely develop facial erythema. Acute arthralgias and arthritis of the hands, knees, and wrists may occur as the sole manifestation of infection in adults. A flu-like illness is also common, as are numbness and tingling of the peripheral extremities. Approximately one-fourth of adults infected with B19 will have a nonrash illness, and another one-fourth of them will be asymptomatic.

## Fifth Disease and Pregnancy

Hydrops fetalis and stillbirth were first associated with B19 infection in 1984. Since then, more than 400 cases of B19 infection have been described during pregnancy. These cases resulted in normal seronegative newborns (most cases), normal seropositive newborns, and spontaneous abortion or stillbirth due to fetal hydrops. Cases of maternal infection and subsequent fetal death have occurred during each trimester. Stillbirth occurred 1 to 16 weeks after maternal infection.

The lack of congenital anomalies among hundreds of infants of B19-infected mothers indicates that B19 probably is not a teratogen. One aborted fetus born to a B19-infected woman had eye anomalies and histologic evidence of damage to multiple tissues. An anencephalic fetus has also been reported in a

B19-infected woman, but the timing of the infection made it unlikely that B19 contributed to the defect. A preliminary report described three liveborn infants with severe perinatal encephalopathy following serologically confirmed maternal B19 infection. In addition, a recent study showed no difference in the frequency of developmental delays in children born of mothers with B19 infection as compared with a control group. Nevertheless, because of the small size of all studies to date, the absence of control groups in some, and relatively brief periods of follow-up, it is possible that a rare teratogenic effect or developmental abnormality has gone undetected.

A prospective study of 186 pregnant women with serologically confirmed B19 infection showed the overall fetal loss rate (16%) was similar to that in an uninfected antenatal sample, although a pronounced excess of fetal loss in the second trimester was observed with the B19-infected mothers. Based on virologic findings in the aborted fetuses, the risk of fetal death from B19 in an infected pregnancy was estimated to be 9%. The majority of the fetal deaths were not associated with fetal hydrops. Using this figure of 9%, together with the estimates of susceptibility and attack rates previously presented, one can calculate a crude upper-limit estimate of the risk of fetal death from B19 in pregnant women of unknown susceptibility who are exposed to this virus in the common settings of the home or school:

Mother exposed to a household member:
50% susceptible × 70% attack rate × 9% = 3.2%

Teacher/staff exposed at school:
42% susceptible × 19% attack rate × 9% = 0.7 %

The crude risks of fetal death if the mother is known to be susceptible are 6.3% (household) and 1.7% (school). These assumptions are based on preliminary or imprecise data and await further refinement.

## Management

For pregnant women with exposure to confirmed or probable cases of B19 infection, or with symptoms compatible with fifth disease, the clinician should obtain B19 IgM and IgG antibody determinations on a single specimen at any time between four days and four weeks after onset of symptoms. If no symptoms are present, the tests should be conducted approximately two weeks after exposure.

If maternal infection is documented by the presence of B19 IgM, several management strategies have been suggested, none of which is validated by controlled trials. These strategies involve various combinations of the following:

1. Serial measurement of maternal serum α-fetoprotein (MSAFP)
2. Serial ultrasound scans
3. Diagnostic tests for fetal infection
4. In utero therapy for fetal hydrops

Although early case reports and a preliminary study suggested that maternal serum alpha-fetoprotein (MSAFP) levels become elevated when the fetus is affected, more recent work shows that MSAFP does not appear to be a regular early marker for poor pregnancy outcome in parvovirus B19-infected pregnancies, and we no longer employ this test.

Serial ultrasound evaluations, looking for fetal hydrops, are the most common approach employed for following pregnant women with documented B19 infection. Early ultrasound indications of fetal hydrops include a dilated heart and ascites; generalized edema and pleural effusions are late signs. There is some controversy over the appropriate duration of ultrasonographic surveillance after the diagnosis of parvovirus infection in the mother. Many clinicians perform serial sonograms looking for evidence of fetal hydrops for 8 weeks, because almost all case reports of parvovirus-associated hydrops have occurred within 8 weeks of maternal infection. However, a single case report (Rodis 1988) describes a fetal death occurring 16 weeks after maternal infection, and a few centers continue serial studies for this period of time.

The prenatal diagnosis of intrauterine infection can be accomplished by either cordocentesis or amniocentesis. Fetal blood may be directly tested for B19 IgM (which may give negative results despite fetal infection) or by B19 virus studies (by DNA hybridization and electron microscopy). The use of polymerase chain reaction (PCR) testing to document intrauterine B19 infection has recently been reported. The PCR assay appeared to be a sensitive indicator of fetal infection with parvovirus B19 when applied to specimens of amniotic fluid and fetal blood. Amniotic fluid may prove to be the optimal sample for PCR, as it is technically easier to obtain than fetal blood. Amniocentesis can be performed earlier in pregnancy, allows for collection of a larger sample, and poses less risk of fetal injury or death.

Suggested management of fetal hydrops due to B19 infection has included fetal transfusion and direct fetal digitalization. Recent reports of spontaneous resolution have demonstrated that fetal hydrops in association with parvovirus B19 infection does not always lead to poor long-term outcomes—an observation in sharp contrast with earlier reports. A conservative approach, combining twice-weekly fetal nonstress tests, serial sonograms, and fetal movement recording, has recently been proposed by Sheikh and coworkers. These authors consider delivery when the fetus is at or beyond 32 weeks of gestation in cases in which hydrops is increasing, arrhythmias are present, or fetal heart rate patterns show no variability or late decelerations. If severe prematurity precludes delivery, perform cordocentesis to reevaluate hemoglobin; if the fetus is severely anemic (hemoglobin of 5 g/dL or less), consider transfusion.

The Public Health Laboratory Service Working Party on Fifth Disease (London) has urged caution regarding recommendations to monitor infected women with frequent ultrasound examinations or MSAFP determinations to detect fetal hydrops and correct it with intrauterine transfusion. A small number of B19-infected fetuses have been saved by these means, but all survivors must be monitored for a long period as they are likely to have been severely infected in utero. It is also unknown, with a few exceptions, whether any of the presumed infected liveborn infants went through a transient hydropic phase in utero, the detection of which might have led to their being unnecessarily subjected to intrauterine transfusion with its associated risks.

At the University of Vermont, the following protocol is employed: Prenatal diagnosis of intrauterine B19 infection by amniocentesis or cordocentesis is limited to those rare instances where a patient presents with fetal hydrops and no serologic documentation of acute B19 infection has taken place. Ultrasound scans are performed every one to two weeks from documentation of maternal infection until 16 weeks after maternal illness occurred. Following the initial scan, serial scans do not begin until approximately 18 weeks' gestation, when intrauterine transfusion becomes a practical option. When fetal hydrops is identified by ultrasonography in a mother with serologically confirmed B19 infection at less than 32 weeks, cordocentesis is performed to assess fetal anemia. Fetal transfusion is considered based on level of anemia and gestational age. Delivery after 32 weeks takes into account the gestational age and fetal condition, much like the approach of Sheikh and coworkers.

## Other Considerations

Pathologists should study any hydropic fetus with nonimmune hemolytic anemia for possible B19 parvovirus infection, especially if hepatitis or nucleopathic changes in the erythroblasts are identified.

Pregnant health care workers should avoid patients with erythema infectiosum until at least 24 hours after onset of rash, as well as patients likely to be viremic for their entire hospitalization. The latter include patients with hereditary or acquired chronic hemolytic anemias who develop aplastic crisis or who are admitted with a fever of unknown origin.

No B19 vaccine for active immunization is available at this time. No studies of prophylaxis with commercially available immune globulin preparations have been conducted, and this usage is not currently recommended by the Centers for Disease Control and Prevention. As yet, researchers have not identified the role of hyperimmune serum globulin in the prevention or modification of fetal B19 infection, although this tactic seems worthy of investigation, based on limited adult experience.

Finally, no Public Health Service guidelines have been developed for counseling pregnant women about the occupational risks of B19 infection. Serologic testing can document the natural immunity of the majority of school and day-care staff. The remaining susceptible women are left with the difficult choice between a small risk of fetal loss and prolonged, recurrent, and unplanned absences from work during community outbreaks of fifth disease. In view of the high prevalence of B19 infection in the community, the low incidence of ill effects on the fetus, and the fact that avoidance of child care or teaching can reduce—but not eliminate—the risk of exposure, routine exclusion of pregnant women from the workplace where fifth disease is occurring is not recommended by most authorities.

## Suggested Readings

Adler SP, Manganello AA, Koch WC, et al. Risk of human parvovirus B19 infections among school and hospital employees during endemic periods. J Infect Dis 1993;168:361–368.

Conry JA, Torok T, Andrews PI. Perinatal encephalopathy secondary to in utero human parvovirus B19 infection. Neurology 1993; 43(suppl):A346. Abstract no. 736S.

Gillespie SM, Cartter ML, Asch S, et al. Occupational risk of human parvovirus B19 infection for school and day-care personnel during an outbreak of erythema infectiosum. JAMA 1990;263:2061–2065.

Humphrey W, Magoon M, O'Shaughnessy R. Severe nonimmune hydrops secondary to parvovirus B19 infection: spontaneous reversal in utero and survival of a term infant. Obstet Gynecol 1991;78:900–902.

Komischke K, Searle K, Enders G. Maternal serum alpha-fetoprotein and human chorionic gonadotropin in pregnant women with acute parvovirus B19 infection with and without fetal complications. Prenat Diagn 1997;17:1039–1046.

Kovacs BW, Carlson DE, Shahbahrami B, et al. Prenatal diagnosis of human parvovirus B19 in nonimmune hydrops fetalis by polymerase chain reaction. Am J Obstet Gynecol 1992;167:461–462.

Morey AL, Nicolini V, Welch CR, et al. Parvovirus B19 infection and transient fetal hydrops. Lancet 1991;337:496.

Pryde PG, Nugent CE, Pridjian G, et al. Spontaneous resolution of nonimmune hydrops fetalis secondary to human parvovirus B19 infection. Obstet Gynecol 1992;79:859–861.

Public Health Laboratory Service Working Party on Fifth Disease. Prospective study of human parvovirus (B19) infection in pregnancy. Br Med J 1990;300:1166–1170.

Ray SM, Erdman DD, Berschling JD, et al. Nosocomial exposure to parvovirus B19: low risk of transmission to healthcare workers. Infect Control and Hosp Epidemiol 1997;18:109–114.

Rodis JF, Borgida AF, Wilson M, et al. Management of parvovirus infection in pregnancy and outcomes of hydrops: a survey of members of the Society of Perinatal Obstetricians. Am J Obstet Gynecol 1998;179:985–988.

Rodis JF, Hovick TJ, Quinn DL, et al. Human parvovirus infection in pregnancy. Obstet Gynecol 1988;72:733–738.

Rodis J, Rodner C, Hansen A, et al. Long-term outcome of children following maternal human B19 parvovirus infection. Am J Obstet Gynecol 1997;176:S3. Abstract no. 7.

Sheikh AU, Ernest JM, O'Shea M. Long-term outcome in fetal hydrops from parvovirus B19 infection. Am J Obstet Gynecol 1992;167:337–341.

Torok TJ, Wang Q-Y, Gary GW, et al. Prenatal diagnosis of intrauterine infection with parvovirus B19 by the polymerase chain reaction technique. Clin Infect Dis 1992;13:149–155.

Zerbini M, Musiani M, Gentilomi G, et al. Symptomatic parvovirus B19 infection of one fetus in a twin pregnancy. Clin Infect Dis 1993;17:262–263.

CHAPTER

# 27

# *Measles in Pregnancy*

*Bryan Larsen*

## Background and Incidence

Measles (rubeola) is a highly contagious infection generally acquired by nonimmune children, although infection among inadequately immunized adolescents remains a problem even in developed countries. In the United States, the majority of cases include those imported from endemic areas, those occurring in groups that express a religious or philosophic-based exception to vaccination, and, more frequently than in the past, those occurring in young adults. The virus is limited in its host range to humans and monkeys. In the absence of adequate vaccination or prior infection, human susceptibility is universal.

The World Health Organization estimates that measles is responsible for 800,000 deaths annually worldwide; it is one of the largest killers among preventable infectious diseases. In 1995, the United States saw a historically low incidence of disease, although a resurgence of the infection had occurred between 1989 and 1991. In 1968, incidence reached an all-time high of 152,209 cases; by 1990, annual incidence had dropped to 27,786. In 1995, only 309 cases were reported to the Centers for Disease Control and Prevention (CDC). This decrease attests to the power of improved immunization practices.

As with any disease that has become uncommon as a result of successful vaccine strategies, prevention of measles requires continued vigilance by the medical community. Complacency about vaccination could lead to resurgences, and unfamiliarity with symptoms of uncomplicated measles infections or their more serious sequelae could lead to poor management of cases.

## Pathophysiology

Measles enters by droplets or by fomites through the upper respiratory tract, with initial replication taking place locally and in the regional lymph nodes. A primary viremia follows, which infects the reticuloendothelial system. A secondary viremia ensues after 5 to 7 days. An incubation period of 9 to 12 days culminates in fever, upper respiratory symptoms, and pathognomonic Koplik's spots (red spots with bluish to white centers on the buccal mucosa) followed 1 to 2 days later by a rash that begins on the head and descends to the body and limbs. Invasion of the respiratory, urinary, and gastrointestinal tracts, along with the central nervous system (CNS), leads to a variety of symptoms and sequelae that are both acute and chronic.

## Diagnosis

The primary means of diagnosing primary measles cases is clinical observation, although atypical manifestations may prove more difficult to recognize. Immunohistochemistry will reveal viral antigen in nasal secretions, urine, or skin biopsy as fluorescent antibody-staining cells, and histologic or cytologic specimens may reveal multinucleated giant cells suggestive of measles virus infection. These indicators decline within a few days of the onset of rash. Viral RNA can be detected by suitably equipped laboratories using reverse-transcriptase polymerase chain reaction (RT-PCR) testing. PCR testing is particularly useful for identifying chronic complications in which few intact viral particles are present, although very high IgG levels appear in the cerebrospinal fluid (CSF) of subacute sclerosing panencephalitic (SSPE) cases.

Serodiagnosis most often relies on a demonstration of IgM antibodies in acute serum samples taken two to three days after the onset of rash and IgG antibody rising in later samples. Antibody in CSF, especially as compared with serum antibody, can be used to demonstrate CNS involvement. Antibody measurement by means of enzyme-linked immunosorbent assay (ELISA) can aid in assessing the level of protection in previously vaccinated individuals. In most cases, however, revaccination is more cost-effective because the presence of protective antibody is not a contraindication to vaccination.

## VIROLOGY

The measles virus belongs to the genus *Morbillivirus* of the Paramyxovirus family. Its genome—a single strand of negative-sense RNA—carries two proteins required for viral replication with its protein nucleocapsid. During the process of maturation, nascent virus acquires a lipid bilayer envelope that contains some host and some viral components. Although host cells may be destroyed by viral replication, some cells may become chronically infected.

Viral replication occurs in a number of cell types, such as epithelium, endothelium, and lymphoid cells, including macrophages and monocytes. Although action of the serum antibody may remove intact virus particles from the bloodstream, incomplete virus in the form of ribonucleoprotein can persist in gray and white matter, leading to a chronic condition unlike the primary measles infection.

## IMMUNITY

A single antigenic type of virus is responsible for natural infection, and infection is considered to confer lifelong immunity through serum antibody response. Antibody transferred passively at low titers (transplacentally derived or parenterally administered) may not prevent measles, but may nevertheless ensure that the patient experiences a milder form of the disease. Recent studies from endemic populations suggest that transplacental antibodies derived from mothers with prior natural infection last longer in the infant than those from mothers with prior measles vaccination. Passive immunization is used in measles-exposed populations at risk of serious illness, including immunosuppressed or immunodeficient individuals. It should also be used when protection is needed during pregnancy.

Vaccination has been available since 1963 and is based on a live-attenuated virus strain usually given as part of measles-mumps-rubella regimen during the first 12 to 18 months of life. Administration of live vaccine is contraindicated during pregnancy, and active vaccination should therefore precede conception by at least three months. Postpartum vaccination of a woman susceptible to rubella provides an opportunity to offer measles vaccine as well. In the absence of a clear history of previous vaccination, the live virus may still be used, as an increased incidence of adverse reactions in those already immune has not been documented.

After vaccination, declining but protective titers remain for about 18 years, with natural exposure providing some boosting of the immune response. Because a small percentage of primary vaccinations are ineffective, some countries recommend revaccination to anticipate this possibility. In the United States, many colleges mandate revaccination before entrance. Table 27-1 summarizes the current vaccine recommendations.

Although most attention is given to the humoral immune response to measles, the virus itself interacts with cell-mediated responses during active disease. The invasion of T and B lymphocytes by the measles virus has been blamed for a transitory loss of delayed hypersensitivity reactions. A recent report suggests that the mechanism may involve down-regulation of interleukin-12 (IL-12) production by monocytes through interaction with CD46, which serves as the measles virus receptor. The importance of suppressed cell-mediated immunity may lie in the increased susceptibility of measles patients to secondary infections, which may be responsible for measles mortality more often than the primary viral disease itself.

## Measles Complications

Measles can be complicated by acute or chronic conditions, and some concomitant illnesses may predispose the patient to complications. For example, in individuals with tuberculosis, measles may follow a more virulent course as well as exacerbate

**Table 27-1.** Recommendations for Measles Vaccination (Nonchildhood)*

| Population | Recommendation/documentation |
|---|---|
| College admission (post-secondary school) | Document receipt of two doses after the first birthday or obtain laboratory evidence of measles immunity, or birth before 1957 (naturally infected) and provide vaccination if needed. |
| Medical personnel beginning employment | Same as for college. |
| Special situations requiring revaccination | Revaccinate persons vaccinated before their first birthday (provide second dose of live measles vaccine).<br>Revaccinate if primary vaccination was given with immunoglobulin (provide second dose of live measles vaccine).<br>Revaccinate if primary vaccination used killed vaccine (available between 1963 and 1967). Provide two doses of vaccine separated by more than 1 month to prevent severe atypical measles.<br>Revaccinate persons vaccinated with unknown vaccine type between 1963 and 1967.<br>Revaccinate if primary vaccination was killed vaccine followed within 3 months by live vaccine (provide two doses of vaccine). |

* Consult local health department officials for additional details and local requirements.

the tuberculosis. Immunosuppressed individuals also are at risk of severe viral illness. A sometimes-fatal giant-cell pneumonia may occur in the absence of rash in immunocompromised children. In addition, inadequate vitamin A nutrition has been associated with increased susceptibility to complications—particularly among children in developing countries—and has prompted the use of vitamin A in active measles cases in both developing and developed countries.

Approximately one-fourth of all people infected with measles will experience complications such as diarrhea (9%), secondary bacterial or viral otitis and pneumonitis (each about 7%), and post-measles encephalitis, which occurs in 50 to 400 of every 10,000 measles cases. Because of its significant mortality (20%) and risk of permanent neurologic sequelae

(20% to 40%), this encephalitis represents the most compelling reason to undertake vigorous vaccination campaigns. The mechanism of pathology in encephalitis cases is believed to be an allergic inflammatory reaction.

One legacy of the early use of killed vaccines is an atypical measles syndrome. This syndrome is essentially an allergic response consisting of fever, an urticarial rash that spreads from limbs to trunk, and atypical pneumonia in young adults.

A very serious and delayed sequel of measles seen mainly in children aged 5 to 10 years is SSPE, which occurs five to seven years after primary measles infection. A recent report describes a 16-year-old gravida with a fatal case of SSPE. This degenerative disease results from the persistence of mutant viral forms from infected cells, which produce significant quantities of ribonucleoprotein in the CNS. Progressive mental deterioration and motor dysfunction may follow personality change, intellectual decline, and inappropriate behavior, culminating within a few years in seizures, coma, and death. The estimated rate of this complication is 0.5 to 2 for every 100,000 cases.

## Pregnancy and Measles

When measles reached the previously unexposed population of Greenland in 1951, a nearly threefold greater mortality was observed in pregnant women compared with nonpregnant women. In addition, measles is considered to produce high rates of fetal loss, although the mechanism appears to be placental compromise rather than fetal damage or viral teratogenicity, as shown by Moroi and coworkers. These investigators found measles virus antigen in syncytial trophoblast and decidua but not in the fetus in a case of fetal death at 25 weeks' gestation.

Overall declining rates of measles in the United States have simultaneously reduced the number of gestational measles cases. Nevertheless, the resurgence of measles in the early 1990s and continued problems with measles in other parts of the world have called attention to the potential for adverse pregnancy outcomes. In 1993, Eberhart-Phillips and colleagues reported 53 cases of gestational measles, in which two maternal deaths and a high rate of fetal loss and prematurity occurred. In 1992, Atmar and colleagues described 12 gravid women with measles and one newly parturient patient whose illnesses suggested a virulent disease course, with one maternal death and seven instances each of maternal hepatitis and pneumonitis. This series also included four premature labors and one spontaneous abortion. Likewise, in 1991, Stein and Greenspoon reported three cases of bacterial pneumonia complicating gestational measles in 1991; one of these patients successfully underwent tocolysis for premature labor but had an unexplained stillbirth seven weeks later.

## Vaccination

Prevention of measles through vaccination is by far the most desirable scenario. As already stated, vaccination must take place when a patient is not pregnant (Table 27-2), although vaccination of her young children will not threaten a pregnant mother. Vaccination against all preventable diseases should be promoted, and the overiding concern about rubella and its dangers should not divert attention from other diseases, including measles. The physician who has a patient expressing a religious or philosophical exception to vaccination should be especially diligent in maintaining communication, as outbreaks may occur in such individuals and their families.

The currently used live virus-containing vaccines are provided in three forms: monovalent (measles), MR (measles-rubella), and MMR (measles-mumps-rubella). Although the measles vaccine is highly effective, a second dose is mandatory to attain an adequate level of protection. Table 27-1 emphasizes the importance of providing two doses of live virus vaccine and lists special situations requiring revaccination.

Measles vaccine has an excellent record of safety but may induce some side effects. As many as 45% of vaccinees may develop a temperature of 103 °F (39.4 °C) or higher, beginning approximately 42 days after vaccination. Transient rashes are reported in 5% of vaccinees; CNS conditions occur in fewer than 1 per 1 million vaccinees.

**Table 27-2.** Precautions for Measles Vaccine Use

| Condition | Recommendation |
|---|---|
| Pregnancy | Live vaccine should not be given during pregnancy. Vaccinated women should not become pregnant for 30 days after vaccination. |
| Febrile illness | Minor febrile illness is not a contraindication. Children with moderate or severe febrile illness can be vaccinated as soon as they recover. |
| Allergies | MMR vaccines contain hen-egg components and traces of neomycin. Vaccination should be undertaken only with extreme caution in persons with a history of anaphylaxis following egg ingestion (refer to special protocol: J Pediatr 1988;113:504–506.). |
| Recent immune globulin treatment | For international travelers, measles vaccine should precede IG administration by 2 weeks; for IG-treated individuals, delay measles vaccine at least 6 weeks but preferably 6 months (whole blood and other antibody-containing products are included in this contraindication). If IG is given within 14 days of measles vaccine, the measles vaccine should be repeated 3 months later (unless the patient has seroconverted). |
| Tuberculosis | Measles vaccine is not contraindicated but may transiently alter tuberculin reactivity. Delay tuberculin test 4 to 6 weeks after measles vaccination. |
| Altered immunocompetence | Patients with immunosuppression (leukemia, lymphoma, generalized malignancy, antimetabolite or alkylating agent therapy, radiation therapy, high-dose corticosteroids, or symptomatic HIV infection) should not receive live virus vaccine. Asymptomatic HIV-infected children and adults who need MMR should receive it. Immediate protection of persons with vaccination contraindications may be achieved with passive IG (0.25 mL/kg or twice the dose in immunocompromised patients up to a maximum of 15 mL). |
| Simultaneous vaccinations | In general, using more than one live or inactivated vaccine at the same time does not impair immune responses, although data are not available for every situation. |

## Management During Pregnancy

When measles infection occurs near the time of delivery, the fetus may become infected at birth or within 12 days after delivery. Children born to infected mothers who have measles in the last week of pregnancy or the first week postpartum should be treated with immune globulin. Immune globulin (0.25 mL/kg IM) also is administered to modify the course of measles in the susceptible gravida within six days of exposure to the virus. Between five and nine days after exposure, secondary viremia will not be prevented but disease may be modified.

Bacterial complications of measles should be treated with appropriate antimicrobial therapy, although no reliable therapy exists for measles encephalopathies. Therefore, management should employ supportive therapy—especially in pregnancy, where symptoms may be exaggerated and may lead to prematurity or pregnancy loss.

### Suggested Readings

Advisory Committee on Immunization Practices (ACIP). General recommendations on immunization. MMWR 1994;43(RR-1):1–38.

Advisory Committee on Immunization Practices (ACIP). Update: vaccine side effects, adverse reactions, contraindications, and precautions. MMWR 1996;45(RR-12):2.

American Academy of Pediatrics Committee on Infectious Diseases. Vitamin A treatment of measles. Pediatrics 1993;91:1014–1015.

American College of Obstetrics and Gynecology. Immunization during pregnancy. ACOG Technical Bulletin Number 160—October 1991. Int J Gynaecol Obstet 1993;40:69–79.

Atmar RL, Englund JA, Hammill H. Complications of measles during pregnancy. Clin Infect Dis 1992;14:217–226.

Eberhart-Phillips JE, Frederick PD, Baron RC, et al. Measles in pregnancy: a descriptive study of 58 cases. Obstet Gynecol 1993;82:797–801.

Enders G. Paramyxoviruses. In: Baron S, ed. Medical microbiology, 4th ed. Galveston, TX: University of Texas Medical Branch, 1996.

Fawzi WW, Chalmers TC, Herrera MG, et al. Vitamin A supplementation and child mortality. A meta-analysis. JAMA 1993;269: 898–903.

http://www.medaccess.com/cdcimun/measles.

Kacica MA, Venezia RA, Miller J, et al. Measles antibodies in women and infants in the vaccine era. J Med Virol 1995; 45:227–229.

Karp CL, Wysocka M, Wahl LK, et al. Mechanism of suppression of cell-mediated immunity by measles virus. Science 1996;273:228.

Modlin JF. Measles virus. In: Belshe RB, ed. Human virology. Littleton, MA: PSG Publishing, 1984:333–360.

Moroi K, Saito S, Kurata T, et al. Fetal death associated with measles virus infection of the placenta. Am J Obstet Gynecol 1991;164: 1107–1108.

Peltola H, Heinonen O. Fequency of true adverse reactions to measles-mumps-rubella vaccine: a double-blind placebo-controlled trial in twins. Lancet 1986;1:939–942.

Stein SJ, Greenspoon JS. Rubeola during pregnancy. Obstet Gynecol 1991;78:925–929.

CHAPTER

# 28

# *Mumps in Pregnancy*

*R. David Miller*
*W. David Hager*

## Background and Incidence

Mumps virus is a member of the paramyxovirus family, which also includes rubeola virus. Mumps is primarily a disease of children aged 5 to 15 and has a worldwide distribution. In the United States, incidence increases in the winter, peaking in March and April. Epidemics tend to occur among nonimmunized persons in confined populations, such as boarding schools and military encampments.

Since the introduction of mumps vaccine in 1967, when 152,209 cases were reported in the United States, the incidence of clinical mumps has declined dramatically. In 1995, only 840 cases were reported. Incidence in pregnancy has been estimated to be from 0.8 to 10 cases per 10,000 pregnancies. A review of the literature shows that clinical mumps is rare and usually benign in neonates. Similarly, death from mumps in adults with intact immune systems is rare.

## Pathophysiology

Mumps is transmitted by droplet nuclei, saliva, and fomites. As no good animal model of this disease has been developed, the precise pathogenesis of infection has not been established. The virus initially replicates in the epithelium of the upper respiratory tract. A viremia follows, after which the agent localizes in glandular or central nervous system tissues. Parotitis is believed to result from the viremia.

Few studies have focused on the pathology of mumps because it is rarely a fatal disease. The histologic changes in the parotid gland and the testis are similar; necrosis affects the acinar and ductal epithelial cells in the salivary glands as well as the germinal epithelium of the seminiferous tubules. The significance of this disease in obstetrics, however, rests with its effects on the fetus.

## Diagnosis

History plays an important role in making a diagnosis of mumps, as the patient presenting with a suspicion of the disease will have been in close contact with a person who has acquired mumps. Mumps patients have a typical viral prodrome of fever, anorexia, malaise, and myalgia. These symptoms are followed within the next 24 hours by infection and swelling of the glands, which resolves in one week or less.

Parotitis is a bilateral infection, although the onset of disease may be asynchronous. The submaxillary and sublingual glands are only rarely involved. Mumps may involve the gonads of the male and rarely will cause aseptic meningitis, mastitis, thyroiditis, myocarditis, nephritis, or arthritis in both sexes.

### Maternal Effects

Mumps in pregnancy is generally a benign illness. Indeed, it is not appreciably more severe in pregnant women than it is in other adult women. Mastitis and thyroiditis can occur in postpartum women, but not more frequently than in nonpregnant women.

### Fetal Effects

Studies comparing women who have mumps during the first trimester with uninfected pregnant women show a significant increase in spontaneous abortion rates. Most of these pregnancy losses occur within two weeks of the infection, so the virus is embryocidal.

No increased risk of prematurity affects women who acquire mumps in the second or third trimester. Although some evidence suggests an increased risk of congenital anomalies such as endocardial fibroelastosis associated with mumps in animal models, data are lacking to support such a relationship in humans. Presence of maternal mumps infection is not an indication for therapeutic abortion.

Congenital mumps or postnatally acquired perinatal mumps has rarely, if ever, been documented virologically or serologically. Several explanations may account for this fact:

- Protection of the neonate by passive maternal antibodies
- Exclusion of mumps virus from the fetus by a hypothetical placental barrier
- Relative insusceptibility of fetal and neonatal tissues to infection by the virus
- Occurrence of infections that are predominantly subclinical

## TREATMENT

Treatment of mumps parotitis is symptomatic. Analgesics and antipyretics are administered, and cold packs may be applied to the parotid gland and breasts, if involved. No evidence suggests that mumps immune globulin has a beneficial effect in treating established disease. Some severe cases of orchitis have been reported to respond to systemic corticosteroids.

### Immunization

The use of live attenuated mumps virus vaccine induces the production of protective antibodies in 98% or more of recipients. The vaccine is usually administered along with measles and rubella vaccines in a two-dose schedule for children. It should never be administered to infants less than 1 year old, to pregnant women, or to immunocompromised patients. The initial MMR (measles-mumps-rubella) vaccination of 0.5 mL is administered at 12 to 15 months of age. The second dose is given at preschool or kindergarten age or before admission to elementary or middle school. Although fever and rash are not infrequently reported in children, major adverse effects such as encephalitis and meningitis are rare.

## Suggested Readings

Advisory Committee on Immunization Practices. Update: vaccine side effects, adverse reactions, contraindications, and precautions. MMWR 1996;45(RR-12):2–4.

Chretien JH, McGinniss CG, Thompson J, et al. Group B beta-hemolytic streptococci causing pharyngitis. J Clin Microbiol 1979;10:263–266.

Garcia AG, Pereira JM, Vidigal N, et al. Intrauterine infection with mumps virus. Obstet Gynecol 1980;56:756–759.

Gershon AA. Chickenpox, measles, and mumps. In: Remington JS, Klein JO, eds. Infectious diseases of the fetus and newborn infant, 3rd ed. Philadelphia: WB Saunders, 1990;432–445.

Lacour M, Maherzi M, Vienny H, et al. Thrombocytopenia in a case of neonatal mumps infection: evidence for further clinical presentations. Eur J Pediatr 1993;152:739–741.

Lim DV, Morales WJ, Walsh AF. Lim Group B strep broth and coagglutination for rapid identification of group B streptococci in preterm pregnant women. J Clin Microbiol 1987;25:452–453.

Monif GR. Maternal mumps infection during gestation: observations on the progeny. Am J Obstet Gynecol 1974;119:549–551.

Nahmias AJ, Armstrong G. Mumps virus and endocardial fibroelastosis. N Engl J Med 1966;275:1449.

Stagno S, Whitley RJ. Herpesvirus infections of pregnancy. N Engl J Med 1985;313:1270–1274.

CHAPTER

# 29

# *Rubella in Pregnancy*

*John H. Grossman III*

## Background and Incidence

Although the number of rubella cases in the United States fell to a low of 225 in 1988, the amount progressively increased thereafter, peaking at 1401 in 1991. In 1992, however, a new low of 160 cases was reported. In 1993, the number increased only slightly, to 190 cases. The incidence of congenital rubella syndrome (CRS) in U.S.-born infants has paralleled these trends. The National Congenital Rubella Syndrome Registry of the Centers for Disease Control and Prevention (CDC) documented two infants born with CRS in 1988 and only one in 1989. In contrast, 25 cases of CRS were reported in 1990 and 31 cases were reported in 1991. In 1992, five reported cases of CRS coincided with the decline in rubella that year. In 1993, no indigenous cases of CRS were reported.

Outbreaks in the United States that cause fluctuations in rubella and CRS prevalence are primarily associated with a failure to vaccinate certain susceptible target groups rather than to any failure of the vaccine itself. For example, retrospective analysis has shown that 12 (57%) of 21 cases of CRS reported in 1990 could have been prevented if the mothers of the infants had been screened and vaccinated. Several outbreaks of rubella in 1993 and 1994 identified additional susceptible groups in correctional institutions and colleges. From an epidemiologic perspective, other important sources of potential outbreaks include immigrants—especially Asians/Pacific Islanders and Hispanics—from countries where rubella vaccination is not routinely performed and groups who take religious exemption from recommended immunization practices (such as settlements of Old Order Amish). In a survey of Amish women in a Pennsylvania county, 20% were susceptible to rubella. Moreover, in a survey of 325 women attending an urban family planning clinic, 10.7% were rubella-susceptible. Consequently, although a national goal of eradicating rubella and CRS has been in place for more than a decade, the potential for outbreaks persists.

## PATHOPHYSIOLOGY

Rubella, a respiratory disease that develops two to three weeks after exposure, is caused by a single-stranded RNA virus belonging to the togavirus family. Infectious virus usually appears in the nasopharynx and upper respiratory tract one week before symptoms develop. Illness is present when a discrete pink-red, maculopapular, three-day rash appears on the face and then spreads to the trunk and extremities. Postauricular and suboccipital lymphadenopathy, fever, and pain in joints may also be present. Some 25% to 50% of all rubella infections are subclinical. Conversely, skin rashes resembling rubella may result from adenovirus, enterovirus, or other respiratory virus infections. Thus laboratory testing is necessary to confirm the diagnosis.

In 1941, Gregg, an Australian ophthalmologist, associated cataracts in children with an epidemic of maternal rubella infection. Long-term follow-up of children born during U.S. epidemics has established the clinical features of congenital rubella syndrome. The eyes, heart, and CNS are most frequently affected at birth. Cataracts, glaucoma, microphthalmia, and chorioretinitis are common ophthalmologic problems. Common manifestations of heart disease include peripheral pulmonic stenosis, patent ductus arteriosus, and septal defects. Mental retardation, microcephaly, and, rarely, encephalitis are neurologic effects of illness. Sensorineural deafness is the most common consequence.

A direct effect of rubella is decreased cell replication, which may result in growth retardation and failure of normal cellular differentiation during embryogenesis. The inflammatory response to infection or autoimmune reactions may also produce tissue damage. Myocarditis, pneumonitis, hepatosplenomegaly, and vascular stenosis may result from these processes. In approximately 20% of individuals, late manifestations of infection develop at 10 to 20 years of age. These problems include endocrinopathies (insulin-dependent diabetes, thyroid abnormalities, hypoadrenalism), hearing loss or additional ocular damage, and, rarely, progressive rubella panencephalitis.

Solid evidence from large studies indicates that first-trimester maternal infection produces a high (70% to 90%) incidence of developmental malformation. Deafness and mental retardation may result when infection occurs as late as the sixth gestational month. Structural defects, however, are not a consequence of third-trimester gestational infection. The absence of clinical manifestations of disease at birth does not exclude the possibility of subclinical damage or subsequent impairment. Consequently, offspring of women who have sustained rubella infections during pregnancy should undergo careful long-term follow-up.

## Diagnosis

The presence of subclinical rubella among adults and newborns underscores the importance of laboratory confirmation in clinically suspicious cases. Although the virus can be isolated from nasopharyngeal secretions, few laboratory facilities provide this service, and rubella isolation usually takes four to six weeks to complete. Serologic testing serves as the cornerstone of efforts to confirm recent infection or immunity. Although reinfection during pregnancy has been reported, detectable rubella antibody constitutes proof of immunity from subsequent systemic infection in most cases. Conversely, serologic conversion using paired acute and convalescent specimens implies recent infection even among asymptomatic individuals. Hemagglutination inhibition—historically the gold standard for serologic testing—has been replaced by less expensive and less labor-intensive commercially available agglutination and enzyme immunoassay tests in clinical laboratories.

In most cases, rubella-specific IgG, whether the consequence of natural infection or immunization, persists for life. Almost all of the 95% of individuals who seroconvert following vaccination with RA 27/3 vaccine demonstrate detectable antibody by enzyme immunoassay at least 18 years after seroconversion. Recent rubella infection is confirmed by the presence of rubella-specific IgM antibody, which appears rapidly and peaks 1 to 1.5 weeks after the onset. Depending on the sensitivity of the assay, detectable IgM may persist for one month or longer.

A recent review reported 19 cases of congenital rubella, none of which was from North America, among women with prior rubella antibody who became reinfected during pregnancy. The causes of these cases are unclear. Laboratory error in antibody determination of immunity, lack of a protective high avidity (IgG1 subclass) antibody, emergence of an antigenically different viral strain, and subclinical maternal immunocompromise are all potential explanations.

Rubella-specific IgM in fetal blood obtained by funipuncture indicates the occurrence of second-trimester intrauterine infection. Fetal seroreactivity has been shown as early as the nineteenth gestational week. Using detection of rubella-specific IgM from funipuncture performed more than two weeks after clinical infection and after 22 weeks' gestation, a recent study of 93 cases reported 95% concordance between fetal and neonatal serologic results. The optimal timing for detecting intrauterine infection using this approach, however, remains uncertain. Although fetal immunoresponsiveness develops during gestational weeks 20 to 24, at least one false-negative serology associated with subsequent congenital infection has been reported when testing took place at the twentieth week.

Although chorionic villus sampling traditionally has been used to diagnose first-trimester intrauterine rubella infections, this method recently has been replaced by ones that detect viral ribonucleic acid using reverse transcriptase–nested polymerase chain reaction amplification (RT-PCR). Although one retrospective study reported 85% concordance between viral culture and RT-PCR, both approaches have detected cases that were missed by the alternative method. Hybridization with cloned, radioactively labeled rubella-complementary DNA probes seems more sensitive for detecting first-trimester infection than chorionic villus sampling, although false negatives may occur with either method. Experience with such approaches remains limited, but they are feasible and continue to represent more sensitive and promising new techniques for selected cases.

## TREATMENT

Rubella vaccines have been available in the United States since 1969. Vaccination produces seroconversion with long-term immunity from infection in 95% of cases. Rashes, arthropathy, and lymphadenopathy are occasional self-limited complications of vaccination. Transient peripheral neurologic complaints also rarely occur.

In 1994, the Committee on Immunization Practices revised its general recommendations and advised that all children should receive a measles-mumps-rubella (MMR) vaccine at 12 to 15 months of age. Women of childbearing age who do not have detectable rubella IgG antibody should be immunized as well, provided that they are not pregnant when they receive the vaccine and will not become pregnant for at least three months after immunization. Primary vaccine failure remains an uncommon cause of rubella and CRS. Subclinical immunocompromise of vaccinees and interference with active immunization due to recent transfusion of blood products or immunoglobulin therapy (but not RhoGAM) represent important clinical causes of vaccine failure.

Rubella vaccination is not recommended during pregnancy because of theoretic concerns about fetal damage. The risks of congenital rubella syndrome from vaccination within three months of conception, however, are considered negligible; therefore, inadvertent rubella vaccination by itself is no longer considered an indication from terminating a pregnancy. The CDC still states that the patient and her physician should make the final decision regarding continuation of the pregnancy. Routine laboratory screening for either pregnancy or rubella antibody is unnecessary before administering vaccine. Clinicians should routinely offer the rubella vaccine whenever they encounter a potentially susceptible woman lacking contraindications for vaccination.

## Prevention

As noted earlier, in most cases, failure to vaccinate rather than vaccine failure has been responsible for the persistence of rubella and CRS in the United States. Crowded or closely contained settings continue to facilitate transmission among susceptible persons. Nevertheless, new social, political, economic, ethical, and religious issues have emerged as epidemiologically important factors that will influence the success of national efforts to eradicate rubella.

The CDC has suggested the following strategies for improving rubella prevention and control:

- Increase vaccination coverage in children.
- Implement laws requiring all students to receive two doses of MMR vaccine.
- Encourage clinicians to use every opportunity to vaccinate susceptible individuals, including women of childbearing age attending family planning and abortion clinics.
- Adopt prematriculation vaccination requirements in colleges.
- Initiate prevention and control programs in all correctional facilities.
- Encourage persons in religious groups who do not seek health care to accept vaccination.
- Target special vaccination programs toward young adults who are likely to be unvaccinated and those who have contact with persons infected with rubella from countries that do not routinely vaccinate against rubella.

## Suggested Readings

Bosma TJ, Corbett KM, Eckstein MB, et al. Use of PCR for prenatal and postnatal diagnosis of congenital rubella. J Clin Microbiol 1995;33:2881–2887.

Centers for Disease Control and Prevention. Recommendation of the Advisory Committee on Immunization Practices (ACIP). MMWR 1994;43(RR-1):1–38.

Centers for Disease Control and Prevention. Rubella and congenital rubella syndrome—United States, January 1, 1991–May 7, 1994. MMWR 1994;43:391.

Eisele CJ. Rubella susceptibility in women of childbearing age. J Obstet Gynecol Neonatal Nurs 1993;22:260–263.

Hwa H, Shyu M, Lee C, et al. Prenatal diagnosis of congenital rubella infection from maternal rubella in Taiwan. Obstet Gynecol 1994; 84:415–419.

Jackson BM, Payton T, Horst G, et al. An epidemiologic investigation of a rubella outbreak among the Amish of northeastern Ohio. Public Health Rep 1993;108:436–439.

Lee SH, Ewert DP, Frederick PD, et al. Resurgence of congenital rubella syndrome in the 1990s: report on missed opportunities and failed prevention policies among women of childbearing age. JAMA 1992;267:2616–2620.

Mellinger AK, Cragan JD, Atkinson WL, et al. High incidence of congenital rubella syndrome after a rubella outbreak. Pediatr Infect Dis J 1995;14:573–578.

Robinson J, Lemay M, Vaudry WL. Congenital rubella after anticipated maternal immunity: two cases and a review of the literature. Pediatr Infect Dis J 1994;13:812–815.

Tanemura M, Suzumori K, Yagami Y. Diagnosis of fetal rubella infection with reverse transcription and nested polymerase chain reaction: a study of 34 cases diagnosed in fetuses. Am J Obstet Gynecol 1996;174:578–582.

CHAPTER

# 30

# *Viral Influenza in Pregnancy*

*Joseph J. Apuzzio*

## Background and Incidence

Viral influenza remains a common and potentially serious problem for pregnant women. Morbidity and mortality from viral influenza were once thought to be higher in pregnant women; in the pandemic of 1918, for example, the mortality rate was higher in pregnant than in nonpregnant women. At that time, however, many of the fatalities in pregnant women probably resulted from secondary infection with bacterial pneumonia, frequently caused by coagulase-positive staphylococci. No antibiotics were available in 1918 to treat that complication.

Today, fatalities related to viral influenza infections continue to reflect primarily complications of pneumonia, but they are not as common as they were in the preantibiotic era. Researchers have estimated that 0.01% to 0.1% of the general population is at risk for death from influenza. Periodically, cases of pregnant women who have died from viral influenza are reported to the Centers for Disease Control and Prevention. Other complications from this type of infection include myocarditis, pericarditis, aseptic meningitis, and postinfection neuritis.

## Etiology

Influenza is caused by an orthomyxovirus that has three distinct types: A, the epidemic type; B, a less common type; and C, the type that is least likely to cause epidemics. The virus contains RNA and has an enveloped helical nucleocapsid enclosing two types of glycoprotein antigens, hemagglutinin (HA) and neuraminidase (NA). NA is concentrated in that region of the viral envelope where the host cell releases newly formed virus particles. Thirteen types of HA and nine subtypes of NA have been identified, allowing antigenic shifts in the virus to cause new epidemics each year. Alterations in the amino acid sequence of these proteins change their antigenic ability and, thus, their recognition by a host cell.

For example, during the 1987–1988 influenza season, influenza A ($H_3N_2$) dominated, with few cases of influenza B being reported. During the 1988–1989 season, type B dominated, with most cases being reported in children. Influenza B epidemics have often resulted in excess mortality compared with type A epidemics. During the 1995–1996 season, influenza A caused the most influenza activity in the United States and worldwide. It was anticipated that during the 1997–1998 flu season, type A ($H_3N_2$), type A ($H_1N_1$), and type B/Beijing/184/93 would be the most common influenza viruses (1).

Virus-laden aerosol droplets spread influenza when an infected person coughs or sneezes and people in the immediate area inhale them. If the virus is not neutralized by a specific antibody from previous exposure or vaccination, replication begins. Because of the aerosol spread, this virus has a high attack rate, especially in such closed environments as classrooms, vehicles, and workplaces.

## Diagnosis

Illnesses may range from occasional asymptomatic infection to more serious and, sometimes, fatal primary influenza pneumonia. The usual clinical course begins within one to four days after exposure, with a sudden rise in temperature—often as high as 39.2 °C (102.5 °F)—accompanied by myalgias, exhaustion, sore throat, nasal congestion, cough, and headache. Because of the severe physical weakness and malaise, the patient may spend several days in bed. Symptoms usually subside within a week, after which she can usually resume her normal routine.

Pneumonia, the most serious complication of influenza, comes in two types. The more frequent is a secondary bacterial infection, with *Staphylococcus aureus*, *Streptococcus pneumoniae*, and *Haemophilus influenzae* being the most common infecting organisms. The second type of pneumonia, which is caused solely by the influenza virus, is uncommon but potentially more lethal. The patient will have paroxysms of coughing, shortness of breath, and scant sputum. Hypoxia may occur and chest X ray could reveal an infiltrate. Aggressive therapy with respiratory support might be necessary, as well as a trial of antiviral agents.

The diagnosis of influenza primarily relies on the history and clinical evaluation. The virus can be grown in the laboratory, but this step usually is not necessary or practical in most clinical situations. Serologic confirmation of the infection is not required in most cases, although complement fixation and hemagglutination tests are available. If pneumonia is suspected, it is important to perform a chest X ray and examine the sputum with a Gram's stain and culture. Appropriate antibiotic therapy, as determined by the results of Gram's staining and culture, should be administered when bacterial pneumonia is suspected.

## TREATMENT

The treatment of uncomplicated viral influenza infection is supportive. Antipyretics, such as acetaminophen for myalgias and fever, and bed rest will comfort the patient. Aspirin may increase the risk of Reye's syndrome in teenagers, especially when type B influenza predominates.

For nonpregnant patients, early treatment with amantadine hydrochloride or rimantadine hydrochloride often diminishes the severity of symptoms and may hasten clinical recovery from influenza A infections. These drugs reduce the titer and duration of viral excretion, as well as the altered pulmonary function that may persist for several weeks after the infection. Neither drug is effective for influenza B.

The use of amantadine or rimantadine is relatively contraindicated in pregnancy, although both drugs are listed in the *Physicians' Desk Reference* as category C during pregnancy.

Although no large-scale studies have examined its use in pregnancy, amantadine is embryotoxic and teratogenic when used in high doses in animals. In an isolated case report, amantadine use during the first trimester was associated with a complex cardiovascular defect in the infant (2). It was hypothesized that agents inhibiting lymphocyte stimulation, such as amantadine and thalidomide, share teratogenic potential. The absence of other case reports may reflect the probable infrequency of use of the drug in pregnant patients. In view of these concerns, symptomatic treatment for influenza in most pregnant women appears to be safer than using amantadine or rimantadine unless one of these agents is needed as a life-saving measure.

Pregnant patients experiencing respiratory failure from influenza pneumonia may benefit from therapy with amantadine and other agents. Kirshon and coworkers reported a favorable outcome for a pregnant patient with influenza pneumonia and respiratory failure who was treated with oral amantadine and ribavirin inhalation therapy (3). Ribavirin has antiviral activity against influenza virus, respiratory syncytial virus, and herpes simplex virus, but it is teratogenic and embryotoxic in animals. No studies have focused on the use of this drug in human subjects. Therefore, its use during pregnancy must be limited to life-saving indications.

## SEQUELAE

Although the influenza virus crosses the placenta and has been considered a cause of fetal malformation, the literature is not clear on this issue. Several studies have indicated a 1% increase in congenital malformation over the control group. Other, larger series, including the Collaborative Perinatal Research Study, have not shown an increased risk of congenital malformation from first-trimester influenza infection (4). Thus it appears unlikely that the disease brings an increased risk of congenital malformation. If it exists, this risk is very small, especially considering the background rate of 3% to 5% for congenital malformations during any pregnancy.

**Table 30-1.** Target Groups for Vaccination

| |
|---|
| Pregnant women in the second or third trimester of pregnancy during the influenza season |
| Residents of chronic-care facilities that house persons who have chronic medical conditions |
| Patients who required medical follow-up or who were hospitalized during the preceding year because of diabetes mellitus, renal dysfunction, hemoglobinopathies, or immunosuppression |
| Patients with chronic disorders of the pulmonary or cardiovascular system, including asthma |

SOURCE: Centers for Disease Control and Prevention. Prevention and control of influenza. Recommendations of the Advisory Committee on Immunization Practices (ACIP). MMWR 1997;46(RR-9):1–25.

## PREVENTION

Because no specific treatment exists for influenza, prevention is appropriate for all pregnant women, especially those at increased risk for influenza-related complications (Table 30-1). The best time to offer vaccination to these patients is in October or November, before the flu season begins. In the United States, high levels of influenza activity are usually not seen before mid-December.

Influenza vaccine is considered safe for pregnant women. New recommendations from the Advisory Committee on Immunization Practices suggest that it should be offered to all pregnant patients, particularly those who have chronic medical conditions that increase their risk of complications from influenza regardless of the trimester of pregnancy (1). A recent study documented the increased risk of hospitalization for cardiorespiratory complications among women with influenza. It was estimated that one to two hospitalizations could be prevented for every 1000 pregnant women vaccinated (1). Consequently, the Advisory Committee on Immunization Practices recommends that all women who will be in the second or third trimester during the influenza season should be offered vaccination (1). If possible, wait until the second trimester of pregnancy before offering vaccination to preclude the theoretic risk of teratogenesis. It may be unwise to wait for the second trimester, however, if influenza activity in the community is imminent or has already begun. Do not give amantadine or rimantadine to pregnant patients for influenza prophylaxis except as a life-saving measure.

Information about influenza is available from the Centers for Disease Control and Prevention by telephone (888-232-3228) or fax (888-232-3299), or from the electronic bulletin board of the Public Health Network (http://www.cdc.gov/ncidod/diseases/flu/weekly.htm).

## References

1. Centers for Disease Control and Prevention. Prevention and control of influenza. Recommendations of the Advisory Committee on Immunization Practices (ACIP). MMWR 1997;46(RR-9):1–25.
2. Nora JJ, Nora AH, Way GL. Cardiovascular maldevelopment associated with maternal exposure to amantadine. Letter. Lancet 1975;2:607.
3. Kirshon B, Faro S, Zurawin R, et al. Favorable outcome after treatment with amantadine and ribavirin in a pregnancy complicated by influenza pneumonia. J Reprod Med 1988;33:399–401.
4. Korones SB, Todaro J, Roane JA, et al. Maternal virus infection after the first trimester of pregnancy and status of offspring to 4 years of age in a predominately Negro population. J Pediatr 1970;77:245–251.

## Suggested Readings

Centers for Disease Control and Prevention. Human infection with swine influenza virus—Wisconsin. MMWR 1988;37:661–663.

Coulson AA. Amantadine and teratogenesis. Letter. Lancet 1975;2:1044.

Elizan T, Ajero-Frobehich L, Fabiyi A, et al. Viral infection in pregnancy and congenital CNS malformations in vivo. Arch Neurol 1969;20:115–119.

McGregor J, Burns J, Levin M, et al. Transplacental passage of influenza A/Bangkok mimicking amniotic fluid infection syndrome. Am J Obstet Gynecol 1984;149:856–859.

Sever J, Larsen J, Grossman J. Handbook of perinatal infection. Boston: Little, Brown, 1989.

World Health Organization. Recommended composition of influenza virus vaccines for use in the 1996–1997 flu season. Wkly Epidemiol Rec 1996;71:57–61.

CHAPTER

# 31

# *Hepatitis B Infection in Pregnancy*

*David A. Baker*

## Background

In the United States, the reported rate of hepatitis B virus (HBV) has declined by more than 50% since 1987. Although new HBV infections occur most commonly in 20- to 39-year-olds, perinatal transmission can take place in certain at-risk groups. Each year, an estimated 20,000 infants are born to hepatitis surface-antigen (HBsAg) positive mothers in the United States.

Transmission of HBV from mother to infant during the prenatal period is one of the most efficient modes of HBV spread and often leads to severe long-term sequelae. The availability of a safe and effective vaccine, however, offers an opportunity to prevent fetal infection and its serious consequences.

## Etiology

HBV infection is caused by a small, double-stranded DNA virus. Several well-defined antigen–antibody systems are associated with HBV infection. Hepatitis B surface antigen (HBsAg) is produced in excess amounts, circulating in blood as 22 nm spherical and tubular particles. HBsAg, which can be identified in serum from 30 to 60 days after exposure to HBV, persists for variable periods. Anti-HBs antibody develops after a resolved infection and confers long-term immunity to the infection.

Antibody to core antigen (anti-HBc) develops in all HBV

infections and persists indefinitely. IgM anti-HBc appears early in infection and persists for six months or longer; it is therefore a reliable marker of acute or recent HBV infection. A third antigen, hepatitis B e antigen (HBeAg), may be detected in samples from persons with acute or chronic HBV infection. The presence of HBeAg correlates with viral replication and high infectivity. Antibody to HBeAg (anti-HBe) develops in most HBV infections and correlates with the loss of replicating virus and with lower infectivity.

## Epidemiology

The major modes of HBV transmission consist of contact with blood, sexual activity, and vertical transmission from mothers to newborns. The newborn will be infected if the mother has acute HBV infection during the third trimester or is a chronic carrier. Perinatal transmission is very high (70% to 90%) if the mother is not only HBsAg-positive but also HBeAg-positive. If the mother is positive only for HBsAg, the chances of transmission in the newborn period decline to only 15%.

The role of the HBV carrier is central in the epidemiology of HBV transmission. A carrier is defined as a person who is HBsAg-positive on at least two occasions, at least six months apart. Although the degree of infectivity correlates strongly with HBeAg positivity, any person who is positive for HBsAg also is potentially infectious. The likelihood of becoming a carrier varies inversely with the age at which infection occurs. During the perinatal period, HBV transmitted from HBeAg-positive mothers causes as many as 90% of infected infants to become carriers, whereas only 6% to 10% of acutely infected adults develop the carrier state.

## Diagnosis

Precise diagnosis relies on the use of serologic tests for the HBV antigens (HBsAg and HBeAg) and for antibodies to HBsAg, HBcAg, and HBeAg. Table 31-1 lists the common serologic patterns of HBV infection. Sensitive and specific techniques have

**Table 31-1.** Commonly Encountered Serologic Patterns of HBV Infection

| HBsAg | Anti-HBs | Anti-HBc | HBeAg | Anti-HBe | Interpretation |
|---|---|---|---|---|---|
| + | – | IgM | + | – | Acute HBV infection, high infectivity |
| + | – | IgG | + | – | Chronic HBV infection, high infectivity |
| + | – | IgG | – | + | Late-acute or chronic HBV infection, low infectivity |
| + | + | + | +/– | +/– | 1. HBsAg of one subtype and heterotypic anti-HBs (common)<br>2. Process of seroconversion from HBsAg to anti-HBs (rare) |
| – | – | IgM | +/– | +/– | 1. Acute HBV infection<br>2. Anti-HBc window |
| – | – | IgG | – | +/– | 1. Low-level HBsAg carrier<br>2. Remote past infection |
| – | + | IgG | – | +/– | Recovery from HBV infection |
| – | + | – | – | – | 1. Immunization with HBsAg (after vaccination)<br>2. Possible remote past infection<br>3. False-positive |

been developed to identify markers in serum of suspected cases. Knowing both the clinical presentation and the serologic pattern permits identification of the specific stage of HBV infection.

In most cases, the patient experiences a prodrome of symptoms that are gradual in onset. The disease may present as a flu-like syndrome, with fatigue, anorexia, nausea, and vomiting. Myalgia, malaise, headache, and pharyngitis also may occur. Approximately two weeks after these symptoms appear, jaundice may become clinically evident along with a low-grade fever.

Clinical manifestations parallel the severity of the disease. In 10% to 20% of patients, signs of hepatomegaly, splenomegaly, and lymphadenopathy may appear. Jaundice may persist for four to six weeks, while symptoms slowly resolve. A slow healing phase may last for as long as three months, but the overwhelming majority of patients eventually recover completely from hepatitis B infection. Approximately 5%, however, will become chronic carriers.

The chronic carrier state appears to be much more common among individuals who acquired the infection vertically and among patients infected while immunosuppressed.

## Treatment

Currently, no specific therapy exists for HBV infection, aside from supportive care.

## Prevention

Because they are frequently exposed to body fluids, health care workers should be considered at high risk and should receive hepatitis B vaccine. In the United States, approximately 15% of health care workers eventually contract HBV infection. The principal source of these infections is the asymptomatic hospital patient who gives no history of HBV exposure and has not been screened for it.

Current recommendations include screening all health care workers for serologic evidence of hepatitis B and immunizing those who are seronegative with hepatitis B vaccine. Both passive prophylaxis with hepatitis B immunoglobulin and active prophylaxis with hepatitis B vaccine are currently available. The vaccine is based on HBsAg, the surface antigen, and has been demonstrated to be safe and highly effective.

## Prevention of Perinatal Transmission

In the United States, an estimated 20,000 births occur to HBsAg-positive women each year, producing approximately 6000 infants who become chronic HBV carriers. In many populations, including the indigent, selective screening fails to identify one-half to two-thirds of infected mothers.

The Centers for Disease Control and Prevention (CDC) and the American College of Obstetricians and Gynecologists recommend that HBsAg screening be added to routine prenatal testing. Women who are at greatest risk for HBV infection who test negative should be counseled about vaccination. Liver function testing is recommended for women for test positive for HBsAg. Family members of HBsAg-positive women should be tested as well. The baby's health care provider should be notified about the mother's HBsAg-positive status, and the infant should receive hepatitis B immune globulin (HBIG) and HBV vaccine after birth. This practice makes it possible to treat newborns of infected women—and such treatment is 85% to 95% effective in preventing development of the HBV chronic carrier state.

Table 31-2 gives the CDC recommendations. Table 31-3 shows the schedule of HBV immunoprophylaxis recommended for preventing perinatal transmisssion. In addition, the CDC recommends universal vaccination of all infants born to HBsAg-negative mothers.

**Table 31-2.** Prevention of Perinatal HBV Infections

1. Routinely test all pregnant women for HBsAg during an early prenatal visit.
2. Administer appropriate doses of hepatitis B immune globulin (HBIG) and HBV vaccine to infants of mothers who are HBsAg-positive.
3. Administer HBsAg test on admission for patients not tested prior to delivery.
4. Do prenatal screening to identify and vaccinate household contacts and sex partners of HBsAg-positive women.

**Table 31-3.** Recommended Schedule of HBV Immunoprophylaxis to Prevent Perinatal Transmission

| Vaccine Dose and HBIG | Age |
|---|---|
| **Infants Born to Mothers Known to Be HBsAg-Positive** | |
| First | Birth (within 12 hours) |
| HBIG* | Birth (within 12 hours) |
| Second | 1 to 2 months |
| Third | 6 months |
| **Infants Born to Mothers Not Screened for HBsAg** | |
| First | Birth (within 12 hours) |
| HBIG* | If mother is HBsAg-positive, give 0.5 mL as soon as possible, and not later than 1 week after birth |
| Second | 1 to 2 months |
| Third | 6 to 18 months† |

* Give HBIG (0.5 mL) IM at a site different from that used for vaccine.
† Infants of HBsAg-positive mothers should be vaccinated at six months of age.
SOURCE: American Academy of Pediatrics. Hepatitis B. In: 1997 red book: report of the Committee on Infectious Diseases, 24th ed. Elk Grove, IL: American Academy of Pediatrics, 1997:258.

## SEQUELAE

Between 6% and 10% of young adults with HBV become carriers. Chronic active hepatitis develops in more than 25% of carriers and often progresses to cirrhosis. Furthermore, HBV carriers' risk of developing primary liver cancer is 12 to 300 times higher than that of other persons. An estimated 4000 people die of hepatitis B-related cirrhosis each year in the United States, and more than 800 die of hepatitis B-related liver cancer.

As noted previously, infants born to HBsAg-positive and HBeAg-positive mothers have a 70% to 90% chance of acquiring perinatal HBV infection, and 85% to 90% of infected infants will become chronic HBV carriers (as opposed to 6% to 10% of infected adults). Estimates are that more than 25% of these carriers will die of primary hepatocellular carcinoma or cirrhosis. Infants born to HBsAg-positive and HBeAg-negative mothers have a lower risk of acquiring perinatal infection. Such infants may develop acute disease, however, and fatal fulminant hepatitis has been reported in this group.

## Suggested Readings

ACOG Committee Opinion No. 111. Guidelines for hepatitis B virus screening and vaccination during pregnancy. Int J Gynaecol Obstet 1993;40:172–174.

Arevalo JA, Washington AE. Cost-effectiveness of prenatal screening and immunization for hepatitis B virus. JAMA 1988;259: 365–369.

Beasley RP, Wang LY, Lee GC, et al. Prevention of perinatally transmitted hepatitis B virus infections with hepatitis B immune globulin hepatitis B vaccine. Lancet 1983;2:1099–1102.

Centers for Disease Control and Prevention. Prevention of perinatal transmission of hepatitis B virus: prenatal screening for all pregnant women for hepatitis B surface antigen. MMWR 1988;37: 341–346.

Dienstag JL, Isselbacher KJ. Acute viral hepatitis. In: Fauci AS, Braunwald E, Isselbacher KJ, et al, eds. Harrison's principles of internal medicine. New York: McGraw-Hill, 1998:1677–1692.

Immunization Practices Advisory Committee (ACIP). Hepatitis B virus: a comprehensive strategy for eliminating transmission in the United States through universal childhood vaccination. MMWR 1991;40(RR-13):1–25.

Immunization Practices Advisory Committee (ACIP). Protection against viral hepatitis. MMWR 1990;39(RR-2):1–26.

Jonas MM, Reddy RK, DeMedina M, et al. Hepatitis B infection in a large municipal obstetrical population: characterization and prevention of perinatal transmission. Am J Gastroenterol 1990;85: 277–280.

Jonas MM, Schiff ER, O'Sullivan MJ, et al. Failure of Centers for Disease Control criteria to identify hepatitis B infection in a large municipal obstetrical population. Ann Intern Med 1987; 107:335–337.

Koretz R. Universal perinatal hepatitis B testing: is it cost-effective? Obstet Gynecol 1989;74:808–814.

Petermann S, Ernest JM. Intrapartum hepatitis B screening. Am J Obstet Gynecol 1995;173;369–373.

Summers PR, Biswas MJ, Pastorek JG II, et al. The pregnant hepatitis B carrier: evidence favoring comprehensive antepartum screening. Obstet Gynecol 1987;69:701–704.

CHAPTER

# 32

# *Hepatitis C, D, and E in Pregnancy*

*D. Heather Watts*

## HEPATITIS C

### Background

An estimated 4 million people in the United States are infected with hepatitis C virus (HCV), and 30,000 acute new infections are acquired annually. Only 25% to 30% of these acute infections are recognized in carriers, however. HCV accounts for 20% of all cases of acute hepatitis in the United States. Evidence of infection is present in 3.2% of African Americans, 2.1% of Mexican Americans, and 1.5% of non-Hispanic whites.

The seroprevalence of antibodies to HCV among pregnant women varies by region and by testing basis. Among predominantly high-risk populations of pregnant women studied in the United States, seroprevalence has ranged from 2.3% to 4.6%. In contrast, population-based studies in Europe and the Caribbean have yielded seroprevalence rates of about 1.3% (range 0% to 4.5%) and in Asia of 0.7% (range 0.09% to 1.3%). Studies indicate that as few as 10% and as many as 65% of pregnant women with hepatitis C antibodies have a history of injection drug use, previous blood transfusion, or other identified risk factors. When tested, from 15% to 64% of antibody-positive women show elevated transaminase levels.

Risk factors for HCV infection include blood transfusion performed prior to 1990, injection drug use, employment in the health care industry, and sexual or household exposure to an infected individual. Since the advent of screening tests for

HCV, the risk of acquisition from donated blood has declined to approximately 1 per 100,000 units, although recipients of blood transfusion before 1990 remain at risk. Injection drug use accounts for half of new infections and at least half of chronic infections. From 50% to 80% of new injection drug users will test positive for HCV antibody within 6 to 12 months.

Other risk factors present in the majority of HCV-positive patients include occupational blood exposure, hemodialysis, multiple sexual partners, history of sexually transmitted diseases (STDs), or use of noninjection illegal drugs. The absolute risk of sexual transmission is unknown but appears to be 5% or less, according to studies of monogamous discordant couples. Multiple partners and concurrent STDs appear to increase the risk of infection. Household transmission appears to be rare. Approximately 10% of individuals who have HCV infection have no identified risk factor.

## Etiology

HCV is an RNA virus of the Flaviviridae family. Individual isolates consist of heterogeneous—but closely related—populations of viral genomes (quasi-species). The genetic diversity of individual infections enables HCV to escape the host's immune surveillance, leading to frequent chronic infection.

The natural history of HCV infection varies according to viral characteristics, geography, alcohol use, coinfections with other viruses such as human immunodeficiency virus (HIV), and other factors. From 65% to 75% of patients who have acute HCV infection are asymptomatic, with the rest developing malaise, weakness, anorexia, and icterus. HCV RNA can be detected in the blood within one to three weeks after exposure, with evidence of liver injury (elevated serum alanine aminotransferase) becoming apparent at an average of 50 days (range 15 to 150 days). Fulminant liver failure with acute HCV infection is rare. Antibodies to HCV can be detected in 50% to 70% of symptomatic patients and in 90% of patients by three months after infection. In 15% of cases, HCV infection is self-limited, with HCV RNA eventually disappearing and liver enzymes becoming normalized.

Eighty-five percent of infected persons develop chronic hepatitis with viremia that persists for more than six months after infection. Both viral levels in the blood and transanimase levels may fluctuate widely in chronic infection. One-third of all individuals with chronic infection may have persistently normal transaminase levels. Most patients who have chronic HCV infection remain asymptomatic for at least 20 years after infection. As many as 20% of them, however, may complain of nonspecific symptoms such as intermittent fatigue or malaise. Less common manifestations of chronic HCV believed to be of immunologic origin include arthritis, keratoconjunctivitis sicca, lichen planus, glomerulonephritis, and mixed cryoglobulinemia.

Chronic infection and inflammation of the liver may lead to fibrosis. Severe fibrosis and necroinflammatory changes on biopsy predict progression to cirrhosis with potential liver failure or portal hypertension. The relationship between serum transaminase levels and degree of histologic inflammation is inconsistent. Chronic HCV infection leads to cirrhosis in at least 20% of patients by 20 years after infection, and cirrhosis increases the risk of hepatocellular carcinoma. The risk of hepatocellular carcinoma appears to be 1% to 5% after 20 years of HCV infection, but rises to 1% to 4% per year if cirrhosis is present.

## Perinatal Transmission

In 12 studies that evaluated the risk of transmission of HCV from HCV-seropositive pregnant women to their infants, the risk identified ranged from zero to 20%, with transmission to 32 (6.9%) of 461 infants. As a proportion of these women may have been seropositive but not viremic, subsequent studies compared the rate of transmission among women with HCV detectable by RNA polymerase chain reaction (PCR) testing during pregnancy with that of women without detectable virus. Transmission occurred among 45 (19%) of 240 women with detectable HCV, compared with 1 (0.9%) of 115 women without detectable HCV. Transmission seemed to correlate with the level of maternal viremia, with the highest risk of transmission occurring among women with a viral load exceeding $5 \times 10^6$ copies/mL. Maternal HIV seropositivity also increased the risk of perinatal transmission of HCV in most studies, and HCV positivity may, in turn, increase the risk of perinatal transmission of HIV (see Chapter 42).

Breast feeding rarely transmits HCV, and current U.S. Public Health Service recommendations do not advise that HCV-positive women should avoid breast feeding. In five studies, HCV RNA was detected in 5 (5%) of 104 breast milk specimens tested, with all five positive specimens found in a single study. Perinatal transmission occurred in only 2 (1.7%) of 119 infants who were breast-fed, despite the high proportion of HCV RNA-positive women participating in these studies. Both infants who acquired infection were breast-fed for at least eight months.

No immunization or immunoglobulin preparation is currently available to prevent perinatal transmission of HCV. Furthermore, no data indicate that cesarean section helps to prevent perinatal transmission of HCV. Routine screening of pregnant women for HCV antibody or RNA is not recommended. If a pregnant patient is HCV-seropositive, it appears prudent to avoid procedures that may introduce maternal blood into the fetal circulation. Avoid amniocentesis, fetal scalp electrodes, and instrumental delivery whenever possible.

Passively acquired maternal antibody may persist in the infant for as long as 12 months after birth; therefore, test an exposed infant for HCV antibody after the baby's first birthday. HCV RNA PCR may be used to determine infant infection status at an earlier age, if indicated. Although the natural history of perinatal HCV infection has not been well described, a single study with an average of 65 months (range 26 to 90 months) of follow-up of seven children suggests that viremia persists for years, although physical examination, growth, bilirubin, and immunoglobulin levels were normal in all seven of these subjects. The five children who underwent liver biopsy all showed some degree of chronic persistent hepatitis. Longer follow-up will be necessary to delineate the possible long-term risks of cirrhosis and hepatocellular carcinoma among those with perinatal infection with HCV.

## Diagnosis

Antibodies to HCV can be detected by enzyme immunoassay (EIA) or recombinant immunoblot assay (RIBA). HCV RNA can be detected in serum using PCR-based assays. As no reliable tests are readily available for detection of HCV antigens in the liver, use biopsy to evaluate the extent of liver injury but not to diagnose HCV infection. EIA tests are suitable for screening both low- and high-prevalence populations and for evaluating patients with liver disease. The sensitivity of second-generation EIA tests is 92% to 95%. If the results of the EIA test are negative, HCV infection is unlikely. If the EIA is positive and supplementary RIBA is positive, past or current HCV infection is likely.

To confirm and assess current disease activity, perform HCV RNA PCR and liver function testing. HCV RNA PCR also may prove helpful if the RIBA gives inconclusive results. If treatment for HCV is considered, liver biopsy is recommended to assess the grade and stage of disease and to evaluate for other forms of liver disease.

## Treatment

To date, only interferon-α and ribavirin have shown antiviral activity against HCV, but neither is recommended during pregnancy. Treatment with interferon-α, consisting of 3 million units given subcutaneously three times weekly for six months, normalized transaminase levels at the end of treatment in 40% to 50% of patients; these levels were sustained six months later in 15% to 20% of these women. Virologic response was 30% to 40% at the end of treatment and 10% to 20% six months later. Some 20% to 30% of patients who received 12 months of treatment maintained normal transaminase levels six months after therapy ended. If the patient's transaminase levels remain elevated and HCV RNA persists after three months of treatment, stop therapy because later response is unlikely.

Side effects with interferon therapy are common and may be severe. One case of delivery of a normal newborn after inadvertent interferon therapy during pregnancy has been reported. Because liver disease may worsen during therapy, stop interferon treatment if a patient's transaminase levels double. Combination therapy with interferon-α and ribavirin may increase the rate of sustained virologic response, although use of ribavirin for treatment of HCV infection remains at an investigational stage only. Currently, treatment is recommended for HCV-infected patients who have persistently elevated transaminases, positive HCV RNA, liver biopsy with portal or bridging fibrosis, and at least moderate inflammation and necrosis. Treatment of patients with normal transaminase levels is not recommended.

### Prevention

Screening of blood and blood products and heat treatment of clotting factors have minimized the risk of transfusion-related HCV infection. Adherence to recommendations for universal precautions for blood and body substance isolation should prevent transmission of HCV between patients and health care workers. Encourage safer sexual practices, including use of latex condoms, for women with multiple sexual partners. Inform HCV-positive women and their partners of the potential risk of sexual transmission, even though data are currently insufficient to recommend routine condom use or other changes in sexual practices in monogamous discordant couples. Although HCV-positive persons should not share razors or toothbrushes with others, other household activities need not be changed. The risk of perinatal transmission appears low, but no specific treatments are currently available to lower the risk other than avoiding exposure of the fetus and infant to maternal blood as much as possible. Breast feeding by HCV-positive women is considered safe.

## HEPATITIS D

### Background

Hepatitis D (delta hepatitis) virus (HDV) is a defective RNA virus that uses hepatitis B surface antigen (HBsAg) for its protein shell. HDV infection can occur only in patients who have HBsAg in their serum from either acute or chronic hepatitis B virus (HBV) infection. In the United States, HDV infection usually affects injection drug users, hemophiliacs, and other patients who have had multiple transfusions, but not male homosexuals or health care workers. HDV also is common in some areas with a high prevalence of HBV carriers, including South America, Central Africa, southern Italy, and the Middle East, but not China or Southeast Asia.

## Etiology

HDV infection can occur as a coinfection with acute HBV infection or as a superinfection to an established chronic HBV infection. With coinfection, HDV infection resolves with clearance of hepatitis B surface antigenemia, and fewer than 5% of patients develop chronic HDV infection because of persistent HBV infection. With superinfection, 70% of patients develop chronic HDV infection because of the persistent HBV infection. Acute hepatitis from HDV tends to be severe, with a mortality rate of 2% to 20%. Chronic infection leads to cirrhosis in 60% to 70% of patients. Progression to cirrhosis usually occurs in 10 to 15 years, but can occur as quickly as 2 years.

## Perinatal Issues

Given that concomitant infection with HBV is required for HDV infection, measures that prevent perinatal transmission of HBV should prevent perinatal transmission of HDV. In one study of 54 pregnant women who were HBsAg-positive, none was positive for HDV infection.

## Diagnosis

HDV infection should be considered in any HBsAg-positive patient who has acute or chronic hepatitis, especially if she experiences severe symptoms, is an injection drug user, or has received multiple blood products. Reliable tests for HDV antigen in the serum are not readily available; thus the diagnosis depends on detection of antibody to HDV in the serum or detection of HDV antigen or RNA in the liver. The diagnosis of acute HDV infection may require testing of acute and convalescent sera, as production of antibody to HDV may be delayed and of low titer. Rising titers of anti-HDV antibody indicate acute infection, whereas stable high titers suggest chronic infection.

## Treatment

Because no cure exists for this infection, treatment of symptomatic HDV infection is supportive.

## Prevention

Immunization and, when indicated, passive immunoprophylaxis with immune globulin are the primary means of preventing HDV infection.

# HEPATITIS E

## Background

Hepatitis E virus (HEV) is a recently described small RNA virus found in the stools of patients during the incubation period and early acute illness with endemic enteric hepatitis. HEV appears to be transmitted by the fecal-oral route, similar to hepatitis A virus (HAV). The former infection affects young adults who have preexisting immunity to HAV. Both outbreaks and sporadic cases occur in developing countries, but such cases have not been documented in the United States, except among travelers returning from endemic areas.

## Etiology

HEV infection usually causes an acute self-limited disease with lower transaminase levels than are seen in other cases of acute viral hepatitis. Outbreaks usually occur in young adults rather than in children, as is the case with HAV infection. HEV infection does not lead to chronic infection or a carrier state, although the duration of protective immunity after infection remains unknown. HEV infection often appears to be more fulminant among pregnant women, and these patients have a higher mortality rate as well. In a large study of fulminant hepatitis in India, HEV was implicated as the cause in 62% of patients. One-fourth of the female patients with fulminant hepatitis were pregnant, suggesting pregnancy as a contributing factor. Care of patients with fulminant HEV hepatitis is supportive, as for other forms of viral hepatitis.

## Perinatal Issues

The primary concern with HEV in pregnancy is the apparent increased risk of fulminant hepatitis and death. In endemic areas, this type of infection has been noted to be a more frequent cause of fulminant hepatic failure than acute fatty liver of pregnancy. The risk of perinatal transmission of HEV has not been well studied, however. The risk of vertical transmission was hypothesized to be low because no chronic carrier state occurs.

Nevertheless, one study of eight infants born to women with acute HEV infection during the third trimester found evidence of HEV infection in six infants. Two infants developed hypothermia and hypoglycemia in the neonatal period and died within 24 hours; one had massive hepatic necrosis; another had icteric hepatitis; and four others had anicteric hepatitis. Although further study is required, it appears that transmission of HEV with infection may occur near delivery. No vaccine or immunoprophylaxis is currently available.

## Diagnosis

HEV can be demonstrated by immunoelectron microscopy in the stools of patients during incubation or early infection. Antibody to HEV can be detected by immunoelectron microscopy and enzyme immunoassay. These tests are primarily available and of value for research purposes.

## Treatment

Treatment of symptomatic HEV is supportive.

## Prevention

Prevention currently focuses on provision of sanitary water, because most outbreaks are related to fecal contamination of the water supply. Ultimate prevention will require development of a vaccine.

## Suggested Readings

## Hepatitis C

Hershow RC, Riester KA, Lew J, et al. Increased vertical transmission of human immunodeficiency virus from hepatitis C virus—coinfected mothers. J Infect Dis 1997;176:414–420.

Hunt CM, Carson KL, Sharara AI. Hepatitis C in pregnancy. Obstet Gynecol 1997;89:883–890.

NIH Consensus Statement Online. (http://odp.od.nih.gov/consensus/statements/cdc/105/105abstr.pdf). Management of hepatitis C. NIH Consensus Development Conference, March 24–26, 1997. Natcher Conference Center, National Institutes of Health, Bethesda, MD.

Palomba E, Manzini P, Fiammengo P, et al. Natural history of perinatal hepatitis C virus infection. Clin Infect Dis 1996;23:47–50.

## Hepatitis D

Jonas MM, Reddy RK, DeMedina M, et al. Hepatitis B infection in a large municipal obstetrical population: characterization and prevention of perinatal transmission. Am J Gastroenterol 1990;85:277–280.

Simms J, Duff P. Viral hepatitis in pregnancy. Semin Perinatol 1993; 17:384–393.

## Hepatitis E

Acharya SK, Dasarathy S, Kumer TL, et al. Fulminant hepatitis in a tropical population: clinical course, cause, and early predictors of outcome. Hepatology 1996;23:1448–1455.

Khuroo MS, Kamili S, Jameel S. Vertical transmission of hepatitis E virus. Lancet 1995;245:1025–1026.

Nanda SK, Yalcinkaya K, Paingrabi AK, et al. Etiologic role of hepatitis E virus in sporadic fulminant hepatitis. J Med Virol 1994;42:133–137.

CHAPTER

# 33

# *Toxoplasmosis in Pregnancy*

*John L. Sever*

## BACKGROUND AND INCIDENCE

Studies of pregnant women in the United States have indicated that approximately 15% to 30% have antibodies to *Toxoplasma gondii* and thus have experienced infection with this organism. Prospective investigations show that the rate of primary infection during pregnancy is approximately 1 in 500 to 1000. Almost all of these infections are asymptomatic.

Among the children of mothers who have experienced a primary infection during pregnancy, about 10% show later evidence of damage, including lower than normal IQ and deafness. In addition, severe congenital toxoplasmosis is apparent at birth in approximately 1 of every 10,000 births.

Chemotherapy is available for *T. gondii*, as are tests for antibody responses and detection of the organism by polymerase chain reaction (PCR) or culture. Unfortunately, the commercial laboratory data frequently do not enable the physician to distinguish a primary infection during pregnancy from a prior infection. In July 1997, the FDA issued a public health advisory concerning limitations of *Toxoplasma* IgM commercial test kits. Awareness of these limitations is extremely important because a primary infection—particularly early in pregnancy—can result in fetal infection and damage, whereas a prior infection is important only if the mother is severely immunocompromised.

# Diagnosis

## Mother

As noted earlier, the great majority of women infected with *T. gondii* are asymptomatic. In one prospective study, the author had the opportunity to examine five women who had documented infection. Only one showed any signs or symptoms possibly related to the infection, and these consisted of mild bilateral occipital lympadenopathy. Occasionally, women with primary infection experience a "monolike" illness or, rarely, *Toxoplasma* infection of the eye with visual impairment.

Tests of IgG antibody are readily available from many laboratories. The fact that 15% to 30% of women have IgG antibody, however, limits the use of this test to documenting past infection or identifying an acute infection by demonstrating a seroconversion. In the United States, 1 in 500 to 1000 women seroconverts during pregnancy. To document the time of these seroconversions, it would be necessary to perform serial antibody tests on antibody-negative women. Unfortunately, in addition to the low rate of seroconversion, standard laboratory tests may be unreliable, making it difficult to use IgG data with any confidence.

Although IgM antibody appears at the time of infection, it may persist at a high titer for several years. Thus its presence does not necessarily indicate recent or current primary infection. Although its absence may help exclude the diagnosis, it must be remembered that IgM antibody may disappear in six months in some patients or may persist for a number of years in other patients.

Problems with reliability and interpretation of IgG and IgM results make these tests difficult to apply clinically. Until improved methods become available, tests should be limited to patients who have clinical symptoms suggesting the diagnosis. The presence of IgG and IgM antibody would then be consistent with a diagnosis of toxoplasmosis.

For special "high-risk" patients, such as individuals with many cats, serial IgG determinations can be performed every one to two months on antibody-negative patients. If a seroconversion occurs, the patient can be treated or counseled.

This approach requires the services of a reliable laboratory for testing specimens. With many laboratories, however, reliability remains a problem.

For patients who may have experienced an infection during pregnancy as indicated by clinical findings, a seroconversion, or high IgG and IgM titers, more specific testing can be obtained from the Toxoplasma Serology Laboratory, directed by Dr. Jack S. Remington at the Palo Alto Medical Foundation, Palo Alto, California [telephone: (415) 853-4828; fax: (415) 614-3292]. That laboratory provides a panel of special tests (for a fee) and a consultation that can aid in documenting recent or current infection. Tests include the Sabin-Feldman dye test for detection of IgG antibodies, IgM ELISA, IgM ISAGA, IgA ELISA, IgE, and AC/HS. If these tests are highly positive, the results are considered strong evidence that infection has occurred recently.

If a woman has serologic evidence of a recent infection, amniotic fluid can be obtained at 18 weeks' gestation or later and sent to the Palo Alto laboratory for determination of in utero infection by the PCR method. Isolation studies are also available to detect viable *Toxoplasma* organisms; these tests require six weeks for completion, however, and have therefore been replaced by PCR tests for most clinical studies.

## Child

Children infected in utero with *T. gondii* may have severe brain damage, hydrocephaly, microcephaly, chorioretinitis, deafness, and other abnormalities. Studies from France have shown that transmission of infection to the fetus is lower in the first trimester (15%) than in the third trimester (60%), but that infection of the fetus early in pregnancy is more likely to cause fetal death or damage.

Laboratory studies from France of fetal blood and amniotic fluid indicate that toxoplasmal organisms can be isolated by mouse inoculation from blood samples of most infected fetuses. In addition, a panel of enzymatic and hematologic laboratory tests, such as a platelet count, run on fetal blood reveals some abnormalities in most infected children. Likewise, ultrasound can detect evidence of some in utero infections. IgM tests of fetal blood are positive only after 22 weeks' gestation and, even then, only 10% to 20% of infected fetuses demonstrate specific IgM antibody. As already noted, PCR tests can be used to detect gene sequences of *T. gondii* in amniotic fluid from proven cases of congenital infection. This approach offers the advantages of speed, sensitivity, and ease of transport of specimens.

## TREATMENT

If a pregnant patient is diagnosed as having acute toxoplasmosis because she exhibits symptoms plus IgM-specific antibody or a seroconversion, treat her with 25 mg of oral pyrimethamine daily plus 1 g of oral sulfadiazine four times daily for 28 days, followed by one-half the dose of each drug for an additional 28 days. In addition, give 6 mg of folinic acid IM or orally three times weekly. If the mother has severe, symptomatic toxoplasmosis, you may have to continue therapy for several months. Note that some groups in France and the United States recommend beginning treatment with spiramycin based on maternal serology and adding pyrimethamine and sulfadiazine if PCR of amniotic fluid confirms infection. Spiramycin is available in the United States only from the FDA following positive results on tests performed at the Toxoplasma Serology Laboratory in Palo Alto, California (cited earlier).

In general, pyrimethamine should not be administered in the first trimester because of possible teratogenic effects associated with the drug. In addition, it is good practice to discontinue sulfadiazine in the last weeks of pregnancy.

A few reports have described pregnant patients who had malignancies, had immunosuppressive diseases, or were receiving immunosuppressive chemotherapy and who had had prior *T. gondii* infection that became reactivated during pregnancy and was transmitted to the infant. Fortunately, these occurrences have been rare. *Toxoplasma* infections of the central nervous system or eyes of immunosuppressed patients can be identified via PCR tests.

## Prevention

Toxoplasmosis is acquired by eating infected raw meat or unpasteurized goat's milk or by exposure to a *T. gondii* oocyst excreted in the feces of infected cats. Instruct pregnant women not to eat raw meat or drink unpasteurized milk. If cats are in the environment, the woman should avoid exposure to the feces, litter, or soil where feces may be present. Another family member should discard litter on a daily basis and clean the box by wiping it with household bleach diluted with 10 parts of water.

### Suggested Readings

Bader TJ, Macones GA, Asch DA. Prenatal screening for toxoplasmosis. Obstet Gynecol 1997;90:457–464.

Daffos F, Forestier F, Capella-Pavlovsky M, et al. Prenatal management of 746 pregnancies at risk for congenital toxoplasmosis. N Engl J Med 1988;318:271–275.

Grover CM, Thulliez P, Remington JS, et al. Rapid prenatal diagnosis of congenital *Toxoplasma* infection by using polymerase chain reaction and amniotic fluid. J Clin Microbiol 1990;28:2297–2301.

Remington JS, McLeod R, Desmonts G. Toxoplasmosis. In: Remington JS, Klein JO, eds. Infectious diseases of the fetus and newborn infant, 4th ed. Philadelphia: W. B. Saunders Company, 1994.

Sever JL, Ellenberg JH, Ley AC, et al. Toxoplasmosis: maternal and pediatric findings in 23,000 pregnancies. Pediatrics 1988;82:181–192.

Sever JL, Larsen JW, Grossman JH. Handbook of perinatal infections. Boston: Little, Brown, 1989:160–167.

CHAPTER

# 34

# *Parasitic Infections in Pregnancy*

*Nancy L. Eriksen*

## Background

Parasitic infections are most prevalent in tropical and underdeveloped areas. Although the incidence of parasitic diseases remains low in the United States, foreign travel increases an individual's susceptibility to these organisms. The influx of immigrants from Central and South America as well as from Southeast Asia in recent years has also led to a much higher U.S. prevalence of these infections. Women taking immunosuppressive drugs and patients with AIDS are at increased risk of infections caused by parasites.

Little information is available about the effects of various human parasites on pregnancy or the effects of pregnancy on parasitic infections. This protocol focuses on parasitic infections common in North America, presenting them in the order of their frequency and describing antiparasitic drugs considered safe in pregnancy (Table 34-1).

## Giardiasis

*Giardia lamblia*, the most commonly detected intestinal parasite in the United States, is found in 3% to 9% of all stool specimens. Associated with contaminated food and water, this endemic infection affects the gastrointestinal tract. Most epidemics have a waterborne origin. The vast majority of patients affected will be asymptomatic or have only mild diarrhea; they generally require no therapy. The most common symptoms are

**Table 34-1.** Therapy for Parasitic Infection in Pregnancy

| Infection | Organism | Route of Infection | Pregnancy Effects | Drug of Choice (FDA Class) | Alternative Drug |
|---|---|---|---|---|---|
| Giardiasis | *Giardia lamblia* | Fecal–oral | Secondary to maternal disease | Paromomycin, 30 mg/kg/day in 3 doses × 5–10 days (B) | Metronidazole, 250 mg t.i.d. × 5 days (B) |
| Pinworms | *Enterobius vermicularis* | Autoinoculation | None known | Pyrantel, 11 mg/kg once up to 1 g dosage, then repeat in 2 weeks | |
| Hookworm | *Ancylostoma duodenale* *Necator americanus* | Skin penetration of larvae from soil | Secondary to maternal anemia | Iron; for severe infections, pyrantel, 11 mg/kg × 3 days (C) | |
| Amebiasis | *Entamoeba histolytica* | Fecal–oral | Secondary to maternal disease | Paromomycin, 30 mg/kg/day in 3 doses × 7 days for moderate infection; metronidazole, 750 mg t.i.d. × 10 days followed by paromomycin for severe infection (B) | For severe infection, dehydroemetine, 1.5 mg/kg/day × 5 days |
| Malaria | *Plasmodium ovale* *P. vivax* Nonresistant *P. falciparum* | Anopheline mosquito | Secondary to maternal disease | Chloroquine, 1 g; then 500 mg at 6, 24, and 48 hours; then weekly until after delivery; reserve primaquine until postpartum | |
| | Chloroquine-resistant *P. falciparum* | | | Quinine, 650 mg t.i.d. × 3–7 days plus sulfadoxine/pyrimethamine, 3 tablets once on day 3 of treatment | |

watery, bulky diarrhea, abdominal pain, flatulence, nausea, weight loss, and malaise. Patients with severe diarrhea and weight loss should be treated; those who are left untreated are at risk for hypokalemia, ketosis, and malnutrition.

Giardiasis can be diagnosed early in its course by looking for trophozoites in the stool specimen. During later stages of the disease, the stool is more formed and contains the cyst form of the organism, which requires concentration techniques to make the diagnosis.

In general, giardiasis has minimal adverse effects on pregnancy outcome unless substantial malabsorption occurs. No cases of transmission of *G. lamblia* to the placenta or to the fetus have been reported. The therapy of choice is paromomycin, 30 mg/kg/day in three divided doses for 5 to 10 days. Because this aminoglycoside is poorly absorbed from the gastrointestinal tract, fecal concentration is high and the therapy has little or no effect on the mother or fetus. This drug is a better choice in pregnancy than the usual drug of choice, quinacrine, 100 mg/day for 5 days. Quinacrine is an FDA class C drug in pregnancy, which means that teratogenic risk cannot be ruled out. An alternative treatment relies on metronidazole, a class B drug, which should be limited to the last two trimesters of pregnancy at a dosage of 250 mg three times daily for 5 days.

## Enterobiasis

*Enterobius vermicularis*, the pinworm, rarely causes symptoms leading to illness. Nevertheless, it can cause intense anal and perianal itching, particularly at night, that can be disabling. The disease is transmitted through autoinoculation, especially with the hand. Ridding the patient's body, family members, and clothing of eggs, larvae, and adult worms can prove difficult. Other than the rare anecdotal case of pinworm salpingitis (with worms actually seen protruding from the fimbriated end of the tube), no gynecologic or obstetric complications are known. Pinworm infection should not be treated during pregnancy unless the woman is incapacitated by itching or is very concerned about the presence of worms. This diagnosis can be confirmed by demonstrating pinworms on adhesive tape, which is applied to the perianal region first thing in the morning.

If treatment is elected, administer pyrantel pamoate in a single dose of 10 mg (base)/kg (maximum dose 1 g of pyrantel base) after the first trimester; repeat this dose two weeks later. The patient's entire family should be treated, and their clothing and bedding should be washed in hot water or chlorine bleach to avoid reinfection by viable eggs. Avoid giving mebendazole and thiabendazole during pregnancy; these agents were associated with teratogenesis in animal studies.

## Hookworm Infection

Hookworm infection was once most commonly seen in the southern United States, where it is still endemic. A series of prevalence studies has also shown that various hookworms are the most common parasites in the stool of Southeast Asian refugees. Infection occurs when the larvae in fecally contaminated soil penetrate the skin of the feet. The larvae migrate throughout the venous system to the lungs, then up to the pharynx, and are swallowed. The most common result of infestation with *Ancylostoma duodenale* or *Necator americanus* is anemia from blood loss in the gastrointestinal tract caused by the adult worms. A single worm consumes 0.2 mL of blood per day. After it detaches, the old wound continues to bleed, adding to the blood loss. The diagnosis depends upon the demonstration of eggs in the fecal smears.

Other than anemia, these parasites do not have any effects on the placenta or fetus. The mainstay of therapy for the intestinal hookworm is iron, with oral iron supplements usually being sufficient treatment for the infected pregnant woman. Heavy infestations that do not respond well to iron should be treated with pyrantel, 11 mg/kg (up to 1 g per day) for three days.

## Amebiasis

Infection with *Entamoeba histolytica* is generally uncommon in the United States. Those affected tend to be new immigrants;

in fact, approximately 10% of immigrants have stool specimens that test positive for this parasite. Infection is acquired by ingesting the cyst form of *E. histolytica* in fecally contaminated food or water.

Although most infected individuals remain asymptomatic, 10% to 50% of patients may present with symptoms of colicky lower abdominal pain and altered bowel habits or loose stool with mucus and/or blood present. As the disease progresses, the patient may have frequent bloody diarrhea and develop intestinal ulcerations. The presence of *E. histolytica* in stool indicates amebiasis. Fresh stool specimens must be examined, and sigmoidoscopy may be helpful in making the diagnosis.

A later stage of infestation is amebic liver abscess. In one case, administering corticosteroids—a treatment for "chronic colitis" (due to amebiasis)—hastened the development of liver abscess.

*E. histolytica* is not transmitted across the placenta. Instead, the effect of this parasitic infection on pregnancy is indirect —it is secondary to chronic diarrhea, anemia, and weight loss. Pregnant women should be treated. The first choice of therapy for asymptomatic to moderately severe amebiasis is paromomycin, 30 mg/kg/day in three divided doses for seven days.

Metronidazole, an alternative that is administered as 750 mg three times per day for 10 days, should be prescribed for patients with severe intestinal disease and for hepatic abscess. Follow metronidazole therapy with paromomycin to eradicate the intraluminal cysts. The alternative for severe disease is dehydroemetine, 1.5 mg/kg/day (maximum 90 mg/day) for five days; this drug can be obtained only from the Centers for Disease Control and Prevention (770-639-3670). Patients receiving dehydroemetine should be monitored in the hospital, as the drug has marked cardiotoxicity. No information is available about its use in pregnancy. Other recommended alternative drugs include iodoquinol and emetine.

## MALARIA

Malaria, an uncommon problem in pregnancy, generally appears as relapse in immigrants or in U.S. residents who have traveled to endemic areas. The majority of cases are caused by four species of the parasite *Plasmodium* (*P. falciparum*, *P. vivax*, *P. malariae*, and *P. ovale*). Malaria is transmitted by the bite of an infected female anopheline mosquito. (Besides the mosquito vector, malaria may be transmitted by transfusion of blood products and sharing of syringes and needles among drug abusers.) After the sporozoites are inoculated by the mosquito, they migrate to the liver, where they invade the hepatic cells. In the liver, the sporozoites are transformed into merozoites. After approximately two weeks, they are released, enter the bloodstream, and invade erythrocytes. Through asexual reproduction, 24 to 32 merozoites are produced within 49 to 72 hours. Rupture of these merozoites into the bloodstream allows them to rapidly attach and invade new red blood cells.

Clinical presentation of malaria includes high fever, chills, abdominal pain, nausea, vomiting, and delirium. Early on, these fevers may be erratic, but they eventually develop a synchronous periodicity related to timing of schizogony. The patient often feels well between the periods of chills and fever. Malaria patients also demonstrate a normochromic, normocytic, hemolytic anemia and thrombocytopenia. The diagnosis of malaria requires demonstrating the *Plasmodium* parasites in stained peripheral blood smears obtained from patients.

The primary effects on the fetus are usually secondary to the severity of the anemia and nutritional status of the mother. Severe illness leads to excess pregnancy wastage and intrauterine growth retardation. In endemic areas, parasitic malaria illnesses strike more pregnant women than nonpregnant women. In one study of malaria in West Africa, even though 40% of the mothers and 16% of placentas were parasitized, no organisms were found in cord blood. On the other hand, congenital malaria is documented in 1% to 4% of nonimmune, infected mothers. In women with HIV infection, breakthrough parasitic and umbilical cord blood infection is more common than in women who are HIV-negative.

Therapy for non–chloroquine-resistant malaria of all types in pregnant women is chloroquine, 1 g, followed by 500 mg at 6, 24, and 48 hours. This dosage should be continued on a once-weekly basis for *P. vivax* and *P. ovale* disease until after delivery. Definitive care of the tissue forms of these organisms is accomplished with primaquine, one tablet (15 mg base) daily for 14 days postpartum.

Patients receiving primaquine should first be screened for glucose-6-phosphate dehydrogenase (G6PD) deficiency. Primaquine should not be administered to pregnant patients because the drug may cross the placenta and cause hemolytic anemia in a G6PD-deficient fetus. Treatment of resistant *P. falciparum* malaria is accomplished with quinine, 650 mg three times daily for three to seven days, plus pyrimethamine/sulfadoxine, three tablets at once on day 3 of treatment. Be careful when using sulfadoxine close to delivery. Also, note that quinine can stimulate uterine contractions and may provoke abortion if given in high doses; it has nevertheless been used successfully to treat seriously ill women in the third trimester.

The CDC has recently reviewed data on the management of life-threatening infectious *P. falciparum* malaria and concluded that the drug of choice in the United States for treatment is parenteral quinine gluconate. Because of this decision, parenteral quinine dihydrochloride is no longer available from the CDC drug service; however, it is available by prescription.

## Prophylaxis in Pregnancy

The most common question about malaria that arises in this country is whether to administer prophylaxis for pregnant women traveling to endemic areas. Information about malaria prophylaxis and treatment is available from the CDC's Division of Parasitic Diseases, National Center for Infectious Diseases, by telephone (770-488-7760) from 8 A.M. to 4:30 P.M., Eastern Time, Monday through Friday (404-639-2888 during other hours and on weekends). The automated information service (404-332-4565) will fax documents containing information about general aspects of malaria, malaria in pregnant women and children, and prescription drugs used for malaria. International travel information is available on the World Wide Web at http://www.cdc.gov/travel/travel.htm.

Malaria infection can be more severe in pregnant patients than in nonpregnant women. For these reasons, and because chloroquine does not appear to harm the fetus when used in doses recommended for malaria prophylaxis, pregnancy is not a contraindication for prophylaxis with chloroquine or hydrochloroquine. In areas free of chloroquine-resistant malaria, a satisfactory therapy is 500 mg of chloroquine salt (300 mg base) weekly beginning one week before and continuing until four weeks after the pregnant woman's return.

Women pregnant or likely to become so should avoid travel to areas with chloroquine-resistant *P. falciparum,* because alternative drugs such as mefloquine, doxycycline, and primaquine should not be used during pregnancy. Women with child-bearing potential who are taking mefloquine for malaria prophylaxis should use reliable contraception until two months after the last dose of mefloquine is taken. Adverse fetal effects of doxycycline and other tetracyclines include discoloration and dysplasia of the teeth and inhibition of bone growth. Use of tetracycline is indicated in pregnancy only to treat life-threatening infections due to multidrug-resistant *P. falciparum.* Primaquine may be passed transplacentally to a G6PD-deficient fetus and cause hemolytic anemia. Whenever radical cure or terminal prophylaxis with primaquine is indicated during pregnancy, chloroquine should be given once a week until delivery, when the decision to give primaquine can be made.

To summarize, in common areas where chloroquine-sensitive *P. falciparum* is present, prophylactic regimens safe for use during pregnancy have been developed. No prophylactic regimen, however, can assure complete protection against malaria; most severe complications appear to be more common in pregnant women, and prophylactic regimens occasionally produce unwanted side effects. In areas where chloroquine-resistant *P. falciparum* is present, no completely safe regimen has been developed for pregnant women, so travel to these areas should be avoided unless the need is imperative. For more discussion about malaria, consult the suggested readings.

## Suggested Readings

Brabin BJ. Epidemiology of infection in pregnancy. Rev Infect Dis 1985;7:579–603.

Centers for Disease Control and Prevention. Recommendations for the prevention of malaria among travelers. MMWR 1990;39(RR-3):1–10.

Centers for Disease Control and Prevention. Treatment of severe *Plasmodium falciparum* malaria with quinidine gluconate; discontinuation of parenteral quinine from CDC drug service. MMWR 1991;40(14):240.

Drugs for parasitic infection. Med Lett 1990;34:23.

Kreutner AK, Del Bene VE, Amstey MS. Giardiasis in pregnancy. Am J Obstet Gynecol 1981;140:895–901.

Lee RV. Protozoan infections in pregnancy. In: Gleicher N, ed. Principles of medical therapy in pregnancy. New York: Plenum, 1985.

MacLeod CL, ed. Parasitic infection in pregnancy and the newborn. Oxford, England: Oxford University Press, 1988.

Roberts NS, Copel JA, Bhutani V, et al. Intestinal parasites and other infections during pregnancy in Southeast Asian refugees. J Reprod Med 1985;30:720–725.

Steketee RW, Wirima JJ, Bloland PB, et al. Impairment of a pregnant woman's acquired ability to limit *Plasmodium falciparum* by infection with human immunodeficiency virus type-1. Am J Trop Med Hyg 1996;55:42–49.

Sweet R, Biggs R, eds. Parasitic disease in pregnancy. In: Infectious diseases of the female genital tract, 2nd ed. Baltimore: Williams and Wilkins, 1990.

Villar J, Klebanoff M, Kestler E. The effect on fetal growth of protozoan and helminthic infection during pregnancy. Obstet Gynecol 1989;74:915–920.

# PART 2

# *Gynecology*

CHAPTER

# 35

# *Screening Tests for Vaginitis*

*Marijane A. Krohn*

## Background and Incidence

Infections of the vagina are typically divided into three categories by etiology:

- Bacterial vaginosis (BV) caused by several microorganisms
- Candidal vaginitis caused by various candidal species
- Trichomoniasis caused by *Trichomonas vaginalis*

BV is an imbalance of microorganisms in the vaginal ecosystem rather than the result of a single infectious agent. Vaginal yeast, 80% to 90% of which is isolated as *Candida albicans*, may be present concurrently with *Lactobacillus*-predominant vaginal flora in women who have no vaginal complaints. Under such conditions, *C. albicans* may be considered part of the normal flora and does not warrant treatment. Among this group of vaginal conditions, trichomoniasis most closely fits the definition of an infection, as it is caused only by *T. vaginalis* and results in inflammation of genital tissue.

No solid data have been gathered about the probability of developing these vaginal conditions during a specified period of time among asymptomatic women who tested negative at the beginning of the observation period. On the other hand, prevalence information from women seeking health care for reasons other than genital complaints suggests that *T. vaginalis* can be isolated from 3% to 10% of women and *Candida* from 10% to 15%. Bacterial vaginosis, diagnosed by a Gram-stained vaginal smear, affects 10% to 20% of asymptomatic women.

The prevalence of these vaginal conditions depends on the type of clinic where the information is collected.

Among women seeking medical care because of lower genital tract symptoms, 60% to 80% will have BV, candidiasis, or trichomoniasis. The remainder may have a sexually transmitted disease or no identifiable infection (15% to 20%).

## Role of Population Under Observation

Screening tests for BV, trichomoniasis, and candidiasis can be classified into two groups: direct observation tests conducted in the physician's office and laboratory tests that require specialized training or equipment. Screening tests that are frequently performed in a physician's office include observation of the appearance of the vaginal discharge, pH, amine odor, and microscopy of vaginal secretions for morphotypes of microorganisms. Laboratory tests for vaginitis include Gram-stained vaginal smears for bacterial morphotypes consistent with BV and assays of specialized growth medium for *T. vaginalis* and *Candida* spp.

The agreement of office-based tests with laboratory-based tests is substantially dependent on the type of women being studied when making the comparisons. When office-based tests are applied to women who are seeking relief for vaginal complaints, agreement with laboratory assays may be good to excellent (60% to 80%). When both kinds of procedures are compared in women seeking health care for reasons other than genital complaints, however, the office-based tests show poorer sensitivity and have less positive predictive value. The positive predictive value of a test compared with a gold standard is highly dependent on the condition's frequency in the observed population. A test with excellent sensitivity and specificity (greater than 95%) will have a positive predictive value of more than 75% when 10% of the population are affected by the condition. Its positive predictive value will drop to 25% when the condition's frequency drops to 1%, even though the test's sensitivity and specificity remain the same.

**Table 35-1.** Characteristics of Vaginal Discharge

| Amount | Color on Swab | Viscosity | Consistency | Distribution | Odor Without KOH |
|---|---|---|---|---|---|
| Minimal | Clear | Moderate | Nonhomogenous | Pooled | None |
| Moderate | White/gray | Thin | Homogenous | Diffuse | Fishy |
| Profuse | Yellow | Thick | Curdy/plaques | Patches | Foul |
| — | Brown | — | Frothy | — | — |
| — | Bloody | — | Other | — | — |

KOH = Potassium hydroxide.
SOURCE: Sweet RL, Gibbs RS, eds. Infectious diseases of the female genital tract, 3rd ed. Baltimore: Williams and Wilkins, 1995.

## Observation of Clinical Signs

Table 35-1 lists the characteristics of vaginal discharge that can be assessed and evaluated among women with vaginal complaints. Systematic recordings of these characteristics will aid in making the initial diagnosis and in determining women's response to treatment. Review of these characteristics in tandem with the results of laboratory tests provides the foundation for improving one's ability to assess vaginal signs.

### Discharge

The discharge associated with BV is typically thin, grayish-white, and homogeneous with a fishy odor. A large proportion of women with candidiasis have normal discharge, though some may have a moderately increased amount accompanied by white or yellow plaques. The discharge associated with trichomoniasis is profuse, yellow or green, frothy, and foul-smelling. Vaginal discharge may be the least reliable of the vaginal signs and the least likely to yield interobserver agreement. When combining characteristics of vaginal discharge with other signs, discharge characteristics may be given less weight because they are less likely to be consistent.

### Odor

The amine odor of vaginal discharge can be assessed after the addition of 10% potassium hydroxide (KOH). Place a swab of vaginal secretions on a slide and add several drops of KOH. The fishy odor associated with BV may become more pronounced under these conditions but should not be present for candidal vaginitis or trichomoniasis.

### pH

Measure vaginal pH by placing a strip of pH paper along the vaginal wall and then comparing the color of the pH strip with the colored standard on the container. A high vaginal pH (greater than 4.5) occurs frequently (80% to 90%) among women with BV or trichomoniasis. Vaginal pH is often normal (4.5 or lower) in cases of candidiasis.

### Microscopy of Vaginal Secretions

Prepare the slide for microscopy by adding 0.9% saline to a smear of vaginal secretions. Observe the slide for cells indicative of BV (bacteria-studded epithelial cells), motile forms associated with trichomoniasis, and budding yeast morphotypes associated with candidiasis. The yeast hyphae are seen more easily on a slide of vaginal secretions after the addition of 10% KOH. You can add a cover slip for the amine odor test for use in microscopy of hyphal forms. Among women with genital symptoms, the sensitivities of clue cells for BV, motile forms for trichomoniasis, and hyphae for candidiasis reach a reported 70% to 85%. Ultimately, the degree of sensitivity will depend upon the skill of the observer.

## Combining Signs into a Diagnostic Algorithm

One of the most important aspects of using clinical observations for diagnosing vaginitis is combining the information about vaginal discharge, pH, odor, and microscopy into a systematic algorithm to predict which vaginal condition is most likely. As compared with laboratory tests, the combination of vaginal signs has the highest sensitivity (70% to more than 80%) for BV and trichomoniasis and is poorest for candidiasis. The

**Table 35-2.** Characteristics of Normal Secretions and Vaginitis

| Feature | Normal | Bacterial Vaginosis | Trichomoniasis | Yeast |
|---|---|---|---|---|
| Appearance | White, floccular; high viscosity | Gray, homogeneous, thin | Gray, yellow, white; homogenous; frothy or milky/creamy | — |
| pH | <4.5 | >4.5 | >4.5 | <4.5 |
| Amine odor | Absent | Present | Absent | Absent |
| Clue cells | Absent | Present | Absent | Absent |
| Trichomonads | Absent | Absent | Present | Absent |
| Mycelia | Absent | Absent | Absent | Present |

SOURCE: Sweet RL, Gibbs RS, eds. Infectious diseases of the female genital tract, 3rd ed. Baltimore: Williams and Wilkins, 1995.

**Table 35-3.** Percent of Clinical Signs in Women with BV Identified by Gram-Stained Vaginal Smear

| Clinical Sign | BV ($n$ = 73) | No BV ($n$ = 520) |
|---|---|---|
| Homogenous discharge | 71 | 24 |
| pH ≥ 4.7 | 84 | 21 |
| Amine odor after KOH | 74 | 22 |
| Clue cells on wet mount | 80 | 24 |
| Three or four signs | 77 | 13 |

SOURCE: Krohn MA, Hillier SL, Eschenbach DA. Comparison of methods for diagnosing bacterial vaginosis among pregnant women. J Clin Microbiol 1989;27:1266–1271.

poor sensitivity of signs for candidiasis may be attributable to the small number of signs that are disturbed; the appearance of discharge, pH, and odor may all be normal among women with candidiasis. The observer must therefore rely on the identification of hyphal forms through the microscopy of vaginal secretions. Table 35-2 provides a method for organizing observations on vaginal secretions and indicates which ones may be present among normal women and those with vaginitis.

The diagnosis of BV by a combination of three of four clinical signs has become more widely accepted than has the diagnosis of trichomoniasis by a combination of signs (Table 35-3). In fact, the sensitivity of clinical signs for diagnosing BV is as high as that of a Gram-stained vaginal smear evaluated microscopically in a laboratory. Nevertheless, using three of four clinical signs as a diagnostic criterion yields fewer false-positive results among women who are negative by the Gram-stained smear.

## Use of Cultures

When using cultures to aid in the diagnosis of BV, trichomoniasis, and candidiasis, you should keep the following factors in mind.

### Bacterial Vaginosis

Using bacterial isolates from specimens sent to the laboratory for culture is not recommended for making a diagnosis. BV

**Table 35-4.** Percent of Bacteria Identified by Culture in Women with BV Diagnosed by Gram-Stained Vaginal Smear

| Bacteria | BV ($n$ = 73) | No BV ($n$ = 520) |
|---|---|---|
| *Gardnerella vaginalis* | 97 | 45 |
| *Mycoplasma hominis* | 74 | 20 |
| *Bacteroides* spp.; *Porphyromonas* spp.; *Prevotella* spp. | 70 | 18 |
| *Peptostreptococcus* spp. | 70 | 25 |

SOURCE: Krohn MA, Hillier SL, Eschenbach DA. Comparison of methods for diagnosing bacterial vaginosis in pregnant women. J Clin Microbiol 1989;27:1266–1271.

represents an imbalance in the frequency and concentration of a group of bacteria that are part of the normal genital microflora. Consequently, the culture-based identification of one bacterium associated with BV will not predict whether a woman has this infection. Women with BV are more likely to have certain bacteria than are women without it, but the specificity of any one bacterium for BV is low.

Instead, you should conduct DNA probe tests for high concentrations of *Gardnerella vaginalis* (more than $10^5$ colony-forming units per milliliter of vaginal fluid) combined with a high pH (greater than 4.5) in an office setting. These probe tests have excellent sensitivity compared with a laboratory assessment of a Gram-stained vaginal smear for BV, but 45% of women who do not have bacterial vaginosis are culture-positive for *G. vaginalis* (Table 35-4).

## Trichomoniasis and Candidiasis

You may have to send vaginal secretion specimens to a laboratory for culture when a woman is suspected to have trichomoniasis or candidiasis in cases where the pattern of clinical signs is not clearly consistent with either condition. Conflicting or inconsistent vaginal signs may be more frequent among women with multiple conditions. DNA probe tests are also available for trichomoniasis and candidiasis and have excellent sensitivity compared with culture results.

Combining careful observations of physical signs with vaginal pH measurement, microscopy, and DNA probe testing is likely to lead to an appropriate diagnosis of BV and trichomoniasis. On the other hand, diagnosing recurrent candidiasis in women who have vaginal symptoms may require the confirmation of a positive culture result.

## Suggested Readings

American College of Obstetricians and Gynecologists. ACOG Technical Bulletin. Vaginitis. Number 226. Int J Gynaecol Obstet 1996;54:293–302.

Briselden AM, Hillier SL. Evaluation of Affirm VP microbial identification test for *Gardnerella vaginalis* and *Trichomonas vaginalis*. J Clin Microbiol 1994;32:148–152.

Ferris DG, Hendrich J, Payne PM, et al. Office laboratory diagnosis of vaginosis: clinician-performed test compared with a rapid nucleic acid hybridization test. J Fam Pract 1995;41:575–581.

Hillier SL, Krohn MA, Nugent RP, et al. Characteristics of three vaginal flora patterns assessed by Gram stain among pregnant women. Am J Obstet Gynecol 1992;166:938–944.

Krohn MA, Hillier SL, Eschenbach DA. Comparison of methods for diagnosing bacterial vaginosis among pregnant women. J Clin Microbiol 1989;27:1266–1271.

Nugent RP, Krohn MA, Hillier SL. Reliability of diagnosing bacterial vaginosis is improved by a standardized method of Gram stain interpretation. J Clin Microbiol 1991;29:297–301.

Sweet RL, Gibbs RS, eds. Infectious vulvovaginitis. In: Infectious diseases of the female genital tract, 3rd ed. Baltimore: Williams and Wilkins, 1995:341–362.

Wathne B, Holst E, Hovelius B, et al. Vaginal discharge: comparison of clinical, laboratory, and microbiological findings. Acta Obstet Gynecol Scand 1994;73:802–808.

CHAPTER

# 36

# Candida *Vaginal Infections*

*Michael R. Spence*

## BACKGROUND

Although oral thrush was described by Hippocrates in the fourth century B.C., it was not until 1839 that the fungal organism causing this disease was identified in buccal lesions. In 1849, a similar fungus was found in vaginal infections. In 1875, the two agents causing vaginal and oral thrush were noted to be identical. The organism subsequently went through many name changes before finally beomg named *Monilia albicans* by Zopf in 1890. This name prevailed until the Eighth Botanical Congress adopted the currently accepted term of *Candida* to describe the genus in 1954.

More than 100 *Candida* species exist, the majority of which are dimorphic fungi pathogenic for humans. These organisms commonly reside in the yeast form as commensals in the reproductive tract, in the gastrointestinal tract, and on the skin. They rarely cause disease unless their numbers increase rapidly because of a disturbance in the status quo. Hence, they truly are opportunistic pathogens.

## EPIDEMIOLOGY

As noted earlier, *Candida* species reside as commensals in humans. As many as 40% of normal women with no evidence of an active disease process likely harbor *Candida* species in their vaginas. Therefore, isolation and identification of *Candida* species by culture in the female reproductive tract are not diagnostic of infection.

Approximately 75% of all women will develop a vaginal fungal (yeast) infection at some time in their lives, and an additional 40% to 50% of these women will have recurrent infections of a similar nature. Because fungal vaginitis is not a reportable disease, no statistics are kept on its occurrence. This lack of data makes it difficult—if not impossible—to determine the prevalence of these infections, much less their incidence. Moreover, because a large number of women self-medicate these infections with over-the-counter products, it is doubtful that we will ever be able to determine how frequently they occur.

Numerous risk factors have been associated with the development of fungal infections of the vagina. These factors include diabetes, acquired immunodeficiency syndrome (AIDS), the taking of broad-spectrum antimicrobial agents, pregnancy, and the use of oral contraceptives (OCs) or intrauterine contraceptive devices.

With respect to the mechanics underlying these risk factors, it has been postulated that diabetics have increased glucose in their vaginal secretions that predisposes the yeast organism to overgrowth and results in the development of an infection. In addition, yeast adhesion is enhanced and phagocytosis is altered by hyperglycemia. Both of these phenomena are associated with increased infectivity.

Tetracycline antibiotics impair the host immune response by altering phagocytosis. They also decrease the numbers of bacteria found in the normal vaginal flora, thereby reducing the number of organisms available to compete with the yeast for the food supply.

OCs and pregnancy are thought to be associated with increased glycogen stores in the vaginal mucosal cells; other possible effects include the alteration of carbohydrate metabolism and the generation of sugar substrates that enhance yeast attachment to epithelial cells. Likewise, fungal proliferation is enhanced by the presence of estrogen and progesterone receptors on the fungi that can be stimulated by the hormones. In addition, use of OCs and pregnancy suppress T-cell immunity, which lowers natural defenses and can spur proliferation of the organisms.

Note, however, that low-dose OCs have not been found to be associated with increased fungal infection, implying that the likelihood of proliferation is related to hormone levels.

Complications that have been associated with vaginal fungal infections include balanitis in the male partner resulting from sexual transmission, chronic persistence or recurrence of the infection due to difficulty in eradicating the fungus, and chorioamnionitis caused by ascending infection.

The species most commonly associated with candidal vaginal infections are *Candida albicans*, *Candida glabrata*, *Candida tropicalis*, *Candida krusei*, *Candida guilliermondii*, and *Candida pseudotropicalis,* although, as noted earlier, more than 100 different species of *Candida* exist. In addition, at least 200 strains of *C. albicans* have been identified. Interestingly, strain typing has demonstrated a concordance between vaginal strains and those found in the rectum and oral cavity of both the patient and her partner. This concordance may play a role in transmission and reinfection. The organisms exist in these sites as commensals, predominantly in the yeast or budding form. Once the events that lead to disease occur, however, these organisms take on the invasive hyphae or pseudohyphae form. The one exception to this rule is *C. glabrata,* which does not have a mycelial phase.

## DIAGNOSIS

One of the major problems in diagnosing and determining the frequency of fungal infections in women is that other physiologic phenomena often mimic these conditions. A woman who has a history of fungal vaginitis and who develops a curdy, white discharge with some pruritus may therefore assume that she has reacquired her "yeast infection." These women often seek care from their local pharmacy and self-medicate without ever receiving an accurate diagnosis.

If the patient does self-medicate but has a self-limiting, increased physiologic discharge at midcycle, her clinical response —disappearance of symptoms—will correspond to her initiation and completion of therapy. The woman then will wrongly believe she has been appropriately treated for an infectious process. This sequence of events has led many women to believe they have a recurrent "yeast infection" every month.

Although many signs and symptoms are associated with the clinical diagnosis of *Candida* infections, the prime symptom of a true infection is pruritus. Erythema, edema, and tenderness are also common clinical signs that are rarely present with a physiologic discharge at midcycle. The discharge of a true yeast infection may take many forms. It may be absent or physiologic in appearance, or it may be thick, white, and curdy with attendant plaques on the vaginal wall. Because clinical diagnosis often can be difficult and fraught with error, the clinician should employ adjunctive diagnostic methods, such as normal saline or strong base (KOH or NaOH) wet preparation methods, rather than relying solely on clinical judgment.

Microscopic examination of vaginal secretions, with either a normal saline or strong base wet preparation, that reveals the presence of the pseudohyphae or mycelial phase is diagnostic of a fungal infection, as opposed to fungal colonization. If only the yeast form appears, the patient either is not infected and carrying a commensal or is infected with *C. glabrata*. Unfortunately, *C. glabrata* does not form a mycelial phase; consequently, a positive result with this diagnostic method cannot be the only criterion used to identify infections caused by this particular organism. In these cases, one can treat empirically or resort to culture.

A Gram's stain of the vaginal secretions often will demonstrate the presence of budding yeast in women carrying the organisms as commensals, but pseudohyphae will appear in women with infection. The organism also has been identified on Pap smears of cervical and vaginal secretions. Another diagnostic method that may prove helpful is a latex fixation for *C. albicans* that has a high correlation with infection.

The organism can be specifically identified by culture employing Sabouraud's, cornmeal, or Nickerson's media. Culture and speciation of the organism may help those patients harboring organisms that do not respond to treatment and patients in whom there is a question of antimicrobial resistance.

As yet, uniform methods for fungal antimicrobial sensitivity have not been established and can be relied upon only if obtained from a few reference laboratories. It has been found that *C. tropicalis* and *C. glabrata* tend to be more hardy and more difficult to treat than *C. albicans*.

## TREATMENT

Vaginal fungal infections can be treated either topically or systemically. Topical preparations are available as creams, suppositories, and vaginal tablets. The duration of use varies from a single dose to 15 days of treatment. The selection of one method of therapy over another is based purely on the patient's preference, as all available data suggest that most therapies have equivalent efficacy. The primary agents commercially available are the polyenes and the azoles.

The only polyene commercially available in the United States for topical treatment of superficial fungal infections is nystatin. This agent, which is administered as a 14-day course of intravaginal tablets, has a cure rate of approximately 80%, similar to cure rates reported with other topical agents. Another polyene widely used for fungal infections is amphotericin. This agent, which is administered systemically, has been reserved for deep-seated, serious infections because of its high toxicity. Although a topical form of amphotericin has been formulated, it remains unavailable in the United States.

Currently, the most commonly employed agents for topical fungal therapy are the azoles, including butoconazole, clotrimazole, miconazole, terconazole, and tioconazole (Table 36-1). Although they come in many different forms, their primary mode of action relies on inhibition of ergosterol synthesis. They appear to be equally effective. Many of the topical azoles are now available as over-the-counter agents. When one compares the generic formulations of the over-the-counter preparations with the brand-name preparations from which they are derived, one often finds a marked difference in price—that is, the generic brands cost much less.

Systemic therapy employing oral ketoconazole, fluconazole, or itraconazole also can be used. Numerous reports of single-dose therapy employing the latter two agents have shown them

**Table 36-1.** CDC-Recommended Regimens for Vaginal Candidal Infection

| Agent | Dosage |
|---|---|
| **Intravaginal** | |
| Butoconazole | 2% cream, 5 g daily for 3 days*† |
| Clotrimazole | 1% cream, 5 g daily for 7 to 14 days*†<br>One 100-mg tablet daily for 7 days*<br>Two 100-mg tablets daily for 3 days*<br>One 500-mg tablet in a single application* |
| Miconazole | 2% cream, 5 g daily for 7 days*†<br>One 200-mg suppository daily for 3 days*†<br>One 100-mg suppository daily for 7 days*† |
| Nystatin | One 100,000-U tablet daily for 14 days |
| Terconazole | 0.4% cream, 5 g daily for 7 days*<br>0.8% cream, 5 g daily for 3 days*<br>One 80-mg suppository daily for 3 days* |
| Tioconazole | 6.5% ointment, 5 g in a single application*† |
| **Oral** | |
| Fluconazole | One 150-mg tablet in a single dose |

* Oil-based preparations that might weaken latex condoms and diaphragms.
† Preparations available as over-the-counter products.
SOURCE: Centers for Disease Control and Prevention. 1998 guidelines for treatment of sexually transmitted diseases. MMWR 1998;47(RR-1):76.

to be as effective as topical therapy. Oral ketoconazole, however, requires more than a single dose to be effective.

A non-azole topical preparation—albeit one that is currently not commercially available—that has been used since the early 1980s and continues to be effective is the boric acid capsule. One 600 mg boric acid capsule inserted intravaginally at bedtime for a period of two weeks usually proves effective in eradicating most of the more aggressive and more difficult-to-treat vaginal fungal infections.

All of the currently available topical therapies as well as the oral therapies appear to be equally effective, with cure rates ranging from 80% to 95%. No one form of therapy appears to have an advantage over another; the choice of treatment therefore depends on the patient's personal preference and finances.

## SUMMARY

Vaginal fungal infections are extremely common conditions that bring many women to gynecologic care on an annual basis. The diagnosis usually relies on symptoms, clinical signs, and confirmatory microscopy. Only rarely are cultures or more sophisticated diagnostic techniques required. Nevertheless, confirmation with microscopy is critically important, as clinical symptoms can be confused with physiologic processes that do not require therapy.

Numerous therapeutic options are available, encompassing a wide range of topical and systemic agents at varying prices. These therapies appear to be equally effective, with all having 80% to 95% cure rates. Hence, the choice of therapy is a matter of individual preference. Thus far, development of resistance to the current therapeutic agents has not been a significant clinical problem.

## SUGGESTED READINGS

Candidiasis. In: Kwon-Chung KJ, Bennett JE, eds. Medical mycology. Philadelphia: Williams & Wilkins, 1992:280–336.

Candidiasis and the pathogenic yeasts. In: Rippon JW, ed. Medical Mycology: The pathogenic fungi and pathogenic actinomytes, 3rd ed. Philadelphia: W. B. Saunders, 1988:532–581.

Centers for Disease Control and Prevention. 1998 guidelines for treatment of sexually transmitted diseases. MMWR 1998;47(RR-1):75–77.

Sobol JD. Vulvovaginal candidiasis. In: Pastorek JG II, ed. Obstetric and gynecologic infectious disease. New York: Raven Press, 1994:523–536.

CHAPTER

# 37

# *Chronic Recurrent Vaginal Candidiasis*

*Steven S. Witkin*
*Paulo C. Giraldo*

## BACKGROUND

The lay press has popularized the unproven idea that *Candida* infections are the underlying cause of a multitude of symptoms in every body part. Consequently, most women who seek help for recurrent symptoms of vaginitis claim to have a "yeast infection." Unfortunately, most of these self-attempted diagnoses are incorrect, with evidence of *Candida* being detected in subsequent examination only 30% of the time. It's not surprising, therefore, that antifungal medications have no effect in most of these patients.

The terms "chronic" and "recurrent" in referring to vulvovaginitis are frequently misinterpreted. This misunderstanding may sometimes confuse the interpretation of the pathophysiology in a particular patient and lead to inadequate treatment. Chronic infection almost always implies an active, persistent infectious process for prolonged periods. This definition does not seem to apply to recurrent candidal vulvovaginitis, which usually occurs in repeated, acute, short-term episodes of variable intensity. Therefore, candidal vulvovaginitis can be recurrent but is not chronic. The recurrences are chronic in a subgroup of women who have acute episodes that repeat themselves over a long period of time.

In addition, it is important to differentiate between colonization and infection of the vaginal epithelium. Many asymptomatic women are continually colonized with *Candida albicans* in their vaginas. The presence of this organism does not imply that the patient has a current, chronic, or even latent infection.

Among private patients at the authors' institution, approximately 5% with an initial episode of candidal vaginitis will have recurrent infection after apparently successful treatment with antifungal medications. To prevent frequent episodes, it is necessary to identify underlying factors predisposing to *Candida* growth and take measures to reduce these risks.

## PATHOPHYSIOLOGY

More than 95% of candidal vaginal infections are caused by *C. albicans*; the remainder are caused primarily by *C. glabrata* and *C. tropicalis*. Although all women have antibodies to *Candida*, these antibodies are nonprotective and do not prevent its growth. Moreover, women with defective B-cell immunity do not exhibit an increased rate of vaginal candidiasis.

Cell-mediated immunity appears to be the major—if not the only—immune mechanism limiting vaginal proliferation of *C. albicans*. Polymorphonuclear leukocytes are not noticeably present in the vagina. Rather, mononuclear lymphoid cells, macrophages, and T lymphocytes appear to serve as the major regulators of vaginal *Candida* growth. Women who have genetic defects that affect T-lymphocyte or macrophage functions therefore have an increased rate of candidal mucous membrane infections.

In healthy women with normally functioning immune systems, infection of mucosal surfaces by *Candida* can be readily treated and rarely recurs. Conversely, a defective in vitro cellular immune response to *Candida* is readily demonstrable in many women with recurrent candidal vaginitis. It sometimes is not appreciated that recurrent *C. albicans* vaginal infections often are opportunistic and occur secondary to a transient deficiency in cell-mediated immunity.

An immune response by T-helper (h) lymphocytes can occur along two pathways. A $Th_1$ response results in the release of cytokines that activate cell-mediated immunity (interferon-$\gamma$, interleukin-1, interleukin-12); a $Th_2$ response, on the other hand, results in the release of different cytokines that stimulate antibody production (interleukin-4, -5, and -10). Women whose T cells manifest a $Th_2$ response upon exposure to *Candida* because of genetic and/or environmental (allergic) factors will be less likely to limit vaginal *Candida* proliferation. As a result, these patients will be increasingly susceptible to repeated episodes of candidal vaginitis.

In approximately 20% of cases, a vaginal allergic response can be implicated as a predisposing factor for recurrent candidal vaginitis. Semen components, contraceptive spermicides, vaginal douches, other chemicals or medicines that may come into contact with the vagina, or *C. albicans* itself can serve as allergens in sensitized women. The vagina's immediate hypersensitivity response causes release of histamine, which stimulates macrophages to produce prostaglandin $E_2$ ($PGE_2$). $PGE_2$ inhibits production of interleukin-2 by T lymphocytes, thereby transiently paralyzing the cell-mediated immune response. Under these conditions, the low levels of *Candida* normally present in many women's vaginas may proliferate and trigger a clinical infection.

Allergy-related candidal vaginitis also can be induced in non-allergic women if the male partner has a genital tract allergic response. In these cases, immunoglobulin E (IgE) antibodies are transferred to the woman by coitus and then bind to her basophils and mast cells. The allergen, which is also present in the ejaculate, reacts with the bound IgE to initiate an allergic response.

Candidal vaginitis most often reappears during the late luteal phase of the menstrual cycle, when the elevated level of progesterone down-regulates the cellular immune response and lessens inhibition of *Candida* growth. For similar reasons, women with endocrinopathies may be especially susceptible to recurrent candidal vaginitis.

Infectivity of *C. albicans* is associated with the germination of the yeast forms. Recent evidence indicates that germination, too, may be regulated by cellular immune system components. Compounds such as $PGE_2$, which increase the intracellular level of cyclic adenosine monophosphate (cAMP), promote *Candida* germination. Thus medications that increase cAMP levels may increase the patient's susceptibility to candidal vaginitis.

Conversely, interferon-γ, a product of activated T lymphocytes, inhibits the development of this condition.

*C. albicans* can be present in the male genital tract. Recurrent infection in the woman, therefore, sometimes may result from failure to eliminate the reservoir of infection in her male partner.

## Diagnosis

Recurrent candidal vaginitis may show the classical symptoms of pruritus, inflammation, and curdlike, cheesy discharge. In some patients, intense pruritus may be the only symptom. Unfortunately, many patients have been treated by numerous physicians, nutritionists, and other health care providers and have tried various home remedies that often complicate and mask presenting symptoms. Therefore, the gross appearance of vaginal secretions is not diagnostic.

In some cases, the clinician may confirm the diagnosis by finding branched, budding pseudohyphae on wet mounts of vaginal secretions in 10% potassium hydroxide. In many symptomatic patients in whom *Candida* infection is suspected but wet mounts are negative, a more sensitive and specific test involves the inoculation of Sabouraud agar slants with a vaginal swab. To identify the yeast as *C. albicans*, inoculate a small colony into serum or glucose beef extract and then examine it for germ tube formation after 90 to 120 minutes.

Use of the polymerase chain reaction (PCR) to detect *Candida* in vaginal specimens of symptomatic women is helpful as well. No relationship has been identified between yeast concentration and clinical symptoms. Some women with high colony counts may be asymptomatic while others may have symptoms; the organism is detectable only by PCR, however. This fact highlights the importance of host factors in candidal infections.

If *Candida* is not detected, the patient should be screened for bacterial vaginosis as well as for *Chlamydia trachomatis*, human papillomavirus, and mycoplasma infections. Patients should be questioned about such classic risk factors as frequent antibiotic or steroid usage, pregnancy, diabetes or other endocrinopathies, poor perianal hygiene, or wearing of tight clothing or nylon or silk undergarments. Typically, most patients will be negative for all of these risk factors.

Ascertain the relationship between sexual activity and vaginal symptoms. Are the symptoms temporally related to coitus with just the patient's current partner or with all partners? Does the sexual partner have symptoms of genital, oral, or digital *Candida* infection? Was he taking any medication or drug to which the woman might be sensitized? What is the means of contraception?

At the authors' institution, women who have recurrent vaginitis are tested for evidence of a vaginal allergic response. We obtain a vaginal wash sample by instilling 5 to 10 mL of sterile saline into the vagina with a needle and syringe (directing the injection flow against the sidewalls), withdrawing the solution, and separating it into pellet and supernatant fractions by centrifugation. ELISA is used to test the supernatant for IgE antibodies to *Candida* and semen and the pellet for bound IgE. In coitus-related vaginitis, we obtain cultures for *Candida* from semen samples and test for total IgE and specific IgE antibodies to the vaginal wash pellet.

Although it is not performed routinely, a lymphocyte proliferation assay on a sample of peripheral blood mononuclear cells isolated from heparinized blood may prove useful when immunosuppression is suspected, such as in women with concomitant oral thrush or condyloma. In such instances, a defective proliferative response to *Candida* and plant mitogens may indicate a more serious underlying disease.

## Treatment

The appropriate comprehensive diagnosis will facilitate the choice of the best treatment option for each patient with presumed chronic recurrent vaginal candidiasis. Treatment has two goals: to alleviate acute infectious symptoms and to avoid subsequent recurrences.

Resistance to antifungal agents does not seem to emerge with candidal vaginal infections. The majority of commercial products successfully treat acute fungal infections in most

**Table 37-1.** Therapy for Chronic Recurrent Candidal Vaginitis

| Drug* | Regimen† |
|---|---|
| **Initial Treatment** | |
| Clotrimazole 1% cream | 5 g intravaginally once daily for 10 to 14 days |
| *or* | |
| Miconazole 2% cream | 5 g intravaginally once daily for 10 to 14 days |
| *or* | |
| Fluconazole | 150 mg orally in a single dose |
| **Followed by Maintenance Therapy** | |
| Clotrimazole 1% cream | 5 g intravaginally once daily for 3 to 5 days before every menstrual period for 6 months |
| *or* | |
| Miconazole 2% cream | 5 g intravaginally once daily for 3 to 5 days before every menstrual period for 6 months |
| *or* | |
| Nystatin 100,000-unit tablets | One tablet intravaginally every fourth night for 6 months |
| *or* | |
| Itraconazole 100-mg capsules | One capsule orally once daily for 6 months |
| *or* | |
| Ketoconazole | 100 mg orally once daily for 6 months |
| *or* | |
| Fluconazole 100-mg tablets | One tablet orally every week for 6 months |

* Other antifungal agents can also be used (e.g., butoconazole, econozole, terconazole, or tioconazole).

† Treatment of acute infection should exceed two to three days.

patients. Currently, no medication is available for clinical use that is completely fungicidal. Although treatment with antifungal agents can reduce the number of vaginal organisms to a level undetectable by culture, complete eradication of the organism in the vagina is not achieved.

Many different approaches have been suggested for the treatment of women with chronic recurrent candidal vulvovaginitis. None, however, will be successful in every case. Table 37-1 shows the various treatment options. Treatment consists of first alleviating the current acute infection and then preventing its clinical recurrence. If the second maintenance phase is not initiated, between 25% and 40% of patients will have a clinical recurrence within six weeks. Most patients will remain symptom-free for at least six months while maintenance treatment continues.

If candidal vaginitis is associated with coitus with one particular partner, the clinician should find out whether the male partner is ingesting any medications or drugs that could enter his semen and elicit a vaginal response. Reports have detailed vaginal allergic reactions to semen that contained products of ingested penicillin or thioridazine. Change or eliminate the offending medication, if possible. Similarly, evaluate the effect on vaginitis recurrence of changing the contraceptive method or spermicide brand.

If the woman has vaginal fluid IgE antibodies to her partner's semen or the man has IgE antibodies in his ejaculate, the use of a condom will eliminate vaginal contact with the allergen. An untested alternative is the use of an oral antihistamine before intercourse.

Vaginal allergic responses to *Candida* appear to be relatively common in women with recurrent candidal vaginitis. In one study conducted by the authors, 18% of 64 patients tested had anticandidal IgE in their vaginal washes. In women who are hypersensitive to *Candida* or to an unidentified component of a vaginal wash sample, the best treatment appears to be to prevent growth of *Candida* by aggressive use of antifungal agents plus use of oral antihistamines to obtain symptomatic relief of vaginal symptoms and reduce the incidence of histamine-mediated inummosuppression.

Hyposensitizing the patient to *Candida*, semen, or any other allergen associated with a vaginal allergic response may ultimately provide the best therapy. Improved methodology and standardization, along with controlled clinical trials, are nevertheless needed to evaluate the effectiveness of these experimental immunizations.

## Suggested Readings

Green RL, Green MA. Postcoital urticaria in a penicillin-sensitive patient: possible seminal transfer of penicillin. JAMA 1985; 254:531.

Kalo-Klein A, Witkin SS. *Candida albicans*: cellular immune system interactions during different stages of the menstrual cycle. Am J Obstet Gynecol 1989;161:1132–1136.

Kalo-Klein A, Witkin SS. Prostaglandin $E_2$ enhances and gamma interferon inhibits germ tube formation in *Candida albicans*. Infect Immun 1990;58:260–262.

Odds FC. *Candida* and candidosis, 2nd ed. Philadelphia: Bailliere Tindall, 1988;273.

Puccetti P, Romani L, Bistoni F. A $TH_1$–$TH_2$-like switch in candidiasis: new perspectives for therapy. Trends Microbiol 1995;3: 237–240.

Rigg D, Miller MM, Metzger WJ. Recurrent allergic vulvovaginitis: treatment with *Candida albicans* allergen immunotherapy. Am J Obstet Gynecol 1990;162:332–336.

Sell MB. Sensitization to thioridazine through sexual intercourse. Am J Psychiatry 1985;142:271–272.

Sobel JD. Recurrent vulvovaginal candidiasis: a prospective study of the efficacy of maintenance ketoconazole therapy. N Engl J Med 1986;315:1455–1458.

Sobel JD, Faro S, Force RW, et al. Vulvovaginal candidiasis: epidemiologic, diagnostic, and therapeutic considerations. Am J Obstet Gynecol 1998;178:203–211.

Sobel JD, Muller G, Buckley HR. Critical role of germ tube formation in the pathogenesis of candidal vaginitis. Infect Immun 1984;44: 576–580.

Witkin SS. Immunology of recurrent vaginitis. Am J Reprod Immunol Microbiol 1987;15:34–37.

Witkin SS, Hirsch J, Ledger WJ. A macrophage defect in women with recurrent *Candida* vaginitis and its reversal in vitro by prostaglandin inhibitors. Am J Obstet Gynecol 1986;155:790–795.

Witkin SS, Jeremias J, Ledger WJ. A localized vaginal allergic response in women with recurrent vaginitis. J Allergy Clin Immunol 1988;81:412–416.

Witkin SS, Jeremias J, Ledger WJ. Recurrent vaginitis as a result of sexual transmission of IgE antibodies. Am J Obstet Gynecol 1988;159:32–36.

CHAPTER

# 38

# *Trichomoniasis*

*Cheryl K. Walker*

## Background

*Trichomonas vaginalis* is a protozoan parasite that was first described in 1836. This organism is unicellular, flagellated, and motile. It forms pseudopods and is slightly larger than a polymorphonuclear neutrophilic leukocyte. *T. vaginalis* prefers an environment of high pH; its maximum growth and metabolic function occur at pH 6.0. Most commonly found in vaginal secretions with pH exceeding 4.5, this organism proliferates during menstruation and is frequently associated with a large number of leukocytes.

Because long-term longitudinal studies of at-risk populations have not been conducted and because many infected women are asymptomatic, incidence rates for this infection have not been defined. Prevalence varies significantly, depending on the population evaluated and the diagnostic method employed. The organism has been found in as few as 3% of college students attending a student health clinic and as many as 37% of women working in the sex industry. Approximately one-fifth of women presenting with symptoms of vaginal infection are believed to have trichomoniasis.

Given that the primary and only significant mode of transmission is sexual intercourse, women who have multiple sexual partners have an increased risk of infection with *T. vaginalis.* Whenever trichomoniasis is diagnosed, the clinician should evaluate the patient for other sexually transmitted infections, such as gonorrhea, chlamydial infection, syphilis, and HIV infection.

## Clinical Presentation

The clinical presentation of persons infected with *T. vaginalis* varies widely, with many women harboring the organism asymptomatically. Vaginal discharge may vary from minimal to copious and may be purulent, homogeneous, yellow-green, or frothy. A patient may be asymptomatic or have significant irritation. Dysuria, urinary frequency, vaginal pruritus, dyspareunia, offensive genital odor, and low back pain can be present as well. The "classic" frothy, yellow, copious discharge with vaginal wall erythema and "strawberry" cervix appears in fewer than 10% of infected women. A disagreeable odor associated with a slight increase in homogeneous nonsticky, yellow-white discharge that pools in the posterior vaginal fornix is the most common presentation.

## Diagnosis

The diagnosis of trichomoniasis can be made in most circumstances by microscopic evaluation of a wet mount of vaginal secretions obtained from the anterior fornix mixed with a drop or two of normal saline. The sensitivity of this method varies from 42% to 92%, depending on the reagents employed, the handling of the specimen, and the compulsiveness of the observer; sensitivity increases to approximately 80% in the hands of experienced microscopists but is only 50% for the average clinician.

Some experts advocate the use of fresh saline without preservative, such as products intended for intravenous administration. If dropper bottles are used, wash and refill them at least monthly to reduce evaporation and prevent the resultant hypertonicity, which can inhibit motility. If test tubes are used to hold the saline, they should be tightly capped and should not contain additives.

Keep specimens warm from the time of collection until microscopic evaluation. Begin the examination by scanning the entire slide at low power and then evaluating suspicious areas under high power. Organisms frequently appear on the periphery of clumps of white blood cells or epithelial cells. If no motile organisms are found, the diagnosis cannot be made with this technique.

The diagnosis of trichomoniasis is made occasionally via a Papanicolaou smear. In a research setting, the sensitivity of this method varies from 52% to 67%—too low to permit its use as a screening method. Moreover, unless the test employs vital stains, its specificity can vary, allowing false-positive results to be reported.

Culture represents another option for diagnosis. Special media, such as modified Diamond's, Feinberg-Whittington, or Kupferberg, are required, making this procedure labor-intensive and costly. It is therefore a poor choice in most clinical settings.

## Treatment

Before the introduction of metronidazole, traditional interventions for trichomoniasis were aimed at providing symptomatic relief. Occasionally, patients would experience a spontaneous cure. In 1959, Durel and colleagues introduced the 5-nitroimidazole metronidazole. Empiric therapy ranged from three to four 250 mg doses per day for 7 to 14 days. Csonka was the first to demonstrate that a single dose of 2 g metronidazole was as effective as prolonged multidose regimens. Two randomized, controlled trials have substantiated the equivalence of the 2 g stat dose and 5- to 7-day regimens. The 2 g regimen is the current standard, being administered either as a single dose or in two divided doses of 1 g each over the course of 8 to 12 hours. Cure rates achieved with this regimen range from 90% to 95%.

Topical metronidazole gel has considerably lower efficacy than oral regimens for treatment of trichomoniasis because it fails to achieve therapeutic levels in the urethra and perivaginal glands. The FDA has approved a regimen of oral metronidazole, 375 mg twice daily for seven days, as an alternative regimen for this infection; no clinical data have been published to support this contention, however. Concurrent treatment with similar dosage of all sexual partners is recommended.

Initially, concerns were voiced about the mutagenic potential of metronidazole, based on rodent data showing that animals developed tumors after chronic high-dose exposure to the drug. Subsequent human studies have not substantiated these early fears.

Until recently, use of metronidazole in pregnancy—particularly during the first trimester—was strongly discouraged because of the potential for increased birth defects. No data have been presented in the English-language literature that support this supposition. The CDC's "1998 Guidelines for Treatment of Sexually Transmitted Diseases" recommends that pregnant women with symptomatic trichomoniasis be treated using the single dose of 2 g metronidazole. Recent studies suggest a possible relationship between *T. vaginalis* infection and pregnancy complications such as preterm premature rupture of membranes and preterm birth. It is not clear whether routine screening and treatment of low- or high-risk pregnant women with trichomonal infection will lower these adverse outcomes.

On occasion, therapy for trichomoniasis may fail. Reinfection by an untreated partner is the most common cause of recurrent infection, and retreatment with the standard dose is recommended in such cases. Persistence of trichomonal infection is less common. Etiologies for persistent infection include nonadherence to the treatment schedule by either the woman or her partner(s), interference with other systemic medications (especially phenytoin and phenobarbitol), and relative antibiotic resistance.

As absolute resistance has never been described, the first approach should rely on treating trichomoniasis with a prolonged metronidazole regimen at increased dosage. A reasonable starting point is 500 mg to 1 g orally twice daily for seven days. Failure at this level of therapy may result from malabsorption of the drug or an inability to deliver adequate amounts of the drug to the infection site. As an intermediate measure, you may increase dosing to 2 g orally for three to five days. If infection persists at this point, obtain a complete blood count and treat the patient with as much as 4 g daily in divided doses for as long as 14 days. Additional benefit may be achieved by intravaginal insertion of two uncoated 500 mg metronidazole tablets twice daily plus high-dose oral therapy. Parenteral metronidazole administration does not appear to confer any benefit.

Regardless of the route of administration or dosage, metronidazole may cause toxic side effects. Instruct patients taking this medication to abstain from alcohol intake during the duration of the treatment course plus one day to avoid an antiabuse-type effect. Metronidazole occasionally produces headache, gastrointestinal upset, and an unpleasant taste. Blood dyscrasias are a rare complication. This drug is a neurotoxin, and its use has been reported to cause peripheral neuropathy, seizures, and Bell's palsy. Finally, because metronidazole can alter bowel flora significantly, pseudomembranous colitis can occur.

## Prevention

Partner identification and treatment are integral components of prevention. As with all sexually transmitted diseases, use of barrier contraceptives—both mechanical and chemical—is recommended strongly to prevent the spread of this infection.

### Suggested Readings

Beard CM, Noller KL, O'Fallon WM, et al. Lack of evidence for cancer due to use of metronidazole. N Engl J Med 1979;301:519–522.

Burtin P, Taddio A, Ariburnu O, et al. Safety of metronidazole in pregnancy: a meta-analysis. Am J Obstet Gynecol 1995;172:525–529.

Centers for Disease Control and Prevention. 1998 guidelines for treatment of sexually transmitted diseases. MMWR 1998;47 (RR-1):74–75.

Csonka GW. Trichomonal vaginitis treated with one dose of metronidazole. Br J Vener Dis 1971;47:456–458.

Hager WD, Brown ST, Kraus SJ, et al. Metronidazole for vaginal trichomoniasis: 7-day vs. single-dose regimens. JAMA 1980;244: 1219–1220.

McCormack WM, Evrard JR, Laughlin DF, et al. Sexually transmitted conditions among women college students. Am J Obstet Gynecol 1981;139:130–133.

Minkoff H, Grunebaum AN, Schwarz RH, et al. Risk factors for prematurity and premature rupture of membranes: a prospective study of the vaginal flora in pregnancy. Am J Obstet Gynecol 1984;150:965–972.

Piper JM, Mitchel EF, Ray WA. Prenatal use of metronidazole and birth defects: no association. Obstet Gynecol 1993;82:348–352.

Spence MR, Hollander DH, Smith J, et al. The clinical and laboratory diagnosis of *Trichomonas vaginalis* infection. Sex Transm Dis 1980;7:168–171.

Thin RN, Symonds MA, Booker R, et al. Double-blind comparison of a single dose and a five-day course of metronidazole in the treatment of trichomoniasis. Br J Vener Dis 1979;55:354–356.

Tidwell BH, Lushbaugh WB, Laughlin MD, et al. A double-blind placebo-controlled trial of single-dose intravaginal versus single-dose oral metronidazole in the treatment of trichomonal vaginitis. J Infect Dis 1994;170:242–246.

Wölner-Hanssen P, Krieger JN, Stevens CE, et al. Clinical manifestations of vaginal trichomoniasis. JAMA 1989;261:571–576.

CHAPTER

# 39

# *Bacterial Vaginosis*

*Jessica L. Thomason*
*N. J. Scaglione*

## BACKGROUND AND INCIDENCE

Bacterial vaginosis (formerly known as nonspecific vaginitis; *Haemophilus*, *Corynebacterium*, or *Gardnerella* vaginitis; nonspecific vaginosis; anaerobic vaginitis; or anaerobic vaginosis) is the most common form of vaginitis in reproductive-aged women. Prevalence varies from 5% of college populations to more than 60% of women treated at sexually transmitted disease clinics. Risk factors associated with increasing incidence include multiple sex partners, lower socioeconomic status, IUD usage, uncircumcised sex partners, smoking, and increasing parity. Bacterial vaginosis (BV) is believed to be a "sexually associated" disease, but obtaining proof of "sexual transmission" is impossible from an ethical standpoint in this modern era.

## PATHOPHYSIOLOGY

The exact etiology of BV is unknown. The theory that a single organism was responsible for the disease has given way to the knowledge that BV is polymicrobial. Massive overgrowth of the vaginal bacterial flora occurs, with anaerobic bacteria such as *Prevotella* sp. and *Mobiluncus* sp. predominating. Both *Gardnerella* and mycoplasmas are generally present in excessively high numbers.

An initiating factor that upsets the normal vaginal bacterial ecosystem is the virtual disappearance of the hydrogen peroxide-producing lactobacilli, which normally are the predominant controlling flora of the vagina. With the loss of this natural host defense, agents like *Gardnerella*, mycoplasmas, and anaerobes proliferate to attain excessively large numbers.

The anaerobes produce catabolic enzymes, such as aminopeptidases and decarboxylases. These enzymes degrade proteins and amino acids to amines. In turn, the amines contribute to the signs and symptoms of BV by elevating the vaginal pH and producing the characteristic odor associated with this syndrome. The decarboxylation of betaine, which is derived from choline, produces trimethylamine, which may produce the rotting fish odor that provides a strong diagnostic clue as to the existence of this syndrome.

Large numbers of the various types of bacteria harbored by BV patients attach to vaginal epithelial cell surfaces to form "clue" cells. These clue cells serve as a principal diagnostic marker for the syndrome.

## Diagnosis

Just as a woman may be asymptomatic with chlamydial or gonococcal infection, so a patient may remain asymptomatic with BV. In fact, more than half of all women with BV will present with no symptoms. Consequently, physicians must rely on objective diagnostic data obtained during the pelvic speculum examination rather than assume that the patient's vaginal discharge must be "normal" if she does not complain of symptoms.

If symptoms occur, the patient will report a profuse, malodorous, nonirritating discharge, which classically has the appearance of a cup of milk (homogeneous) poured into the vagina. This discharge may adhere to, but can easily be wiped from, the vaginal walls. In addition, the woman may complain of an offensive odor, which is especially prevalent after intercourse.

Certain indicators of the disease are both sensitive and specific (Table 39-1).

**Table 39-1.** Diagnosis of Bacterial Vaginosis

| |
|---|
| **Highly Specific Signs*** |
| Clue cells present |
| Fishy amine odor |
| *Mobiluncus* bacteria motility |
| **Less Specific Signs** |
| Vaginal pH > 4.5 |
| Lactobacilli fewer than background bacteria |
| Homogeneous discharge |

* For highly specific signs, the best sensitivity and specificity are obtained when clue cells and amine odor are detected.

### *Clue Cells*

The disease is best diagnosed by microscopic examination (wet preparation) of freshly collected vaginal secretions for clue cells. These vaginal epithelial cells are so densely covered with attached bacteria that the cell borders are no longer clearly discernible. These cells are virtually pathognomonic for the syndrome and can be observed at 400× magnification.

### *Fishy Amine Odor*

This odor can best be elicited by adding 10% to 20% potassium hydroxide to freshly collected vaginal secretions. It is considered virtually pathognomonic for BV. The same volatile amines are released when vaginal secretions are alkalinized by seminal fluid during intercourse in BV-infected patients. A recent highly sensitive and specific test using this indicator of disease has become commercially available (see the "Laboratory Test Results Revealing Bacterial Enzymes and Products" section later in this chapter).

### Mobiluncus *Bacteria*

The highly characteristic motility of the crescent-shaped *Mobiluncus* species is pathognomonic for BV. Motility is wavelike, with rapid movements of short duration occurring in a straight line or slightly arched direction, though the organism rarely moves out of the view field. Characteristic corkscrew or spinning activity becomes evident as one end of the bacterium appears to attach to epithelial cells or to the glass slide. The bacterium then may break away and move in its characteristic wavelike pattern before stopping again.

Seeing these bacteria in the vaginal secretions of a patient assures diagnosis of BV. Unfortunately, only some 50% of patients with BV have *Mobiluncus* bacteria visually present at wet preparation examination, making this objective sign highly specific but not very sensitive.

Other objective signs that indicate BV are less sensitive.

### pH Greater Than 4.5

Normally, vaginal (not endocervical) pH is approximately 4.0, except during menses. In BV, the pH is elevated by the amines to exceed 4.5. Many conditions, such as recent intercourse or douching, can falsely elevate pH. Although a finding of a vaginal pH of less than 4.5 virtually excludes the diagnosis of BV, a finding of a vaginal pH greater than 4.5 by itself does not establish the diagnosis. Use of other objective criteria is necessary.

### Absence of Lactobacilli

On Gram's stain, patients with BV exhibit a large number of small rods and coccobacillary bacterial morphotypes rather than the lactobacilli that predominate in normal healthy vaginal flora. This valuable indicator of abnormal vaginal flora appears to be only an early change in the BV disease process. Some women do not go on to develop BV, and their lactobacilli return to normal predominance. Determining the relative concentration of the bacterial morphotypes is an acceptable laboratory method for diagnosing BV.

### Homogeneous Discharge

The weakest and most subjective of the original classic signs of BV is homogeneous discharge. Variation in quantity of this discharge adds to difficulty of evaluation, making this sign less reliable.

### *Laboratory Test Results Revealing Bacterial Enzymes and Products*

The ability of an enzyme to detect proline aminopeptidase from bacteria present in high quantity in the secretions of patients with BV has recently been used to develop an accurate, rapid diagnostic tool for BV. This test combines the classic "amino" odor with pH on a test card. Vaginal secretions are rubbed directly onto the card, thereby eliminating the need for a microscopic evaluation of vaginal discharge. Preliminary data reveal this test to be both highly sensitive and highly specific. For the first time, a practical, efficient, and rapid way exists for making an accurate diagnosis of BV without using microscopic skills. Other laboratory tests found to have utility for research purposes only include gas-liquid chromatography and DNA probes for various bacteria.

### *Vaginal Culture for* Gardnerella *or Anaerobes*

Because as many as 40% of healthy women may have high numbers of *Gardnerella* or anaerobes present as normal flora, detection of these organisms is *not* a reliable predictor of BV and culture is therefore *not* advised. Furthermore, although anaerobic bacteria diminish with cure, *Gardnerella* levels can persist.

## Treatment

All women having symptoms of BV should be treated, regardless of pregnancy status. Treatment of asymptomatic women is becoming less controversial as more data are gathered showing serious infectious sequelae of untreated BV. Clinicians must make their own choices in determining treatment of the woman without symptoms by judging the risk/benefit ratio for that patient. (*Example:* Asymptomatic pregnant teen with a previous preterm birth—recommend treatment.) The following guidelines are suggested.

## Gynecologic

In asymptomatic women about to undergo elective vaginal or abdominal surgical procedures, treat to decrease the risk of postsurgical infections. Treat asymptomatic women about to undergo outpatient ambulatory invasive procedures, such as endometrial biopsy or hysterosalpingography. Consider treating asymptomatic woman at risk for pelvic inflammatory disease (PID). (*Example:* Treat postabortal women.)

## Obstetric

Consider treating the asymptomatic patient with a history of preterm labor, premature rupture of membranes (PROM), or previous delivery of an infant of low birthweight.

## Sex Partners

Although sexual intercourse is believed to be a primary method of transmitting BV, unequivocal proof of this relationship is lacking. Currently, treatment of sex partners is advised only in cases involving recurrent BV.

## Medication

The only medications considered effective for treating BV are metronidazole and clindamycin. Recommended treatment regimens for the nonpregnant woman include metronidazole, 500 mg orally daily for seven days, or intravaginal products. Clindamycin 2% cream, one applicator intravaginally at bedtime for five to seven days, and metronidazole 0.75% gel, one applicator intravaginally twice daily for three to five days or once daily for five days, are equally efficacious. Alternative regimens include clindamycin, 300 mg orally twice daily for seven days; metronidazole (Flagyl ER), 750 mg daily for seven days; and, with less efficacy, metronidazole as a single dose of 2 g.

Beginning at the earliest part of the second trimester, pregnant patients may be treated safely with metronidazole, 250 mg orally three times daily for seven days or 500 mg orally twice daily for seven days. Alternative regimens include clindamycin,

300 mg orally twice daily for seven days, or a much less well-tolerated oral single dose of 2 g metronidazole.

Douching and vaginal medications designed to lower vaginal pH may relieve symptoms but do not cure BV. Although once thought to be effective, antibiotics such as amoxicillin and sulfa are now considered less useful alternatives.

## Sequelae

Although vaginitis generally is considered benign, serious sequelae have been associated with BV. Obstetric patients are at significant risk for preterm labor, PROM, and preterm delivery. More recently, postpartum endometritis following vaginal or operative delivery and chorioamnionitis have been identified as serious sequelae.

Gynecologic infectious sequelae include an increased frequency of laparoscopically proven PID and posthysterectomy cuff cellulitis. In addition, patients with BV are at significant risk for recurrent urinary tract infections and nonpuerperal endometritis. Moreover, patients with BV have a higher incidence of cervical dysplasia.

### Suggested Readings

Centers for Disease Control and Prevention. 1998 guidelines for treatment of sexually transmitted diseases. MMWR 1998;47(RR-1):70–74.

Hillier SL, Nugent RP, Eschenbach DA, et al. Association between bacterial vaginosis and preterm delivery of a low-birth-weight infant. N Engl J Med 1995;333:1737–1742.

James JA, Thomason JL, Gelbart SM, et al. Is trichomoniasis often associated with bacterial vaginosis in pregnant adolescents? Am J Obstet Gynecol 1992;166:859–863.

Livengood CH III, Thomason JL, Hill GB. Bacterial vaginosis: treatment with topical intravaginal clindamycin phosphate. Obstet Gynecol 1990;76:118–123.

Spiegel CA, Amsel R, Holmes KK. Diagnosis of bacterial vaginosis by direct Gram stain of vaginal fluid. J Clin Microbiol 1983;18:170–177.

Thomason JL, Anderson RJ, Gelbart SM, et al. Simplified Gram stain interpretive method for diagnosis of bacterial vaginosis. Am J Obstet Gynecol 1992;167:16–19.

Thomason JL, Gelbart SM, Anderson RJ, et al. Statistical evaluation of diagnostic criteria for bacterial vaginosis. Am J Obstet Gynecol 1990;162:155–160.

Thomason JL, Gelbart SM, Scaglione NJ. Bacterial vaginosis: current review with indications for asymptomatic therapy. Am J Obstet Gynecol 1991;165:1210–1217.

Thomason JL, Gelbart SM, Wilcoski LM, et al: Proline aminopeptidase activity as a rapid diagnostic test to confirm bacterial vaginosis. Obstet Gynecol 1988;71:607–611.

CHAPTER

# 40

# *Vulvodynia*

*Mark D. Pearlman*
*Hope K. Haefner*

## BACKGROUND

Vulvodynia, a catch-all term for vulvar pain, is derived from the Greek word *odynia,* meaning pain. As defined by the International Society for the Study of Vulvar Diseases (ISSVD) in the early 1980s, vulvodynia is chronic vulvar discomfort that is especially characterized by complaints of burning, stinging, irritation, or rawness.

Because vulvar pain can derive from many sources, classification of vulvodynia can prove confusing. It has been described as "primary" (with onset from first tampon or sexual experience) or "secondary" (with onset coming months or years after first tampon or sexual experience); it has also been classified as either "pure" (occurring only with touch) or "mixed" (occurring with touch and at other times).

Clinically, it may be more useful to consider two major categories of vulvodynia: organic and idiopathic. *Organic* vulvodynia includes the many conditions that have a known cause (Table 40-1). *Idiopathic* vulvodynia, the subject of this chapter, includes all manifestations that have no apparent cause. In turn, idiopathic vulvodynia can be divided into two subcategories: dysesthetic or "essential" vulvodynia (pain not typically confined to the vestibule) and vulvar vestibulitis (pain confined to the vestibule). Dysesthetic vulvodynia more commonly affects perimenopausal and postmenopausal women, whereas vulvar vestibulitis patients tend to be younger.

**Table 40-1.** Organic (Identifiable) Causes of Vulvar Pain

| Infections | Trauma | Systemic Diseases | Preinvasive/Invasive Conditions | Irritants | Other Conditions |
|---|---|---|---|---|---|
| Bartholin's gland abscess | Sexual assault | Behçet's disease | Vulvar intraepithelial conditions | Soaps | Allergic or contact dermatitis |
| Candidal vaginitis | Other physical injuries | Crohn's disease | Invasive squamous cell carcinoma | Sprays | Eczema |
| Herpes genital infection | | Sjögren's syndrome | | Douches | Hidradenitis suppurativa |
| Herpes zoster | | Systemic lupus erythematosus | | Antiseptics | Lichen planus |
| Human papillomavirus infection | | | | Suppositories, creams | Lichen sclerosus |
| *Molluscum contagiosum* | | | | 5-Fluorouracil (5-FU) | Pemphigus |
| Trichomonal infection | | | | Trichloroacetic acid (TCA) | Pemphigoid |
| | | | | Podophyllin | Psoriasis |
| | | | | Laser treatment | Squamous cell hyperplasia |

## Prevalence

Very few studies have attempted to estimate the prevalence of vulvodynia. Goetsch evaluated the prevalence of vulvar pain in a general obstetrics and gynecology practice and also investigated the variation in normal vulvar sensation. During a six-month period, 210 patients were questioned about symptoms and examined for evidence of vestibular tenderness. Seventy-eight (37%) of the women demonstrated some signs of vulvar tenderness and 31 (15%) fit the clinical definition of vulvar vestibulitis syndrome.

## Presentation

The largest subset of idiopathic vulvodynia patients have vulvar vestibulitis. The vulvar vestibule is the area just outside the vagina extending from the hymen outward to a region where the epithelium becomes stratified, known as Hart's line. Vestibulitis typically presents with pain on tampon insertion or sexual intercourse. Although women with this presentation typically are in their twenties, this form of disease may be seen as early as the teen years and as late as menopause. Women with severe symptoms may also experience burning or throbbing at other times, such as when wearing tight clothing, jogging, or riding a bicycle or horse. In more severe cases, patients will experience these symptoms while sitting or walking, or even without any movement.

Duration of vulvar vestibulitis may vary from weeks to several years. Symptoms often begin after a woman has experienced some type of "infection" or trauma. Burning, stinging, irritation, or rawness at the vaginal opening (vestibule) with intercourse are the most common complaints. Interstitial cystitis, other bladder syndromes, and urethritis may be present as well.

## Etiology

A number of specific causes of vulvodynia exist (see Table 40-1). In the majority of patients presenting with vulvodynia, however, no cause can be identified. In many cases, the cause can be multifactorial, complicating the evaluation.

## Diagnosis

Vulvodynia is suggested by the patient's history. The examination should include gentle pressure with a cotton swab over several regions of the vestibule, and the severity of tenderness should be recorded. Look for obvious ulcerations, genital warts, or Bartholin's gland enlargement. Several tests may help to rule out organic causes of vulvodynia:

- Wet preparation, KOH, vaginal pH, and fungal culture to evaluate for *Candida* and other causes of vulvovaginitis
- Herpes culture, if ulcerations are present
- Colposcopy/vulvoscopy to identify tissue abnormalities such as vulvar intraepithelial neoplasia (VIN)
- Biopsy (under local anesthesia) of discrete vulvar lesions or obvious abnormalities

## Treatment

Vulvodynia can prove difficult to treat. Specific conditions like those listed in Table 40-1 may be more amenable to treatment (and are covered in other chapters of this book). Nonspecific conditions, such as vulvar vestibulitis, present a great challenge. Improvement may take weeks to months. Spontaneous remission of symptoms has occurred in some women; in other patients, multiple therapy attempts involving medical management have failed to relieve all symptoms. No single treatment program is successful in all women, and rapid resolution of symptomatic vulvodynia is unusual even with appropriate therapy. Many patients become frustrated with the failure to identify a specific cause for their symptoms, and they may change providers frequently in an effort to relieve their suffering.

Both dysesthetic vulvodynia and vulvar vestibulitis are commonly treated with norepinephrine reuptake inhibitors, such as amitriptyline. These drugs have been used to treat many other chronic pain conditions lacking an obvious cause. Norepinephrine reuptake inhibitors may work by inhibiting certain pain fibers that innervate the vulva. Common side effects include drowsiness, dry mouth, memory loss, and weight gain. Less common side effects include blurred vision, confusion or delirium, constipation (especially in older women), decreased sex drive, palpitations, and difficulty in swallowing. To minimize these unwanted effects, an incremental dosing protocol is very useful. In younger patients, amitriptyline, 10 mg to 25 mg at bedtime increased weekly by 10 mg to 25 mg increments to a maximum of 100 to 150 mg, has been useful. In older women particularly, or those with debilitating side effects, a regimen that begins at 5 to 10 mg and increases by 10 mg weekly is recommended. Often, a good response is seen at 50 mg nightly, but doses as high as 100 mg may be required.

Other treatments include topical lidocaine and various measures to control pain and itching, such as use of hydroxyzine hydrochloride (Atarax).

Patients should be advised to do the following:

1. Keep the vulva dry.
2. Avoid vulvar irritants.
3. Rinse the vulva with plain cool water after voiding.
4. Use mild soap (such as Neutrogena or Basis) on the vulva when bathing.
5. Wear loose clothing, especially during exercise.
6. Rinse clothing thoroughly to remove chemical soap or detergent irritants.
7. Use only 100% natural (unbleached) cotton menstrual pads.

In addition to antidepressants, many treatment options have been tried, despite the lack of a clear etiology for vulvodynia. These therapies have included oral gabapentin (Neurontin), transcutaneous electrical nerve stimulation (TENS), topical steroids, long-term topical antifungal therapy, local interferon injections, a low-oxalate diet with calcium citrate supplementation, pulse dye laser therapy (considered experimental), and surgical excision. With the exception of surgical excision, no long-term studies have proved the effectiveness of these therapies.

Interferon injections have been tried to treat vulvar vestibulitis regardless of the presence of human papillomavirus. Because long-term improvement with this approach has not been optimal, this therapy is rarely used. The low-oxalate diet approach was developed in response to a suggestion that the vulvar burning associated with vestibulitis might be associated with elevated levels of oxalates in the urine. One group of investigators has described improvement in patients following such a diet, combined with calcium citrate supplements. Their results have not been duplicated, however.

Biofeedback and/or physical therapy, which have been employed to treat various disorders characterized by chronic pain, are being used currently to treat vulvodynia with good success. These techniques are particularly helpful when the patient has concomitant vaginismus, which is not uncommon in this population. Biofeedback helps vulvodynia patients develop self-regulation strategies for confronting and reducing pain. Generally, women with vulvar vestibulitis have an increased resting tone and a decreased contraction tone. With a biofeedback machine, the patient can view numbers on a meter or colored lights to assess nerve and muscle tension. With practice, she can develop voluntary control over the biologic systems involved in pain, discomfort, and disease. The time required and frequency of visits varies according to the individual, but success rates of 60% to 80% have been reported with an experienced therapist.

Physical therapy has also produced some success. After a thorough evaluation and assessment of muscle tone and strength, posture, and mobility, a therapist with experience in managing vulvodynia can prescribe specific exercises aimed at correcting imbalances.

Surgical excision of the vulvar vestibule has met with success in as many as 60% to 80% of reported cases, but it should generally be considered a last-resort measure. Surgery should be reserved exclusively for women with long-standing and severe vestibulitis after all other management options have failed. $CO_2$ laser ablation of the vestibule has not been successful and has, in some cases, worsened or caused vulvodynia.

## Sequelae

Most patients with chronic idiopathic pain suffer from some level of depression. It is therefore necessary to address the emotional and psychosexual aspects of any form of vulvodynia. Accurate information and support are crucial for helping women cope with this condition. Referral to a qualified therapist is often an important component of successful management.

## Suggested Readings


Abramov L, Wolman I, David MP. Vaginismus: an important factor in the evaluation and management of vulvar vestibulitis syndrome. Gynecol Obstet Invest 1994;38:194–197.

Baggish MS, Sze EH, Johnson R. Urinary oxalate excretion and its role in vulvar pain syndrome. Am J Obstet Gynecol 1997; 177:507–511.

Bergeron S, Binik YM, Khalife S, et al. Vulvar vestibulitis syndrome: a critical review. Clin J Pain 1997;13:27–42.

Bergeron S, Bouchard C, Fortier M, et al. The surgical treatment of vulvar vestibulitis syndrome: a follow-up study. J Sex Marital Therapy 1997;23:317–325.

Bornstein J, Kaufman RH. Perineoplasty for vulvar vestibulitis. Harefuah 1989;116:90–92.

Friedrich EG Jr. Vulvar vestibulitis syndrome. J Reprod Med 1987;32:110–114.

Glazer HI, Rodke G, Swencionis C, et al. Treatment of vulvar vestibulitis syndrome with electromyographic biofeedback of pelvic floor musculature. J Reprod Med 1995;40:283–290.

Goetsch MF. Vulvar vestibulitis: prevalence and historic features in a general gynecologic practice population. Am J Obstet Gynecol 1991;164:1609–1614; discussion 1614–1616.

Jones KD, Lehr ST. Vulvodynia: diagnostic techniques and treatment modalities. Nurse Pract 1994;19:34–46.

Mann MS, Kaufman RH, Brown D, et al. Vulvar vestibulitis: significant clinical variables and treatment outcome. Obstet Gynecol 1992;79:122–125.

McKay M. Dysesthetic ("essential") vulvodynia. Treatment with amitriptyline. J Reprod Med 1993;38:9–13.

McKay M. Vulvodynia. A multifactorial clinical problem. Arch Dermatol 1989;125:256–262.

McKay M. Vulvodynia. Diagnostic patterns. Dermatol Clin 1992;10: 423–433.

Paavonen J. Diagnosis and treatment of vulvodynia. Ann Med 1995;27:175–181.

Paavonen J. Vulvodynia—a complex syndrome of vulvar pain. Acta Obstet Gynecol Scand 1995;74:243–247.

Schover LR, Youngs DD, Cannata R. Psychosexual aspects of the evaluation and management of vulvar vestibulitis. Am J Obstet Gynecol 1992;16:630–636.

Solomons CC, Melmed MH, Heitler SM. Calcium citrate for vulvar vestibulitis. A case report. J Reprod Med 1991;36:879–882.

Stewart DE, Reicher AE, Gerulath AH, et al. Vulvodynia and psychological distress. Obstet Gynecol 1994;84:587–590.

Van Lankveld JJ, Weijenborg PT, ter Kuile MM. Psychologic profiles of and sexual function in women with vulvar vestibulitis and their partners. Obstet Gynecol 1996;88:65–70.

White G, Jantos M, Glazer H. Establishing the diagnosis of vulvar vestibulitis. J Reprod Med 1997;42:157–160.

CHAPTER 41

# *HIV Infection and AIDS in the Gynecology Patient*

*Rhoda Sperling*

## Background

Human immunodeficiency virus (HIV) infection and the acquired immunodeficiency syndrome (AIDS) represent an enormous health problem for women. According to the World Health Organization, 42% of the estimated 21 million adults living with HIV/AIDS worldwide are women. In the United States, an estimated 107,000 to 150,000 women are living with HIV infection; many of these women have not yet developed advanced immunosuppression and AIDS. As of December 30, 1996, the Centers for Disease Control and Prevention (CDC) had received reports of 85,000 cases of AIDS among female adults, 48,186 of whom had died. Minority women are disproportionately affected by AIDS; of reported cases in the United States, 56% involve black women and 20% affect Hispanic women.

In the United States, factors associated with a woman testing HIV-seropositive include a history of any of the following: (1) intravenous drug use (IVDU); (2) unprotected intercourse with HIV-infected men or men with high-risk behavior (IVDUs or bisexual men); (3) prostitution or multiple sexual partners; (4) residence in a country with a high prevalence of HIV infection; or (5) blood transfusions between 1978 and 1985. During unprotected intercourse with an infected partner, women appear to be more easily infected than men. Epidemiologic studies have identified cofactors that can facilitate HIV-1 transmission, including genital ulcer disease, anal-receptive intercourse, and severity of HIV-related immunosuppression in a sexual partner.

## Pathophysiology

The etiologic agent of AIDS is a retrovirus designated as human immunodeficiency virus type 1 (HIV-1). The T-helper lymphocyte (CD4+ T lymphocyte) represents the primary target for HIV infection, because the virus shows a marked affinity for the CD4+ surface marker. The CD4+ T lymphocyte coordinates a number of important immunologic functions, and a loss of these functions results in a progressive impairment of the immune response.

## Diagnosis

Clinicians should be aware of the spectrum of illness represented by HIV infection and should be prepared to recognize the following presentations.

### Primary Infection

An acute clinical illness associated with HIV-1 seroconversion occurs in 50% to 70% of cases. The incubation period from exposure to time of onset typically lasts two to four weeks (average 21.4 days). This generally self-limiting illness resolves in one to three weeks. It can be associated with an appreciable degree of morbidity, and patients may require hospitalization.

The main clinical feature of primary HIV-1 infection reflects both the lymphocytopathic and neurologic tropism of HIV-1. Patients typically present with an acute illness characterized by fever, lethargy, malaise, myalgias, headaches, retro-orbital pain, photophobia, sore throat, lymphadenopathy, and maculopapular rash. Seroconversion in primary infection is prompt. Second-generation anti-HIV-1 enzyme-linked immunosorbent (ELISA, EIA) assays tend to become positive from 14 to 21

**Table 41-1.** HIV-Related Conditions

| |
|---|
| Bacillary angiomatosis |
| Candidiasis, oropharyngeal |
| Candidiasis, vulvovaginal—persistent, frequent, or poorly responsive to therapy |
| Cervical dysplasia (moderate or severe)/cervical carcinoma in situ |
| Constitutional symptoms, such as fever (38.5 °C) or diarrhea lasting one month or longer |
| Hairy leukoplakia |
| Herpes zoster (shingles) involving at least two distinct episodes or more than one dermatome |
| Idiopathic thrombocytopenic purpura |
| Listeriosis |
| Pelvic inflammatory disease, particularly if complicated by tubo-ovarian abscess |
| Peripheral neuropathy |

days after onset of symptoms. The median time from initial infection to the development of detectable anti-HIV-1 antibodies is 2.1 months, with 95% of individuals developing antibodies within 5.8 months of their initial infections.

## Clinical Latency

During the period of clinical latency, active viral replication occurs and CD4+ T lymphocytes undergo a progressive decline. Many conditions, although not pathognomonic for AIDS, may be associated with progressive immunosuppression and are classified by the CDC as HIV-related (Table 41-1). These conditions include recurrent vulvovaginal candidiasis, cervical dysplasia, pelvic inflammatory disease (PID), unexplained fever lasting more than 30 days, unexplained weight loss, herpes zoster involving two distinct dermatomes, and idiopathic thrombocytopenic purpura. All of these conditions may be reported by a woman seeking medical care from an obstetrician-gynecologist. If any of these conditions are diagnosed, the clinician should encourage the patient to undergo HIV testing.

## AIDS

Effective January 1, 1993, the CDC expanded the surveillance case definition for AIDS. The expanded case definition classifies a woman as having AIDS if she is an HIV-infected adult with:

1. A CD4+ T-lymphocyte count of less than 200 cells/mm$^3$ or less than 14% of total lymphocytes;
2. Pulmonary tuberculosis;
3. Recurrent bacterial pneumonia (more than one episode in a one-year period); or
4. Invasive cervical cancer.

These criteria have been added to the 23 other clinical conditions that the 1987 CDC guidelines previously specified as criteria for patients having AIDS (Table 41-2). The decision to include cervical cancer as an AIDS-defining condition was controversial, as it was based on information taken from small, uncontrolled case series. The available epidemiologic evidence suggests an increased prevalence of cervical dysplasia, the precursor of cervical cancer, in HIV-infected women. In addition, it suggests an adverse effect of HIV infection on the progression, clinical course, and treatment of both cervical dysplasia and cancer.

## MANAGEMENT

### Patient Monitoring—Immunologic Profile

The T-helper (CD4+) cell count is a commonly used surrogate marker for assessing HIV-related disease progression. Individuals who have absolute T-helper cell counts of less than 200 cells/mm$^3$ are at high risk for the early development of the opportunistic infections that define AIDS. Clinically, T-cell counts are used to determine the point at which prophylactic therapies should begin. In nonpregnant adults, routine primary prophylaxis is recommended for *Pneumocystis carinii* infection when the CD4+ cell counts are less than 200 cells/mm$^3$, for *Toxoplasma gondii* infection when toxoplasma IgG-seropositive adults have CD4+ cell counts of less than 100 cells/mm$^3$, and for *Mycobacterium avium* complex (MAC) infection when the CD4+ cell count is less than 50 cells/mm$^3$.

**Table 41-2.** Conditions Included in the 1993 CDC AIDS Surveillance Case Definition

| |
|---|
| Candidiasis of bronchi, trachea, or lungs |
| Candidiasis, esophageal |
| Cervical cancer, invasive |
| Coccidioidomycosis, disseminated or extrapulmonary |
| Cryptococcosis, extrapulmonary |
| Cryptosporidiosis, chronic intestinal (more than one month's duration) |
| Cytomegalovirus disease (other than liver, spleen, or nodes) |
| Cytomegalovirus retinitis (with loss of vision) |
| Encephalopathy, HIV-related |
| Herpes simplex, chronic ulcer(s) (more than one month's duration) or bronchitis, pneumonitis, or esophagitis |
| Histoplasmosis, disseminated or extrapulmonary |
| Isosporiasis, chronic intestinal (more than one month's duration) |
| Kaposi's sarcoma |
| Lymphoma, Burkitt's (or equivalent term) |
| Lymphoma, immunoblastic (or equivalent term) |
| Lymphoma, primary, of brain |
| *Mycobacterium avium* complex or *M. kansasii*, disseminated or extrapulmonary |
| *Mycobacterium tuberculosis*, any site (pulmonary or extrapulmonary) |
| *Mycobacterium*, other species or unidentified species, disseminated or extrapulmonary |
| *Pneumocystis carinii* pneumonia |
| Pneumonia, recurrent |
| Progressive multifocal leukoencephalopathy |
| *Salmonella* septicemia, recurrent |
| Toxoplasmosis of brain |
| Wasting syndrome due to HIV |

## Patient Monitoring—Viral Load

Studies have demonstrated that plasma viral load can predict the progression of HIV infection to AIDS. Combination therapy with antiretrovirals can reduce plasma HIV RNA and increase CD4+ cell counts. Clinicians now routinely use plasma viral load determinations to decide when to initiate therapy and to determine the adequacy of the patient's response to therapy.

The tests most commonly used for viral load determinations are branched deoxyribonucleic acid (bDNA) and reverse transcriptase polymerase chain reaction (RT-PCR) assays; the results of these tests are reported as the plasma RNA copy number per milliliter.

## Antiretroviral Therapy

The goal of antiretroviral therapy is to control viral replication. For nonpregnant adults, the standard of care continues to evolve as the understanding of the pathophysiology of HIV grows. The number of effective drugs continues to expand rapidly.

Antiretroviral regimens that reduce high viral loads are associated with better outcomes and fewer opportunistic infections or deaths. Therapeutic agents that inhibit different parts of the HIV-1 viral replication cycle are used in combination; these combination regimens are often able to achieve (at least for a short time) plasma viral levels undetectable by current assays. The likelihood of successful viral suppression resulting in a "cure," with complete HIV-1 eradication and immune reconstitution, remains in doubt. In fact, replication-competent HIV-1 virus has been isolated from memory CD4+ T lymphocytes in patients who had been virologically suppressed for more than two years.

Currently, 11 antiretroviral drugs have received FDA approval, including five nucleoside reverse transcriptase inhibitors (zidovudine, didanosine, zalcitibine, lamivudine, and stavudine), two non-nucleoside reverse transcriptase inhibitors (nevirapine and delaviridine), and four potent protease inhibitors (ritonavir, indinavir, nelfinavir, and saquinavir). Four investigational drugs (abacavir, efavirenz, amprenavir, and adefovir dipovoxil) are in advanced stages of clinical evaluation.

Choices for multidrug regimens are not a simple reflection of possible combinations. Practical issues such as drug compatibilities, adverse effects, and cross-resistance constrain the options available. The initial therapies that are most commonly utilized in clinical practice are three-drug regimens that combine two nucleoside reverse transcriptase inhibitors with a potent protease inhibitor.

The initiation of antiretroviral therapy represents a long-term commitment. Factors to consider before recommending that a patient initiate highly active antiretroviral therapy (HAART) include the following:

- The relative ability of available regimens to inhibit HIV-1 replication for prolonged periods of time (durability of the response)
- The relative ability of available agents to delay or prevent the emergence of drug-resistant HIV variants
- The relationship between the emergence of drug resistance and treatment failures
- The short-term and long-term adverse effects
- The impact on quality of life of adhering to these regimens
- The patient's ability and/or motivation to adhere to a complex treatment regimen

Adherence to a prescribed regimen is crucial to maintaining inhibition of viral replication and reducing the risk of drug resistance. For asymptomatic patients with low plasma RNA levels (for example, less than 5000 to 10,000 copies/mL) and high CD4+ cell counts (for example, more than 350 to 500 cells/mm$^3$), deferral of treatment and close follow-up may be appropriate, given the complexity of treatment and the risk of adverse effects.

## Associated Gynecologic Manifestations of HIV Disease

Women may experience HIV-associated gynecologic problems, many of which also occur in uninfected women but with less frequency or severity. Problems that have been reported to date include vulvovaginal candidiasis, genital ulcer disease, genital tract HPV disease, and PID.

### Vulvovaginal Candidiasis

Mucosal candidiasis (vaginal, oropharyngeal, and esophageal) is common among women with HIV infection. In one series from a university-based AIDS program, 59% of women reported that they experienced frequent vaginal candidal infections even before other signs of immune system compromise became evident. In addition, they reported the progression of candidal infection from vagina to oropharynx to esophagus, which was associated with decreasing CD4+ cell counts.

In a recent clinical trial, weekly oral prophylaxis with 200 mg of fluconazole proved effective in reducing the frequency of recurrent mucosal candidiasis in women with CD4+ cell counts of 300 cells/mm$^3$ or less. In this study, clinical or in vitro resistance to fluconazole was rare and did not increase in the fluconazole group.

## Genital Ulcer Disease

Genital ulcer disease is another common condition among women with HIV infection. A retrospective cohort study of 307 women reported a 14% prevalence of genital ulcers during a 20-month follow-up period. Twelve (28%) of the 43 women tested positive for herpes simplex virus-2 (HSV-2); five (12%) of 43 had unusual or mixed bacteriologic pathogens; and 26 (60%) of 43 had no identifiable pathogen despite diagnostic tests. Other investigators have observed idiopathic genital ulcers, without evidence of an infectious or neoplastic origin. An ongoing multicenter trial is attempting to assess the prevalence of idiopathic genital ulcers in women infected with HIV-1 and to elucidate the effectiveness of thalidomide treatment. Thalidomide has already been proved an effective treatment of idiopathic aphthous ulceration of the mouth and oropharynx in HIV-infected adults.

In patients infected with HIV-1, herpes recurrences appear to be more frequent, more prolonged, and more severe, especially with advancing immunosuppression. A mucocutaneous herpes episode lasting longer than one month is considered to be an AIDS-defining condition. Acute episodes of HSV infection usually respond to administration of oral acyclovir. Persons who experience frequent or severe episodes can receive daily suppressive acyclovir therapy. Acyclovir-resistant isolates have been reported; in such cases, treatment with intravenous foscarnet or cidofovir is recommended.

## Human Papillomavirus Infections (HPV)

HPV infections are more common among HIV-seropositive women with all levels of immunosuppression. When compared with control populations, HIV-infected women have increased rates of anogenital HPV disease (both asymptomatic shedding and visible condyloma), higher prevalence rates of cervical dysplasia, and higher failure rates following standard treatment of cervical dysplasia. Some investigators have also reported that these patients have an increased risk for multifocal dysplasia and higher risk for progression of dysplasia to cervical cancer. Despite the recent inclusion of cervical cancer in the AIDS case definition, high rates of cervical cancer have not been reported to date among AIDS cases.

Specifically, studies from the United States have estimated the prevalence of CIN in HIV-infected women at 15% to 42%. In contrast, rates of cervical dysplasia in urban populations are typically 3% to 5%.

Higher failure rates after standard treatment for cervical dysplasia have been a consistent finding in many populations studied. In one study of women infected with HIV-1 who were treated by loop electrosurgical excision (LEEP), persistent or recurrent CIN was documented in 56% of HIV-infected women, as compared with 13% of women with unknown serostatus within six months of initial treatment. Multiple investigators have reported high failure rates following standard cryosurgery as well.

Preliminary reports suggest that HIV-infected cervical cancer patients may present with more advanced cancer than HIV-negative patients, thus raising the possibility that HIV-related immunodeficiency might accelerate the invasive process. A recently published multivariate analysis from the same centers, however, found that HIV status was not an independent predictor of advanced cervical cancer. According to this analysis, in both HIV-infected and HIV-negative women, lack of cytologic screening and prolonged duration of symptoms were the only independent predictors.

The clinical management of HIV-infected women must include routine Pap smear evaluations. The Agency for Health Care Policy and Research recommends that a Pap smear be obtained twice in the first year after diagnosis of HIV infection and, if the results are normal, annually thereafter. Prospective trials are under way that will assess the risk for disease progression following standard treatment for dysplasia and study the utility of adjuvant treatments. Until these results become available, patients should be managed according to accepted standards.

## Pelvic Inflammatory Disease

High rates of HIV seroprevalence have been reported in women admitted to hospitals for treatment of PID. Indeed, the same behavior that places a patient at risk of acquiring sexually transmitted HIV may also place her at risk of acquiring PID.

Data from retrospective studies have suggested that PID may follow a more aggressive course in HIV-infected women. A CDC-funded prospective, multicenter trial of PID that compared HIV-infected women and controls with respect to microbiologic etiology, initial presentation, and response to therapy has been completed. Preliminary analyses have demonstrated that seropositive women appeared more severely ill at initial presentation, with significantly higher proportions of women being diagnosed with endometritis, fever, pelvic masses, and higher abdominal tenderness scores. After 48 to 72 hours, however, responses to standard treatment did not differ between the two groups. Future analyses from this study will focus on possible differences in the risk for clinical relapse and differences in microbiologic etiology.

### Suggested Readings

Adachi A, Fleming I, Burk RD, et al. Women with immunodeficiency virus infection and abnormal Papanicolaou smears: a prospective study of colposcopy and clinical outcome. Obstet Gynecol 1993; 81:372–377.

Carpenter CC, Fischl MA, Hammer SM, et al. Antiretroviral therapy for HIV infection in 1996. JAMA 1996;276:146–154.

Carpenter CC, Fischl MA, Hammer SM, et al. Antiretroviral therapy for HIV infection in 1998: updated recommendations of the International AIDS Society—USA Panel. JAMA 1998;280:78–86.

Centers for Disease Control and Prevention. 1993 revised classification system for HIV infection and expanded surveillance case definition for AIDS among adolescents and adults. MMWR 1992; 41(RR-17):1–19.

Centers for Disease Control and Prevention. The 1997 USPHS/IDSA guidelines for the prevention of opportunistic infections in persons infected with human immunodeficiency virus. MMWR 1997; 46(RR-12):1–46.

Centers for Disease Control and Prevention. Report of the NIH Panel to Define Principles of Therapy of HIV Infection and guidelines for the use of antiretroviral agents in HIV-infected adults and adolescents. MMWR 1998;47(RR-5):1–82.

Centers for Disease Control and Prevention. Risk for cervical disease in HIV-infected women—New York City. MMWR 1990; 39:846–849.

Fruchter RG, Maiman M, Arrastia CD, et al. Is HIV infection a risk factor for advanced cervical cancer? J Acquir Immune Defic Syndr Hum Retrovirol 1998;18:241–245.

Fruchter RG, Maiman M, Sedlis A, et al. Multiple recurrences of cervical intraepithelial neoplasia in women with the human immunodeficiency virus. Obstet Gynecol 1996;87:338–344.

Hoegsberg B, Abulafia O, Sedlis A, et al. Sexually transmitted diseases and human immunodeficiency virus infection among women with pelvic inflammatory disease. Am J Obstet Gynecol 1990;163:1135–1139.

Imam N, Carpenter CC, Mayer KH, et al. Hierarchical pattern of mucosal *Candida* infections in HIV-seropositive women. Am J Med 1990;89:142–146.

Jacobson JM, Greenspan JS, Spritzler J, et al. Thalidomide for the treatment of oral aphthous ulcers in patients with human immunodeficiency virus infection. N Engl J Med 1997;336: 1487–1493.

Kurman RJ, Henson DE, Herbst AL, et al. Interim guidelines for management of abnormal cervical cytology. The 1992 National Cancer Institute workshop. JAMA 1994;271:1866–1869.

LaGuardia KD, White MH, Saigo PE, et al. Genital ulcer disease in women infected with human immunodeficiency virus. Am J Obstet Gynecol 1995;172:552–562.

Maiman M, Fruchter RG, Clark M, et al. Cervical cancer as an AIDS-defining illness. Obstet Gynecol 1997;89:76–80.

Maiman M, Fruchter RG, Guy L, et al. Human immunodeficiency virus infection and invasive cervical carcinoma. Cancer 1993; 71:402–406.

Pantaleo G, Graziosi C, Fauci AS. New concepts in the immunopathogenesis of human immunodeficiency virus infection. N Engl J Med 1993;328:327–335.

Safrin S, Dattel BJ, Hauer L, et al. Seroprevalence and epidemiologic correlates of human immunodeficiency virus infection in women with pelvic inflammatory disease. Obstet Gynecol 1990;75:666–670.

Schuman P, Capps L, Peng G. Weekly fluconazole for the prevention of mucosal candidiasis in women with HIV infection. Ann Intern Med 1997;126:689–696.

Wright TC Jr, Koulos J, Schnoll F, et al. Cervical intraepithelial neoplasia in women infected with the human immunodeficiency virus: outcome after loop electrosurgical excision. Gynecol Oncol 1994;55:253–258.

CHAPTER

# 42

# HIV Interactions with Other Sexually Transmitted Diseases

*Daniel V. Landers*
*Geraldo Duarte*

## Background

The most common mode of transmission for human immunodeficiency virus type-1 (HIV) worldwide is heterosexual intercourse. Published studies suggest that a number of behavioral and biologic cofactors may significantly enhance the efficiency of transmission by this route. Emerging as one of the most important of these cofactors is the presence of other sexually transmitted diseases (STDs). Epidemiologic studies have identified enhanced risk of HIV acquisition in association with both ulcerative and nonulcerative STDs, including chancroid, syphilis, genital herpes, gonorrhea, chlamydial infection, trichomoniasis, and genital warts.

Clinical studies of genital tract HIV viral load and inflammation in the genital tract suggest that certain biologic mechanisms are at work in this relationship. Experimental laboratory models have been used to produce in vitro data on direct and indirect effects of STDs on HIV replication and infectivity, providing investigators with the means to study the molecular mechanisms involved in STD–HIV interactions. Also, widespread screening and treatment of STDs have led to a significant reduction in HIV acquisition during intervention trials. This result suggests that STDs not only are associated with an increased risk of HIV acquisition, but also may have a direct role in causation. In this chapter, we review the epidemiologic, biologic, molecular, and clinical data on STD–HIV interactions and potential interventions.

## Epidemiology

Epidemiologic studies may identify risk factors or other variables that may be associated with an outcome; these studies must be carefully controlled, however, so as to avoid assignment of spurious risk and misleading conclusions. As an STD, HIV infection shares demographic and behavioral risk factors with other STDs. These factors must be controlled to identify true biologic risk.

Further confounding of study results can occur because of the high coinfection rate associated with multiple STDs. Large, prospective, longitudinal cohort studies are needed to determine true associations between individual STDs and risk of HIV acquisition. The heterogeneity in gender and sexual behavior of populations acquiring STDs hampers efforts to identify specific risk factors for HIV acquisition. In preparing this review, the authors therefore focused on studies that used multivariate analyses to control for confounding variables. Furthermore, we gave greater weight to longitudinal and prospective case-control studies than to cross-sectional studies, because cause-and-effect relationships can be identified accurately only by longitudinal studies. True causality requires intervention trials showing that expected outcomes are altered by appropriate intervention.

## HIV and Genital Ulcer Disease

In 1992, Judith Wasserheit reviewed 25 reports that used multivariate analyses with at least some measure of sexual behavior to address STD-associated HIV transmission risk. Her review included 17 cross-sectional and 8 prospective or nested case-control studies representing 15 different study populations. She noted that two of three prospective or nested case-control studies and four of seven cross-sectional studies detected a significant association between HIV transmission and genital ulcer disease (GUD), primarily chancroid. The two longitudinal studies involved heterosexual populations in Kenya and Zaire. These prospective studies controlled for sexual behavior, and two of three showed an increased risk of HIV seroconversion. The male-to-female risk was increased, with an odds ratio (OR) of 3.3; the female-to-male OR was 4.7. The third study had a low incidence of genital ulcers in its population and did not detect an enhanced risk associated with genital ulcers.

The highest risk estimate appeared in a cross-sectional study of men based on physical diagnosis of GUD; in this study, the OR was 18.2 for circumcised men. The three case-control studies in which no significant association was found between GUD and HIV seropositivity were performed in women, and two of these relied on a history of GUD without clinical or laboratory verification. More recently, GUD has been associated with HIV in two prospective, longitudinal cohort studies (OR: 2.9–4.7; CI: 1.3–15.6) and two cross-sectional studies (OR: 2.0–3.9; CI: 1.0–7.4).

## HIV and Syphilis

The associated HIV risk attributable to the individual ulcerative STDs is not well established, because most studies group both syphilis and genital herpes as GUDs. Nevertheless, a significant association between syphilis and HIV infection was found in two of two prospective and seven of nine case-control studies that controlled for behavioral risk factors. Risk estimates were slightly higher for heterosexual men (median OR: 6.0) than for women (median OR: 4.0). Since these reports were made, five more cross-sectional studies have been published showing an association between HIV seropositivity and syphilis, with ORs ranging from 1.65 to 6.0.

## HIV and Herpes

The association of HIV seropositivity and genital herpes has been addressed in three prospective (in males only) and three cross-sectional studies. No association was reported in two of three prospective and one of three cross-sectional studies, including one cross-sectional study of female sex workers in the Philippines. Three additional cross-sectional studies have been published in the past three years, two of which showed an association between genital herpes and HIV.

## HIV and Nonulcerative STDs

Nonulcerative STDs, such as chlamydial infection, gonorrhea, and trichomoniasis, are more prevalent than GUDs and thus may present a greater attributable HIV risk. Many investigators have reported an association of chlamydial infection with HIV serconversion. In two of four prospective studies, both of which focused on African sex workers, a significant association was found, with a median OR of 4.5 (95% CI: 3.2–5.7). Three of eight cross-sectional studies showed a significant association between chlamydial infection and HIV seropositivity; three case-control studies did not detect an association. Gonorrhea was associated with an increased risk of HIV seroconversion in 2 of 7 prospective and 9 of 13 case-control studies that controlled to some extent for sexual behavior. In one prospective, longitudinal study, trichomoniasis was detected three times more often among female sex workers seroconverting to HIV than among those not seroconverting. In two subsequent longitudinal studies, however, no significant association was found between trichomoniasis and HIV seroconversion. Only one of four case-control studies showed trichomoniasis associated with HIV seropositivity.

It is apparent that epidemiologic studies in this area of research are plagued by confounding variables and shared risk factors that make it difficult to interpret even prospective, longitudinal studies. Moreover, many of these studies include a mixture of men and women that dilutes any gender-specific effects. For example, if having gonorrhea in the endocervix was a significant risk factor for HIV acquisition and a cohort of couples was studied for seroconversion over time, only females who were uninfected with *Chlamydia* (but without gonorrhea) and who seroconverted could be included in the analysis; enormous numbers of subjects would therefore be required to demonstrate statistical significance.

## HIV and Vaginitis

Bacterial vaginosis (BV), though not an STD in the classic sense, is associated with sexual activity and represents a disturbance in the normal vaginal ecosystem. A large cross-sectional study demonstrated that BV is associated with an enhanced risk of HIV acquisition. The relative risk for HIV acquisition in the presence of severe BV (by Gram's stain scoring) was 2.08 (range of 1.48 to 2.94). Two longitudinal cohort studies have also reported on the relationship between BV and HIV, one using nonstandard diagnostic criteria and the other Gram's stain. The relative risk of HIV acquisition was not significantly enhanced in either study.

The theoretic concern that the loss of endogenous lactobacilli might lead to an increase in pH and possible enhanced transmission of HIV is not supported by results of current epidemiologic studies. Two cross-sectional studies have associated BV with HIV seropositivity (ORs of 2.08 and 4.0, respectively).

Because BV is not a single organism but rather a summation of the effects of altered vaginal flora resulting in (1) excess anaerobes, (2) the presence of *Gardnerella vaginalis,* (3) elevated pH, and (4) a paucity of lactobacilli, this diagnosis may include a heterogeneous population of individuals with different patterns of altered microflora. It is conceivable that the presence of specific anaerobes in high concentrations rather than BV per se, as diagnosed by Gram's stain, may lead to increased risk of HIV acquisition or transmission. This enhancement may not be detected, however, because the diagnostic methodology for BV is not specific for any particular anaerobe (for example, *Prevotella bivia*).

Vulvovaginal candidiasis is also not technically an STD, although epidemiologic associations between this condition and HIV have been reported. In one of two longitudinal (OR of 3.3) and one of two cross-sectional studies, vaginal candidiasis has been associated with HIV seroconversion or seropositivity.

## Clinical and Laboratory Observations

In assessing enhancement of HIV risk by the presence of other STDS, two clinically relevant situations must be considered. The first is the HIV-infected individual with an STD who exposes a partner uninfected by HIV or an STD. The second is the HIV-infected individual who exposes an HIV-negative partner who has an STD. In the first situation, the effects of the concurrent STD on HIV infectivity and replication may influence the size and characteristics of the viral inoculation. In the second, the STD may alter host defenses in the partner's genital tract and increase that individual's susceptibility to HIV acquisition. Some clinical data appear to be relevant to both of these situations. Moss and colleagues studied 106 HIV-positive men and found that detection of HIV-infected cells in urethral secretions was independently associated with gonococcal infection (OR of 3.2). These researchers also found that treatment of urethritis was associated with a twofold reduction in urethral HIV DNA.

Other investigators have identified significant associations between cervical inflammation and cervical HIV DNA. More recent reports confirm that HIV RNA—presumably representing actively replicating virus—has been found in increased concentrations in the seminal plasma of men with both chlamydial and gonococcal urethritis and that these levels drop significantly after treatment of the urethritis. These studies and others raise suspicions that genital tract inflammation involving both inflammatory cells and their soluble cell products (cytokines and others) may directly increase the amount of HIV to which an uninfected partner is exposed. This potential for enhanced risk may be affected by treatment with antiretroviral agents, which in turn may lower both the genital tract viral load and the plasma viral load.

As for HIV-negative partners with an STD, alterations in host defenses may render them more susceptible by increasing the number of HIV target cells and thus enriching the environment with proinflammatory cytokines that enhance HIV replication or chemokines with potential to serve as coreceptors for viral entry. This tendency may apply to female-to-male HIV transmission, but especially applies in cases of male-to-female transmission. An increase in inflammation and associated inflammatory cells in the genital tract has been associated with some STDs. Recently Levine and coworkers reported increased numbers of endocervical CD4 lymphocytes in women with an STD (gonorrhea, chlamydial infection, or trichomoniasis). Several STDs have been associated with recruitment of inflammatory leukocytes to the genital tract and the presence of proinflammatory cytokines.

In 1995, Ho and colleagues demonstrated that the polymorphonuclear neutrophil leukocytes (PMNs) and peripheral blood mononuclear cells (PBMCs) up-regulate HIV expression in vitro and that these effects could be enhanced by the presence of *Chlamydia trachomatis*. Two years later, the authors' group at the University of Pittsburgh found that certain biovars of *C. trachomatis* may induce different patterns of up-regulation of HIV expression in vitro and that these effects can be enhanced by the presence of inflammatory leukocytes. These changes in HIV replication correlated with cytokine levels, including those of the proinflammatory cytokines TNF-α and IL-6. *Neisseria gonorrhoeae* has also been shown to enhance HIV replication in vitro—an effect that could be enhanced by the presence of inflammatory leukocytes. Additional laboratory studies have demonstrated a virucidal effect of *Lactobacilli acidophilus* on HIV and a significant reduction in HIV replication by peroxide-producing *Lactobacillus crispatus* in vitro.

## Interventions and Control

In 1995, a published report demonstrated the effect of STD treatment on HIV transmission. It described results of a community-based syndromic approach to treating symptomatic STDs that was carried out in 12 communities of Tanzania, each comprising approximately 1000 adults. The rate of HIV seroconversion was 1.2% in the intervention community and 1.9% in the control community, representing a 40% reduction. The estimated risk ratio was 0.58 (95% CI: 0.42–0.79; $P < 0.007$). This difference was attributed to a reduction in the duration, and hence the prevalence, of symptomatic STDs.

In another study in Tanzania, a community-based randomized trial was undertaken to assess the impact, cost, and cost-effectiveness of averting HIV infection through improved management of STDs by primary health care workers. The investigators estimated that treatment of 632 STD cases averted 232 HIV infections (40% reduction). This strategy was also estimated to be highly cost-effective and to compare favorably with the childhood immunization program.

In a randomized, controlled trial of STD control by home-based, mass antibiotic treatment, there was no effect on HIV acquisition.

## Summary

An increasing rate of HIV acquisition is occurring among individuals who are at risk for other STDs. The synergy between HIV and STDs relates to both behavioral and biologic factors. Consequently, the integration of HIV and STD services must become a worldwide priority. This program must include efforts to (1) induce behavior modification to change sexual practices, (2) promote condom use, and (3) achieve better control of STDs. Every HIV prevention program should include STD screening, control, and treatment. STD patients must receive counseling about their increased risk of HIV acquisition, and HIV-infected individuals must be informed of the importance of viral load, STDs, and transmissibility. Finally, the complex interrelationship of STDs and HIV requires further research to define specific biologic and epidemiologic mechanisms that enhance HIV transmission.

In May 1997, the Advisory Committee for HIV and STD Prevention reviewed data on the relationship between curable STDs and the rise of sexual transmission of HIV. The committee made the following recommendations:

1. Early detection and treatment of curable STDs should be a major part of HIV prevention programs at the national, state, and local levels.
2. Where STDs that facilitate HIV are prevalent, screening and treatment programs should be expanded.

3. In implementing these strategies, HIV and STD prevention programs in the United States should be the joint responsibility of private- and public-sector partners.

## Suggested Readings


Advisory Committee for HIV and STD Prevention. HIV prevention through early detection and treatment of other sexually transmitted diseases. United States. MMWR 1998;47(RR-12):1–24.

Cohen CR, Duerr A, Pruithithada N, et al. Bacterial vaginosis and HIV seroprevalence among female commercial sex workers in Chiang Mai, Thailand. AIDS 1995;9:1093–1097.

Cohen MS, Hoffman IF, Royce RA, et al. Reduction of concentration of HIV-1 in semen after treatment of urethritis: implications for prevention of sexual transmission of HIV-1. Lancet 1997;349: 1868–1873.

Duarte G, Cosentino LA, Creighton DJ, et al. *Neisseria gonorrhoeae* and associated inflammatory neutrophils upregulate HIV-1 expression in vitro. Abstracts of Annual Meeting of the Infectious Diseases Society for Obstetrics and Gynecology. Infect Dis Obstet Gynecol 1998; 6:82–83.

Grosskurth H, Mosha F, Todd J, et al. Impact of improved treatment of sexually transmitted diseases on HIV-1 infection in rural Tanzania: randomised controlled trial. Lancet 1995;346:530–536.

Hillier SL. The vaginal microbial ecosystem and resistance to HIV. AIDS Res Hum Retroviruses 1998;4(suppl 1):S17–S21.

Ho JL, He S, Hu A, et al. Neutrophils from HIV-seronegative donors induce HIV replication from HIV-infected patients' mononuclear cells and cell lines: an in vitro model of HIV transmission facilitated by *Chlamydia trachomatis*. J Exp Med 1995;181:1493–1505.

Klebanoff SJ, Coombs RW. Viricidal effect of *Lactobacillus acidophilus* on human immunodeficiency virus type 1: possible role in heterosexual transmission. J Exp Med 1991;174:289–292.

Laga M, Manoka A, Kivuvu M, et al. Non-ulcerative sexually transmitted diseases as risk factors for HIV-1 transmission in women: results from a cohort study. AIDS 1993;7:95–102.

Landers DV, Mills JP, Moncada J, et al. Cytokine secretion in *Chlamydia trachomatis* induced upregulation of HIV-1 in vitro. Paper presented at International Congress of Sexually Transmitted Diseases, October 1997, Seville, Spain. Abstract 0321.

Levine WC, Pope V, Bhoomkar A, et al. Increase in endocervical CD4 lymphocytes among women with nonulcerative sexually transmitted diseases. J Infect Dis 1998;177:167–174.

Martin HL, Nyange PM, Richardson BA, et al. Hormonal contraception, sexually transmitted diseases, and risk of heterosexual transmission of HIV-1. J Infect Dis (in press).

Moss GB, Overbaugh J, Welch M, et al. Human immunodeficiency virus DNA in urethral secretions in men: association with gonococcal urethritis and CD4 cell depletion. J Infect Dis 1995;172:1469–1474.

Plourde PJ, Pepin J, Agoki E, et al. Human immunodeficiency virus type 1 seroconversion in women with genital ulcers. J Infect Dis 1994;170:313–317.

Plummer FA. Heterosexual transmission of human immunodeficiency virus type 1 (HIV-1): interactions of conventional sexually transmitted diseases, hormonal contraception, and HIV-1. AIDS Res Human Retrov 1998;14(suppl 1):S5–S10.

Sewakambo N, Gray RH, Ronald H, et al. HIV-1 infection associated with abnormal vaginal flora morphology and bacterial vaginosis. Lancet 1997;350:546–550.

Wasserheit JN. Epidemiological synergy. Interrelationships between human immunodeficiency virus infection and other sexually transmitted diseases. Sex Transm Dis 1992;19:61–77.

Wawer MJ, Sewankambo NK, Serwadda D, et al. Control of sexually transmitted diseases for AIDS prevention in Uganda: a randomised community trial. Rakai Project Study Group. Lancet 1999;353:525–535.

CHAPTER

# 43

# *Mucopurulent Cervicitis*

*Newton G. Osborne*

## Background

Mucopurulent cervicitis (MPC) is a distinct clinical entity seen predominantly in sexually active women who are in their reproductive years and who are not in the bleeding phase of the menstrual cycle. This entity is characterized by a yellow, mucopurulent, endocervical discharge with polymorphonuclear (PMN) leukocytes. Although it is considered the counterpart of nongonococcal urethritis (NGU) in men, *Chlamydia trachomatis*, *Neisseria gonorrhoeae*, or both organisms can be recovered from the cervices of affected women in as many as 70% of MPC cases. Herpetic cervicitis has also been associated with mucopurulent cervicitis.

Although the true incidence of MPC remains uncertain, recent reports suggest that as many as 36% of women with high concentrations of leukocytes in their vaginal secretions may have chlamydial cervicitis. Sexually active adolescents have a particularly high risk of cervicitis, especially as a result of *C. trachomatis* infection, and the risk of subsequent chlamydial cervicitis following treatment is high.

The true incidence of MPC does not appear to have changed significantly since Brunham and coworkers reported in 1984 that, among women selected randomly for testing in a clinic for sexually transmitted diseases (STDs), 40% were diagnosed as having MPC according to strict criteria. Majeroni and associates reported that as many as 36% of women in a primary care clinic who had more leukocytes than epithelial cells on a wet mount harbored either *C. trachomatis* or *N. gonorrhoeae*.

Studying sexually active adolescents, Oh and colleagues reported cumulative positive rates of 20.8% for chlamydial infection and 17.1% for gonorrhea. Both of these studies were reported in 1996. Also in 1996, Paavonen reported that *C. trachomatis* remains a major cause of MPC and pelvic inflammatory disease (PID) among women in Finland.

## Etiology

At least three organisms are recognized as causing cervicitis in women: *C. trachomatis*, *N. gonorrhoeae*, and herpes simplex virus (HSV). As much as 70% of MPC is caused by *C. trachomatis*, *N. gonorrhoeae*, or a mixed infection with both organisms. Nongonococcal urethritis, the male counterpart of MPC, is caused by *C. trachomatis* in as many as 50% of cases. As many as 75% of women identified as sex partners of men with chlamydial urethritis have cultures positive for *C. trachomatis*, and a significant percentage of these women have findings considered diagnostic of MPC. Other organisms may be involved as secondary invaders in both urethritis and MPC.

## Diagnosis

Criteria for diagnosis of MPC include the following:

- The presence of yellow-green mucopus on a white cotton-tipped applicator that has been applied to the endocervical canal (positive swab test)
- Observation of 10 or more PMN leukocytes per microscopic oil immersion field in a Gram-stained smear of the endocervical exudate
- The presence of cervicitis, as evidenced by cervical friability with erythema or edema within a zone of cervical ectopy

*Chlamydia trachomatis* can be identified by DNA probes, nucleic acid amplification techniques, any one of several enzyme imunoassay techniques, or culture on specially pretreated cells. Detection of HSV of the endocervix can best be made by tissue culture. *Neisseria gonorrhoeae* is identified by DNA probes, direct fluorescent antibody techniques, or culture in special media.

Women with MPC may be asymptomatic or they may complain of abnormal vaginal discharge, postcoital bleeding, or dyspareunia. On clinical examination, the columnar epithelium of the endocervix may be friable and may bleed easily on contact with a cotton-tipped swab or when a spatula or brush is applied for a Pap smear. The cervix may be tender to instrument application, palpation, or movement. The mucopurulent discharge can be observed after clearing any obscuring material from the portio.

Following the diagnosis of MPC, appropriate steps should be taken to identify *C. trachomatis*, *N. gonorrhoeae*, or HSV. One key to preventing the spread of chlamydial, gonococcal, and herpetic infections is being able to identify the organisms with methods that are both sensitive and specific. Recent advances have made it possible to detect *C. trachomatis* more effectively than was possible previously with cultures and traditional antigen-detection methods. Nucleic acid amplification techniques, such as polymerase chain reaction (PCR) and ligase chain reaction (LCR) tests, have the ability to detect as many as 20% more positive specimens than can be identified with culture. In addition, the sensitivity of amplified tests permits the detection of *C. trachomatis* in multiple sites, such as the endocervix, urethra, or urine. Other methods for rapid detection of cervical chlamydial antigen remain under evaluation.

## Clinical Findings

Women with MPC may be completely asymptomatic. If symptoms are present, they may include abnormal discharge, postcoital spotting, and dyspareunia. Although some cases of asymptomatic disease may resolve spontaneously, most persist or ascend progressively to culminate in either silent or acute salpingitis.

At the time of clinical examination, certain signs may assist in making the diagnosis. The columnar epithelium of the endocervix often is friable and bleeds on contact with a swab or when an Ayre's spatula is used to obtain a cytologic specimen. The classic mucopus should become evident after the cervical portio has been cleared of debris. Tenderness may be seen upon palpation or with cervical motion.

## Treatment

Appropriate antibiotic treatment for infection by *C. trachomatis* or *N. gonorrhoeae* should begin as soon as possible after the identification of either of these organisms or if strong evidence indicates that a genital infection is present. An intramuscular injection of a ß-lactamase-resistant, second-generation cephalosporin (such as ceftriaxone, cefoxitin, or cefotetan) followed by doxycycline, 100 mg every 12 hours for one week, is still considered the treatment of choice. The IM dosage for ceftriaxone is 250 mg.

For patients who may not comply with the seven-day oral regimen, for pregnant women, or for women who are allergic to cephalosporins or to the tetracyclines, 1 g of azithromycin may be given orally as a single dose, or erythromycin base, 500 mg orally every six hours, may be prescribed for seven days. Azithromycin is a macrolide antibiotic that is rapidly absorbed following oral administration; it achieves a higher concentration in tissues than in plasma or serum. This agent is effective against *C. trachomatis* as a single dose because of its long terminal half-life of 68 hours. In addition, azithromycin is effective against other organisms associated with NGU, such as *Mycoplasma hominis* and *Ureaplasma urealyticum;* it cannot be relied on to treat infection by *N. gonorrhoeae* or *Treponema pallidum*, however. Because azithromycin may mask manifestations of incubating gonorrhea or syphilis, adequate diagnostic tests must be performed for these diseases prior to administering this drug. Appropriate antimicrobial therapy and follow-up tests for gonorrhea and syphilis must be initiated if these infections are identified in patients with MPC.

No evidence suggests that azithromycin treatment is associated with adverse pregnancy outcome. Because its effects in pregnancy have been studied only in laboratory animals (mice and rats), however, erythromycin remains the treatment of choice for MPC in pregnancy. Azithromycin should be used in pregnancy or administered to nursing mothers only if clearly needed. It should be administered one hour before or two hours after meals. The main side effect associated with this therapy is gastrointestinal disturbance in some patients.

It is important to counsel sex partners of women affected with MPC and encourage them to seek medical attention and treatment for both gonorrhea and chlamydial infection to prevent reinfection and sequelae of reinfection. Untreated and reinfected women are at risk of developing urethritis, endometritis, salpingitis, salpingo-oophoritis, ectopic pregnancies, and tubal infertility. Salpingitis may be silent in these women, even with severe damage to the fallopian tubes.

Mucopurulent cervicitis must be considered in any woman who presents with an abnormal vaginal discharge, postcoital spotting, or dyspareunia or who is found to have easily induced cervical bleeding on physical examination. The presence of mucopus on the cervix or evidence of inflammation on a Pap smear should alert the health care professional to rule out endocervical infection with *C. trachomatis*, *N. gonorrhoeae*, or HSV. Early diagnosis and therapy will prevent the consequences of ascending infection and avoid further transmission of these sexually acquired pathogens.

## SEQUELAE

Untreated MPC leaves a woman at risk for a wide variety of diseases caused by genital *C. trachomatis* and *N. gonorrhoeae*. Chlamydial infection, for example, has been associated with the presence of atypical cells on cervical cytologic examinations. Treatment of the infection usually will resolve the atypia.

Failure to treat MPC promptly will allow *C. trachomatis* or *N. gonorrhoeae* to invade the urethra and cause acute urethritis, “sterile pyuria,” or troublesome dysuria. Chlamydial infection has been associated with the urethral syndrome, characterized by symptoms of cystitis in the absence of abnormal microscopic findings in the urinary specimen.

If genital chlamydial infection or gonorrhea remains untreated, the infecting organisms may ascend into the uterus and fallopian tubes and cause endometritis, salpingitis, or salpingo-oophoritis. *Chlamydia trachomatis* may cause an insidious type of salpingitis that presents with minimal to moderate symptoms, yet harms the tubal mucosa severely enough to result in permanent damage. Other possible consequences of salpingitis include tubo-ovarian abscesses and ectopic pregnancy. Perihepatitis may also result from gonococcal or chlamydial infection.

## Suggested Readings

Black CM. Current methods of laboratory diagnosis of *Chlamydia trachomatis* infections. Clin Microbiol Rev 1997;10:160–184.

Brunham RC, Paavonen J, Stevens CE, et al. Mucopurulent cervicitis—the ignored counterpart in women of urethritis in men. N Engl J Med 1984;311:1–6.

Centers for Disease Control and Prevention. 1998 guidelines for treatment of sexually transmitted diseases. MMWR 1998;47(RR-1):52–53.

Majeroni BA, Schank JN, Horwitz M, et al. Use of wet mount to predict *Chlamydia trachomatis* and *Neisseria gonorrhoeae* cervicitis in primary care. Fam Med 1996;28:580–583.

Oh MK, Cloud GA, Fleenor M, et al. Risk for gonococcal and chlamydial cervicitis in adolescent females: incidence and recurrence in a prospective cohort study. J Adol Health 1996;18:270–275.

Osborne NG, Hecht Y, Gorsline J, et al. A comparison of culture, direct fluorescent antibody test, and quantitative indirect immunoperoxidase assay for detection of *Chlamydia trachomatis* in pregnant women. Obstet Gynecol 1988;71(3 Pt 1):412–415.

Paavonen J. *Chlamydia trachomatis*: a major cause of mucopurulent cervicitis and pelvic inflammatory disease in women. Curr Probl Dermatol 1996;24:110–122.

Wagar EA. Direct hybridization and amplification applications for the diagnosis of infectious diseases. J Clin Lab Anal 1996;10:312–325.

Woolley PD, Pumphrey J. Application of "Clearview Chlamydia" for the rapid detection of cervical chlamydial antigen. Int J STD AIDS 1997;8:257–258.

CHAPTER

# 44

# *Uncomplicated Anogenital Gonorrhea*

*Daniel V. Landers*

## Background and Incidence

An estimated 600,000 new infections by *Neisseria gonorrhoeae* occur each year in the United States. Although this incidence represents a continued decline of gonococcal infections in this country, it remains significantly higher than that of other developed countries.

The majority of uncomplicated anogenital gonorrhea cases occur in the 15- to 29-year-old age group. Sexually active 15- to 19-year-olds have twice the incidence rate seen in 20- to 24-year-olds. Nevertheless, the highest total incidence is found among 20- to 24-year-olds, reflecting the higher proportion of sexually active individuals in this age group. Seasonal variations of approximately 20% in the incidence of gonorrhea also occur in the United States, with the peak in late summer.

Many risk factors have been associated with gonococcal infections, including low socioeconomic status, urban residence, non-Asian and non-white race and ethnicity, early onset of sexual activity, unmarried marital status, illicit drug use, prostitution, and history of gonococcal infections. Contraceptive choices may affect risk as well. Spermicides, diaphragms, and condoms have been found to reduce the risk of acquiring this infection.

## Etiology

Transmission of gonorrhea is almost entirely by sexual contact. The risk of transmission from male to female from a single sexual encounter is estimated at 80% to 90%, compared with a risk of 20% to 25% for transmission from female to male.

Although uncomplicated anogenital gonorrhea often remains asymptomatic, it can be associated with many different clinical manifestations. Most women develop symptoms within 10 days of infection or else remain asymptomatic.

The primary site of urogenital gonococcal infection in women is the endocervix. Mucopurulent cervicitis (MCP)—the hallmark of clinical infection of the endocervix associated with *N. gonorrhoeae* or *Chlamydia trachomatis*—is characterized by a purulent or mucopurulent endocervical exudate. This exudate may be visible at the endocervical canal or in an endocervical swab specimen. Unfortunately, MCP is most often asymptomatic and, in most cases, neither *N. gonorrhoeae* nor *C. trachomatis* can be isolated.

MCP may persist despite repeated courses of antimicrobial therapy in the absence of gonorrhea or chlamydial infection. Some experts suggest that easily induced cervical bleeding and/or an increased number of polymorphonuclear (PMN) leukocytes observed on endocervical Gram's stain should raise suspicions of gonoccocal infection. Although isolated colonization of the urethra is uncommon, such infection may often be seen in association with endocervical infection. Occasionally, Bartholin's, Skene's, and periurethral glands may be involved in gonococcal infections.

As many as 50% of women with gonococcal cervicitis have a concurrent gonococcal rectal infection with or without a history of acknowledged rectal sexual contact. Anal examination may frequently be normal or it may reveal erythema, discharge, or both. Anoscopy may reveal mucoid or purulent exudate, edema, and mucosal friability.

## Diagnosis

Definitive diagnosis of gonorrhea depends on identifying the causative agent, *N. gonorrhoeae*, a Gram-negative intracellular diplococcus. Isolation in culture continues to be the standard means of diagnosis. Newer DNA-based tests may provide improved diagnostic utility but are more expensive and not widely available at this time.

Culture is best accomplished by using selective media containing antibiotics. Modified Thayer-Martin medium has a diagnostic sensitivity of 96% in cultures from the endocervix. Sensitivity can be increased by duplicate endocervical swabbings or consecutive endocervical and anal swabbings. To collect specimens, first cleanse the cervix to remove external exudate and then insert a swab 1 to 2 cm up to the internal os and rotate it gently for 5 to 10 seconds.

Gram's stain can be useful as a substitute for culture (when the latter is unavailable) or as an adjunct to culture. Finding gram-negative diplococci with typical morphology identified or closely associated with PMN leukocytes is considered diagnostic. Gram's stain is used primarily when the index of suspicion of infection is high.

Nucleic acid detection assays, such as the nonamplification method (GenProbe), and, more recently, amplification methods, such as polymerase chain reaction (PCR) and ligase chain reaction (LCR) tests, have been developed for use in the diagnosis of *N. gonorrhoeae* infection. These detection systems boast a high degree of sensitivity and specificity (near 100%) and may accurately identify *N. gonorrhoeae* from vaginal (clinician- or self-collected) swabs. Although their expense and limited availability are major disadvantages at present, these DNA-based tests may eventually become the test of choice.

## Treatment

Antimicrobial therapy for gonococcal infections reflects in vitro resistance patterns. The rising incidence of infection from penicillinase-producing or tetracycline-resistant *N. gonorrhoeae* (PPNG and TRNG) or strains with chromosomally mediated resistance to multiple antibiotics has led the Centers for Disease Control and Prevention (CDC) to alter its treatment recommendations over the years. As of February 1997, quinolone-

**Table 44-1.** Treatment of Uncomplicated Gonoccocal Infections of the Cervix, Urethra, and Rectum

| | |
|---|---|
| Cefixime | 400 mg orally in a single dose |
| | *or* |
| Ceftriaxone | 125 mg IM in a single dose |
| | *or* |
| Ciprofloxacin | 500 mg orally in a single dose |
| | *or* |
| Ofloxacin | 400 mg orally in a single dose |
| **Add to Any of the Above Regimens:** | |
| Azithromycin | 1 g orally in a single dose |
| | *or* |
| Doxycycline | 100 mg orally twice a day for 7 days |

SOURCE: Centers for Disease Control and Prevention. 1998 guidelines for treatment of sexually transmitted diseases. MMWR 1998;47(RR-1):59–65.

resistant strains (MIC greater than 1.0 μg/mL) occurred in less than 0.05% of 4639 isolates collected by the CDC's Gonoccocal Isolate Surveillance Project.

Guidelines also have been influenced by the high frequency of chlamydial infections in individuals with gonorrhea and the absence of a rapid, inexpensive, and accurate test for these infections. The current CDC recommendations for treatment of uncomplicated anogenital gonorrhea therefore call for a single oral dose of 400 mg cefixime or a single IM dose of ceftriaxone or a single dose of a fluoroquinolone (ciprofloxacin or ofloxacin) followed by a single dose of 1 g azithromycin or a seven-day course of oral doxycycline (Table 44-1). According to the CDC's 1998 guidelines, cefixime and ceftriaxone have similar antimicrobial spectra, but the 400-mg oral dose may not provide as high (97.1% versus 99.1%) or as sustained a bactericidal level as a 125-mg IM dose of ceftriaxone. The former agent's obvious advantage is the ease of oral administration.

Ciprofloxacin and ofloxacin also show effectiveness against most strains of *N. gonorrhoeae* in single doses of 500 mg and 400 mg, respectively. Other single-dose quinolone regimens —including enoxacin, 400 mg; lomefloxacin, 400 mg; and norfloxacin, 800 mg orally—appear to be safe and effective for uncomplicated gonorrhea. Data for these drugs are less extensive, however. None of the quinolones seems to offer a significant selective advantage over the others. The safety of the quinolones in pregnant or lactating women or in women younger than 18 years of age has not been established.

A single dose of 2 g spectinomycin has long been an alternative treatment for gonorrhea in the pregnant cephalosporin-allergic patient or in patients who cannot tolerate either the quinolones or cephalosporins. Other alternative regimens included in the CDC guidelines have been shown to be effective in less extensive studies. All alternatives to ceftriaxone are followed with a seven-day course of oral doxycycline. Although tetracycline represents a possible substitute for doxycycline, compliance may be worse with this drug because it must be administered four times daily instead of twice daily. Also, tetracycline currently costs slightly more than generic doxycycline. Doxycycline or tetracycline is added to cover coexisting chlamydial infection; neither agent by itself is considered adequate therapy for gonococcal infection.

## Follow-up

Because treatment failure after the ceftriaxone/doxycycline regimen is rare, the CDC considers follow-up cultures ("test-of-cure") nonessential. A more cost-effective strategy may rely on reexamination with culture one to two months after treatment ("rescreening"). This approach detects both treatment failure and reinfections. Patients treated with regimens other than ceftriaxone/doxycycline should have follow-up cultures taken four to seven days after completion of therapy.

Persons exposed to gonorrhea within the preceding 60 days should be examined, cultured, and treated presumptively. All patients with gonorrhea should have a serologic test for syphilis and should be offered confidential counseling and testing for HIV infection. Most patients with incubating syphilis will be cured by a regimen containing ceftriaxone, another ß-lactam, or tetracyclines. Patients treated with other regimens (for example, spectinomycin, ciprofloxacin, or norfloxacin) should receive a serologic test for syphilis in one month.

## Treatment Failure

Persistent symptoms after treatment should be evaluated by culture for *N. gonorrhoeae*, and any gonococcal isolate should be tested for antibiotic sensitivity. Because of reinfection (rather than treatment failure), infections occurring after treatment with one of the recommended regimens are common.

## Prevention

As with all sexually transmitted diseases, reducing the incidence of gonorrhea depends on educating patients and raising public awareness of modes of transmission and means of prevention. Among contraceptive choices, condoms are most effective in preventing transmission and acquisition of *N. gonorrhoeae*. Use of a diaphragm, cervical cap, and, to a lesser degree, topical bactericidal agents may reduce risk of acquisition in women. Practices such as douching, washing, or urinating after intercourse have not been shown to reduce risk of acquiring *N. gonorrhoeae* significantly. In fact, douching may be associated with potentially harmful effects.

Most important to any prevention effort is the tracing and treating of sexual contacts. This task is easier in areas where reporting gonococcal infections is mandatory, as in the United States. Private physicians, as well as public health departments, should make every attempt to refer or treat partners of infected individuals.

Efforts continue toward developing a vaccine for the prevention of gonorrhea and gonococcal pelvic inflammatory disease. Thus far, however, no effective vaccine appears on the immediate horizon.

## Suggested Readings

Bassiri M, Mårdh P-A, Domeika M. Multiplex Amplicor PCR screening for *Chlamydia trachomatis* and *Neisseria gonorrhoeae* in women attending non-sexually transmitted disease clinics. J Clin Microbiol 1997;35:2556–2560.

Centers for Disease Control and Prevention. 1998 guidelines for treatment of sexually transmitted diseases. MMWR 1998;47 (RR-1):59–65.

Hook EW III, Ching SF, Stephens J, et al. Diagnosis of *Neisseria gonorrhoeae* infections in women by using the ligase chain reaction on patient-obtained vaginal swabs. J Clin Microbiol 1997;35: 2129–2132.

Institute of Medicine (U.S.) Committee on Prevention and Control of Sexually Transmitted Diseases. Eng TR, Butler WT, eds. The hidden epidemic: confronting sexually transmitted diseases. Washington, DC: National Academy Press, 1997.

Moran JS, Levine WC. Drugs of choice for the treatment of uncomplicated gonococcal infections. Clin Infect Dis 1995;20(suppl 1): S47–S65.

CHAPTER

45

# *Disseminated Gonococcal Infection*

*David E. Soper*

## Background and Incidence

Disseminated gonococcal infection (DGI) is a rare but important complication of *Neisseria gonorrhoeae* mucosal infection. Although the exact incidence is not known, approximately 1% of women with an uncomplicated gonococcal infection will develop DGI. The disseminated form is the most common cause of septic arthritis or tenosynovitis in adults. DGI is more common in pregnant women than in nonpregnant women.

## Pathophysiology

Dissemination occurs when the *N. gonorrhoeae* organisms infecting the genital tract, pharynx, or rectum invade the bloodstream. This bacteremia leads to infection of the skin, synovia, and joints and accounts for the clinical manifestations of the disease. Associated strains of *N. gonorrhoeae* usually are of transparent colony phenotype; they have growth requirements for arginine, hypoxanthine, and uracil, and they have a low-molecular-weight protein I. These factors may be associated with an increase in the invasiveness of the infecting microorganism.

Host factors also play an important role in the development of disseminated gonococcal infection. Patients with deficiencies in one of the late-acting complement components (C5, C6, C7, or C8) responsible for the bactericidal action of serum are predisposed to disseminated infection. Hormonal influences may be important as well, given that most cases in women occur close to menstruation or during pregnancy.

## DIAGNOSIS

*N. gonorrhoeae* infection may be considered a two-stage process: an initial bacteremia associated with skin lesions, followed by a secondary phase associated with septic arthritis. Patients may present with degrees of severity ranging from uncomplicated cases with skin lesions alone to metastatic infections such as endocarditis.

The primary manifestations are fever, usually with temperatures between 38 °C (100.4 °F) and 39 °C (102.2 °F), and skin lesions (Table 45-1). The skin lesions begin as erythematous macules, 1 to 5 mm in diameter, and rapidly become pustular. They appear on the extremities, commonly near the small joints of the hands or the feet. It is important to look for these lesions between the fingers and toes.

Tenosynovitis, involving the extensor and flexor tendons and sheaths of the hands and feet, is another common finding. Erythema, swelling, and tenderness are found along the tendon sheath. Marked pain is associated with tendon motion.

Arthritis is the third most common clinical manifestation. The knee is the joint most typically affected, followed by the elbow, ankle, and small joints of the hand. Erythema, edema, pain, and effusion are the most frequent manifestations of a septic joint. Endocarditis and meningitis—the most serious complications—occur only rarely.

**Table 45-1.** Clinical Manifestations of DGI

| |
|---|
| Fever, typically < 103 °F |
| Skin lesions: |
| Pustular macules |
| Purplish, with erythematous base |
| Tenosynovitis |
| Arthritis (usually a single joint) |
| Endocarditis (rare) |

**Table 45-2.** Positive Cultures from Various Sites in DGI Patients

| Site | Culture Positive | Gram's Stain |
|---|---|---|
| Skin lesions | 10% | 10% |
| Joint fluid | 20%–30% | 10%–30% |
| Blood | 10%–30% | — |
| Mucosa* | 80%–90% | — |

* Pharynx, urethra, cervix, or rectum.

SOURCE: Mills J, Brooks GF. Disseminated gonococcal infection. In: Holmes KK, Mårdh PA, Sparling PF, et al., eds. Sexually transmitted diseases, 3rd ed. New York: McGraw-Hill, 1997.

The clinician should consider a diagnosis of DGI in any patient who complains of tenosynovitis, polyarthritis, or peripheral pustular skin lesions. The differential diagnosis includes other bacteremias and noninfectious causes of tenosynovitis and arthritis. Meningococcemia may mimic gonococcal infection. In such cases, however, the skin lesions are more likely to be petechial or purpuric, and tenosynovitis is rarely associated with meningococcal infection.

Laboratory diagnosis of DGI relies upon Gram's stain and culture. The local mucosal site is the most common source of a positive culture (Table 45-2). Blood cultures are positive in only some 10% to 30% of patients. A positive blood culture is more likely to be obtained when the polymorphonuclear neutrophil (PMN) leukocyte count of the synovial fluid is 40,000 or greater. When the PMN leukocyte count is 20,000 or less, culture of the synovial fluid will likely be negative.

## TREATMENT

Antimicrobial therapy is the mainstay of DGI treatment (Table 45-3). Selected patients may be treated as outpatients. On the other hand, women who cannot reliably comply with treatment, pregnant women, women with septic arthritis, and women in whom the diagnosis is unclear should be hospitalized for observation and therapy. Although most strains of *N. gonorrhoeae* causing disseminated disease are very susceptible

**Table 45-3.** DGI Treatment Regimens

**Initial Therapy**
Ceftriaxone, 1 g IM or IV every 24 hours

**Alternative Initial Therapy**
Cefotaxime, 1 g IV every 8 hours
*or*
Ceftizoxime, 1 g IV every 8 hours

**Therapy for Patients Allergic to ß-Lactam Drugs**
Ciprofloxacin, 500 mg IV every 12 hours
*or*
Ofloxacin, 400 mg IV every 12 hours
*or*
Spectinomycin, 2 g IM every 12 hours

**Completion Therapy**
For each regimen, continue treatment for 24 to 48 hours after improvement begins; therapy may then be switched to one of the following for a full week:
Cefixime, 400 mg orally twice daily
Ciprofloxacin, 500 mg orally twice daily
Ofloxacin, 400 mg orally twice daily

SOURCE: Centers for Disease Control and Prevention. 1998 guidelines for treatment of sexually transmitted diseases. MMWR 1998;47(RR-1):64.

to penicillin, a few cases caused by penicillinase-producing strains of *N. gonorrhoeae* have been reported.

If an outpatient regimen is used, the patient should return for follow-up examinations in 24 hours and one week after the initiation of therapy. Symptoms should resolve rapidly once therapy begins. Skin lesions should disappear within a few days. Tenosynovitis markedly improves within 24 hours, and septic arthritis is much improved within 48 hours. Failure of symptoms to respond rapidly to appropriate antibiotic therapy should alert you to the possibility of an incorrect diagnosis, such as Reiter's syndrome. Adjunctive anti-inflammatory drug therapy is not recommended, as it may cloud the patient's symptomatic response to antibiotic therapy and obscure the final diagnosis.

Recovery of *N. gonorrhoeae* from any site constitutes strong evidence of the presence of DGI. The therapeutic response of patients to antibiotic therapy alone—even in the face of negative cultures—provides good evidence that the diagnosis is correct. It is important to note that the patient with DGI may have a negative cervical culture; the pharynx and rectum therefore should be cultured as well.

Contact tracing is an important element of both diagnosis and therapy. The sexual partner may have a positive culture when the index case does not, and epidemiologic treatment is important to prevent reinfection of the patient or infection of others with a strain of *N. gonorrhoeae* likely to cause disseminated infection. Because the sex partner is likely to be asymptomatic, it is extremely important that a specimen for culture of *N. gonorrhoeae* and *C. trachomatis* be obtained and treatment instituted. Treatment of both partners for chlamydial infection should be included.

## Suggested Readings

Centers for Disease Control and Prevention. 1998 guidelines for treatment of sexually transmitted diseases. MMWR 1998;47(RR-1):63–64.

Hook EW, Holmes KK. Gonococcal infections. Ann Intern Med 1985;102:229.

Mills J, Brooks GF. Disseminated gonococcal infection. In: Holmes KK, Mårdh PA, Sparling PF, et al., eds. Sexually transmitted diseases. New York: McGraw-Hill, 1990.

CHAPTER

# 46

# *Syphilis in Adult Women*

*George D. Wendel, Jr.*
*Larry C. Gilstrap III*

## Incidence and Pathophysiology

Syphilis is a complex, chronic systemic infection caused by the spirochete *Treponema pallidum*, which is usually transmitted through intimate or sexual contact. The incidence of syphilis increased markedly in the 1980s in the United States, primarily because of increases in large urban areas plagued by drug abuse and prostitution. Not surprisingly, an increase in the incidence of congenital syphilis followed, because most of the infections occurred in reproductive-age men and women (see Chapter 15). In 1997, the incidence of primary and secondary syphilis was 3.2 per 100,000 persons (8551 cases) in the United States, and 1049 cases of congenital syphilis were reported to the Centers for Disease Control and Prevention (CDC).

Currently, decreases in the prevalence of infectious syphilis are occurring in heterosexual men and women, with marked declines also noted in gay males, presumably because of greater use of safe sex practices to prevent HIV infection. The ratio of the total cases of primary and secondary syphilis in men to women is now nearly 1:1.

The infectious organism in syphilis, *T. pallidum*, exhibits a characteristic spiral motion and flexing about its midportion, which allows for easy identification by dark-field microscopy. The organism enters the body through minute abrasions in skin or a mucosal surface and begins to replicate locally. As a result, the common sites of the initial lesions of syphilis are those most likely to sustain microscopic frictional trauma during intimate contact: the fourchette, the cervix, the anus, the lips, and the nipples.

## Laboratory Diagnosis

The most accurate method for confirming the clinical diagnosis of syphilis is visualization of *T. pallidum* by dark-field microscopy in material taken from a moist genital lesion or a regional lymph node aspirate. Serologic tests for syphilis constitute the most common means for confirming infection, especially in cases of latent syphilis. Nonspecific antibody can be measured by the rapid plasma reagin (RPR) test or the Venereal Disease Research Laboratory (VDRL) test, either of which can be used for screening and for following up on the response to therapy. These tests are reported as nonreactive or reactive; they are also given a titer, which generally reflects the degree of current infection and allows for comparison with post-treatment titers.

Specific antitreponemal antibody testing is used to confirm infection following a reactive RPR or VDRL test; either the microhemagglutination assay for antibodies to *T. pallidum* (MHA-TP) method or the fluorescent treponemal antibody-absorption (FTA-ABS) technique may be used for this purpose. These tests also are reported as nonreactive or reactive but without titers. Because they remain positive even after therapy, they cannot be used as an index of response to treatment or for primary diagnosis.

False-positive tests (reactive nontreponemal tests and nonreactive treponemal tests) occur transiently in 1% of patients and are generally of low titer. They are often attributed to laboratory error, subclinical autoimmune disease, intravenous drug abuse, or HIV infection.

## Clinical Diagnosis

### Primary Syphilis

The initial clinical manifestation of syphilis is the chancre, usually accompanied by a regional adenopathy. One or more lesions develop at the site of inoculation approximately three weeks after exposure, though they can take 10 to 90 days to appear. The chancre is a painless, red, round, firm ulcer with a granular base that has well-formed, raised edges. A "press prep" of material squeezed from a chancre will, under dark-field microscopy, usually show motile spirochetes, thereby confirming the diagnosis. Serologic testing is reactive in 80% to 90% of patients with primary infection because of a several-day delay in the production of antibody after primary infection. Chancres spontaneously heal in three to eight weeks without treatment.

## Secondary Syphilis

After several weeks, the local manifestations of primary syphilis progress to dissemination, characteristic of the secondary stage of infection. Chancres may be present at this stage. Nearly all patients will progress to this state approximately six weeks after the development of primary syphilis. The secondary stage is characterized by diffuse, symmetric skin lesions and systemic abnormalities. The dermatologic manifestations of secondary syphilis are numerous, explaining its familiar designation as the "great imitator." Generalized lymphadenopathy, hepatitis, nephrosis, and alopecia also may occur.

The genital manifestations of secondary syphilis are moist cutaneous external lesions called condylomata lata and mucous patches, the latter often resembling genital herpes simplex virus infection. Both types of lesions are moist, highly infectious, and easily diagnosable by dark-field examination. Serologic testing for syphilis is reactive in almost all immunocompetent adults at this stage. Immunocompromised HIV-infected women may have high-titer nontreponemal tests or seronegative infections.

## Latent Syphilis

After 3 to 12 weeks, the untreated lesions of secondary syphilis resolve, and the patient progresses to the latent stage of infection. The diagnosis at this stage is made by a reactive serologic test for syphilis without the signs or symptoms of primary or secondary disease. This stage often is divided into early latent syphilis and late latent syphilis based on the duration of illness, using one year's duration as the reference point. This classification is useful because infectivity for sexual or fetal transmission is significant during the early period, when approximately 25% of patients will experience a clinical recurrence similar to that of the secondary stage. In late latency, patients run a greater risk of having or progressing to tertiary syphilis or neurosyphilis.

## Late or Tertiary Syphilis

After prolonged latency of many years, late complications of syphilis will develop in 20% to 30% of untreated patients. Today, these entities are quite rare, as fewer patients escape early diagnosis and treatment. Additionally, because of the long latency period, most signs of late syphilis are rarely encountered in young, reproductive-age women. Benign late syphilis, characterized by gumma, occurs in 15% of patients. Cardiovascular syphilis, characterized by aortitis, develops in a least 10% of patients. Late neurosyphilis, which causes meningovascular disease, paresis, and tabes dorsalis, affects 7% of untreated adults.

## Neurosyphilis

Unfortunately, neurosyphilis cannot be diagnosed accurately by any single testing technique. Moreover, the decision about when to perform a lumbar puncture for cerebrospinal fluid (CSF) analysis in patients with latent syphilis remains controversial. The CDC recommends that all adults with latent syphilis be evaluated clinically for tertiary disease such as aortitis, neurosyphilis, gumma, and iritis. Perform a lumbar puncture in any patient with latent syphilis of unknown or greater than one year's duration in specific situations (Table 46-1).

Invasion of the CSF by *T. pallidum* and accompanying CSF abnormalities are common in adults with early (primary, secondary, or early latent) syphilis. As most patients with early

**Table 46-1.** Indications for Lumbar Puncture in the Management of Syphilis

| |
|---|
| **Latent Syphilis of Uncertain or More Than One Year's Duration** |
| Neurologic signs or symptoms: |
| Auditory |
| Cranial nerve |
| Meningeal |
| Ophthalmic (for example, uveitis*) |
| Treatment failure |
| Evidence of active late syphilis: |
| Aortitis |
| Gumma |
| Iritis |
| HIV infection |
| **Primary and Secondary Syphilis** |
| Neurologic signs or symptoms: |
| Auditory |
| Cranial nerve |
| Meningeal |
| Ophthalmic (for example, uveitis*) |

* Ocular slit-lamp examination for syphilitic eye disease recommended.

syphilis and abnormal CSF findings do not develop neurosyphilis, no clear evidence indicates that these patients need additional therapy. A lumbar puncture is not recommended generally in cases of early syphilis with or without HIV infection, unless signs or symptoms of neurdogic involvement are present.

CSF tests, when performed, should include a cell count, a quantitative protein determination, and a VDRL test. The CSF leukocyte count usually is elevated—that is, greater than 5 WBC/mm$^3$—when neurosyphilis is present. The CSF WBC is also a sensitive measure of the effectiveness of treatment. The CSF VDRL test should be considered diagnostic of neurosyphilis when positive; however, because it may be negative when neurosyphilis is present, it cannot rule out neurosyphilis. Some experts rely on the CSF FTA-ABS test, which is less specific for neurosyphilis—that is, it produces more false positives—but is believed to be highly sensitive in excluding the diagnosis.

**Table 46-2.** Recommended Regimens for Treatment of Syphilis

| |
|---|
| **Early Syphilis*** |
| Benzathine penicillin G, 2.4 million units IM as a single injection |
| **Syphilis of More Than One Year's Duration†** |
| Benzathine penicillin G, 2.4 million units IM weekly for three doses |
| **Neurosyphilis** |
| Aqueous crystalline penicillin G, 3 to 4 million units IV every 4 hours for 10 to 14 days, followed by benzathine penicillin G, 2.4 million units IM |
| Aqueous procaine penicillin G, 2.4 million units IM daily, plus probenecid, 500 mg orally four times daily, both for 10–14 days, followed by benzathine penicillin G, 2.4 million units IM |

* Primary, secondary, and latent syphilis of less than one year's duration.

† Latent syphilis of unknown or more than one year's duration, cardiovascular syphilis, or late syphilis.

## Treatment

Penicillin is the preferred drug for treating syphilis patients (Table 46-2). Penicillin is the only clinically-tested therapy that has been widely used for patients with all stages of infection, including pregnant women (see Chapter 15). In general, barring reinfection, therapy with long-acting benzathine penicillin G can eradicate early syphilis in 98% of immunocompetent adults. The goal of treatment of primary and secondary syphilis is resolution of lesions, prevention of transmission, and prevention of late sequelae. Treatment of latent infection prevents occurrence or progression of late sequelae.

Penicillin desensitization is the optimal mode of therapy for patients allergic to penicillin (after documentation of this allergy by skin testing). Oral and intravenous penicillin desensitization regimens are available, and the oral regimen has been widely used on a clinical basis. Table 46-3 describes a protocol for oral desensitization with penicillin. Alternative doxycycline and tetracycline regimens are less effective but should cure more than 90% of patients (Table 46-4). Ceftriaxone, erythromycin, and azithromycin may be effective as well. Close follow-up and compliance are necessary when using alternative regimens.

**Table 46-3.** Oral Desensitization Protocol for Women with Penicillin Allergy and Syphilis

| Penicillin V Suspension Dose* | Dose Strength† (U/mL) | Measured Dose† (mL) | Total Dose (U) | Cumulative Dose (U) |
|---|---|---|---|---|
| 1 | 1000 | 0.1 | 100 | 100 |
| 2 | 1000 | 0.2 | 200 | 300 |
| 3 | 1000 | 0.4 | 400 | 700 |
| 4 | 1000 | 0.8 | 800 | 1500 |
| 5 | 1000 | 1.6 | 1600 | 3100 |
| 6 | 1000 | 3.2 | 3200 | 6300 |
| 7 | 1000 | 6.4 | 6400 | 12,700 |
| 8 | 10,000 | 1.2 | 12,000 | 24,700 |
| 9 | 10,000 | 2.4 | 24,000 | 48,700 |
| 10 | 10,000 | 4.8 | 48,000 | 96,700 |
| 11 | 80,000 | 1.0 | 80,000 | 176,700 |
| 12 | 80,000 | 2.0 | 160,000 | 336,700 |
| 13 | 80,000 | 4.0 | 320,000 | 656,700 |
| 14 | 80,000 | 8.0 | 640,000 | 1,296,700 |

Observe 30 minutes for allergic signs or symptoms before parenteral administration of penicillin. Then observe for at least one hour after injection or infusion for signs of urticaria, angioedema, or anaphylaxis.

* Interval between doses: 15 minutes; elapsed time: 3 hours and 45 minutes.

† Undiluted penicillin V suspension is 80,000 U/mL. The penicillin V suspension is first diluted to 1000 or 10,000 U/mL and then administered orally in 30 mL of water.

**Table 46-4.** Alternative Syphilis Treatment Regimens for Penicillin-Allergic Patients

**Early Syphilis***

Tetracycline, 500 mg orally four times daily for 2 weeks
Doxycycline, 100 mg orally two times daily for 2 weeks
Erythromycin, 500 mg orally four times daily for 2 weeks
Ceftriaxone, 1 g IV daily for 8 to 10 days†

**Syphilis of More Than One Year's Duration‡**

Doxycycline, 100 mg orally two times daily for 4 weeks
Tetracycline, 500 mg orally four times daily for 4 weeks

**Neurosyphilis**

Non-penicillin treatment not recommended
Desensitization and parenteral penicillin

* Primary, secondary, and latent syphilis of less than one year's duration.

† Probably effective; limited clinical experience.

‡ Latent syphilis of unknown or more than one year's duration, cardiovascular syphilis, or late syphilis.

After treatment of early syphilis, the Jarisch-Herxheimer reaction occurs in more than 60% of patients. This reaction manifests as an acute febrile reaction that occurs within 24 hours of therapy and produces systemic symptoms such as headache, myalgia, and flushed lesions. Antipyretics may be recommended, but no proven methods exist to prevent this reaction. Warn pregnant patients to watch for decreases in fetal activity and preterm labor.

## Early Syphilis

Early syphilis treatment failures can occur with any regimen, but are infrequently observed with penicillin regimens. Quantitative serologic titers probably fall more slowly than previously believed. Patients should be reexamined clinically and serologically at 6 and 12 months after treatment. Nontreponemal antibody titers should decline fourfold (two dilutions) by 6 months with primary or secondary syphilis and by 12 to 24 months with latent syphilis.

Patients with signs and symptoms that persist or recur or who have a fourfold increase in nontreponemal titer should be considered treatment failures or reinfections. Unless reinfection is certain, these individuals should undergo a CSF examination by lumbar puncture, evaluation for HIV infection, and retreatment. Although the optimal management has not been definitively identified, retreatment with penicillin G. benzathine, 2.4 million U IM weekly for three weeks, is reasonable after excluding neurosyphilis.

## Late Latent and Tertiary Syphilis

Patients with late latent syphilis of more than one year's duration, gumma, or cardiovascular syphilis ideally should have a CSF examination prior to treatment. This decision can be tailored to the particular patient, because in the older asymptomatic patient, the lumbar puncture result is likely to be normal. A CSF examination is indicated in specific cases (see Table 46-1).

The recommended regimen for treating infection at this stage is benzathine penicillin G given weekly as three doses in consecutive weeks (see Table 46-2). The alternative regimen of doxycycline or tetracycline daily for four weeks for penicillin-allergic patients is applicable to patients in whom penicillin skin testing and desensitization are unavailable (see Table 46-4). Repeat the quantitative serologic test at 6, 12, and 24 months. Clinical response is uncertain and depends on the nature of the lesions.

### Neurosyphilis

Clinical evidence of neurologic involvement, such as ophthalmic and auditory symptoms or cranial nerve palsies, warrants CSF examination (see Table 46-1). The treatment of neurosyphilis is not well established but requires prolonged parenteral penicillin (see Table 46-2). Experience with non-penicillin regimens for neurosyphilis remains too limited to recommend their use. If CSF pleocytosis was present initially, examine spinal fluid every six months until the cell count is normal. If it does not decrease in six months or does not reach normal levels by two years, consider HIV testing and retreatment.

## Syphilis in HIV Patients

All sexually active patients with syphilis should undergo testing for HIV antibody, because coinfection is frequent and clinical management may need to be adjusted to deal with both infections. In areas with high HIV prevalence, retest patients with early syphilis again in three months. Always consider neurosyphilis in the differential diagnosis of neurologic abnormalities in HIV-infected persons. Abnormal serologic tests with unusually high, unusually low, and fluctuating non-treponemal antibody titers have been noted in HIV-infected patients.

Penicillin regimens should be used whenever possible for all stages of syphilis in HIV-infected patients; however, the CDC does not recommend any change in the dosage for early syphilis (see Table 46-2). A recent CDC-sponsored multicenter trial of adults with and without HIV infection found no clinical benefit to enhancing recommended syphilotherapy with a 10-day course of amoxicillin and probenecid.

Syphilis serologic tests appear to be accurate and reliable for the diagnosis and follow-up of most adults with HIV infection. Closer follow-up is necessary, however, to ensure adequate clinical and serologic response to treatment. HIV-infected patients should receive more frequent follow-up, including serologic testing at 2, 3, 6, 9, and 12 months for primary and secondary syphilis and at 6, 12, 18, and 24 months for latent syphilis.

## Management of Sex Partners

Sexual partners of individuals with early syphilis should be evaluated clinically and serologically. Sexual transmission is uncommon without mucocutaneous lesions or after the first year of infection. If the contact occurred within three months, the partner may be infected but seronegative and should be presumptively treated. If the contact occurred more than three months ago, the partner should be treated presumptively if serologic testing is not available or follow-up is uncertain. For partner notification and management, consider adults with latent syphilis of uncertain duration and with high titers (1:32 or higher) to have early syphilis.

Administer presumptive treatment according to the guidelines for early syphilis. One recommended treatment for gonorrhea (ceftriaxone and doxycycline or erythromycin) probably is effective for incubating syphilis. If a noncephalosporin antimicrobial is administered to treat gonorrhea, the patient should undergo serologic testing for syphilis in three months.

### Suggested Readings

Centers for Disease Control and Prevention. 1998 guidelines for treatment of sexually transmitted diseases. MMWR 1998;47 (RR-1):28–41.

Fraser CM, Norris SJ, Weinstock GM, et al. Complete genome sequence of *Treponema pallidum*, the syphilis spirochete. Science 1999;281:375–388.

Hook EW, Marra CM. Acquired syphilis in adults. N Engl J Med 1992;326:1060–1069.

Nakashima AK, Rolfs RT, Flock ML, et al. Epidemiology of syphilis in the United States, 1941–1993. Sex Transm Dis 1996;23:16–23.

Rolfs RT. Treatment of syphilis, 1993. Clin Infect Dis 1995;20(suppl 1):S23–S38.

Rolfs RT, Joesoef MR, Hendershot EF, et al. A randomized trial of enhanced therapy for early syphilis in patients with and without human immunodeficiency virus infection. N Engl J Med 1997;337:307–314.

St. Louis ME, Wasserheit JN. Elimination of syphilis in the United States. Science 1999;281:353–354.

CHAPTER

# 47

# Chancroid

*H. H. Allen*

## Background

Chancroid is a common sexually transmitted disease in many parts of the developing world, especially in Africa. Its global incidence far exceeds that of syphilis. The disease is less common in North America, however. Between 1971 and 1980, a mean of 878 cases were reported annually in the United States, with most cases occurring in the southern part of the country; the peak incidence of 5047 was recorded in 1987. Outbreaks in Greenland; Winnipeg, Canada; Sheffield, England; and New Orleans, Louisiana, emphasize the disease potential in temperate climates.

## Etiology and Epidemiology

The infectious organism in chancroid, *Haemophilus ducreyi*, was discovered by Augosto Ducrey in 1889 at the University of Naples as the cause of soft chancre. He examined the exudate and identified the short component streptobacilli but could not culture them.

Today, *H. ducreyi* remains a difficult organism to grow in culture; as a result, suspected cases are not often confirmed in clinics. Because certain physicians, especially those in sexually transmitted disease (STD) clinics, are more aware of the disease, geographic clustering is a prominent feature of reports. The actual incidence and overall rate in North America, therefore, are difficult to assess. Estimates of the male–female ratio for chancroid range from 3.1 to 25.1. Because prostitutes are important transmitters of the disease, a few women can infect a large number of men.

Efforts to eliminate chancroid have not proved successful in any reported areas over the past decade. Case findings and culture efforts in some areas where outbreaks have occurred have not been helpful in pinpointing the source of infection. Attempting to find women who harbored *H. ducreyi* without symptoms or signs was also fruitless. A few women without symptoms were found with cervical ulcers; the role played by such asymptomatic carriers remains unclear.

Chancroid has been associated with increased HIV infection rates. It has been reportedly associated with syphilis in 10% to 15% of cases and herpes genital infection in as many or more patients.

## Pathogenesis

The mechanism by which the *H. ducreyi* organism adheres to and produces tissue destruction is not well understood. This gram-negative organism lacks an extracellular capsule and surface appendages. It seems clear that its virulence and pathogenicity vary considerably. Outer membrane protein and lipopolysaccharide differences may explain this characteristic. The organism has only two penicillin-binding proteins. A fastidious organism, *H. ducreyi* is very difficult to grow in culture.

## Clinical Presentation

The incubation period of chancroid generally spans 2 to 10 days, but may last as long as 35 days. No prodromal illness occurs prior to the appearance of the ulcer, and no systemic signs of infection emerge after the ulcer appears. The ulcer usually is painful with undermined irregular edges. Very little erythema appears around the edges unless secondary infection is present. The base bleeds easily. Although a single ulcer is the most common presentation, multiple ulcers and even extragenital ulcers do occur.

Disseminated infections have not been described. Inguinal adenitis is present in only some 30% of cases and is unilateral in approximately two-thirds of those cases. McCarley and colleagues found that most gland enlargement subsides with adequate antibiotic treatment. Some authorities have recommended that lymph nodes of 5 cm or more be aspirated through normal tissue to prevent suppuration.

## Diagnosis

Chancroid must be considered in the differential diagnosis of any patient with a painful genital ulcer. Clinical diagnosis based on the appearance of the ulcer often is inaccurate. Reports comparing bacteriologic with clinical diagnosis show that accuracy of diagnosing lesions caused by *H. ducreyi* has varied from 33% to 53%. In areas where chancroid was prevalent and the clinicians more experienced, however, diagnostic accuracy reached as high as 75%. These reports emphasize the necessity of definitive laboratory testing, because a wide variety of aerobic and anaerobic bacteria can be isolated from ulcers that clinically resemble chancroid.

Aids in making the diagnosis include the following:

- Clinical suspicion when a genital ulcer is seen
- Cultures from the genital ulcer material (aspirates from inguinal nodes are less reliable)
- Transporting the swab in Amies or Stuart transport medium (a sterile swab transported on chocolate agar has been shown to be effective as well)

The organism is difficult to grow, but culturing in Nairobi medium has proved fairly successful.

Direct examination of Gram's staining has not given consistent results. In addition, the Ito-Reenstierna skin test and the complement fixation test have produced both false-negative and false-positive reactions; poor sensitivity and specificity preclude their clinical use. Researachers have noted qualitative and quantitative differences in the immune response to *H. ducreyi*, although the factors controlling this response are not clearly understood.

Circulating immune globulins (IgM and IgG) have been detected in patients with a clinical diagnosis of chancroid. Immunobinding and enzyme immunoassays have been used to investigate culture-confirmed and clinically suspected cases of chancroid, but these techniques do not appear to have clinical diagnostic value. The geographic differences in the protein on the outer membrane make it difficult to select a cross-reacting antigen. Polymerase chain reaction (PCR) testing for culture confirmation and direct detection of organisms in material from genital ulcers have not proved to have practical value.

## Treatment

Antibiotic resistance of *H. ducreyi* has been observed to trimethoprim, gentamicin, tetracycline, chloramphenicol, streptomycin, kanamycin, penicillin, ampicillin, and sulfonamides. The genetics and mechanisms of the antibiotic resistance by various strains of *H. ducreyi* are believed to be plasmid-mediated. The organism appears to be susceptible to macrolides (erythromycin and azithromycin) and to ceftriaxone, and most strains are susceptible to some quinolones (ciprofloxacin and trovafloxacin).

The recommended treatment regimens for chancroid infection are azithromycin, 1 g; erythromycin, 500 mg orally four times a day for seven days; or ceftriaxone, 250 mg in one intramuscular dose. Alternative regimens include ciprofloxacin, 500 mg orally every 12 hours for a total of three days, or amoxicillin, 500 mg, plus clavulanic acid, 125 mg, orally every 8 hours for seven days.

Because of the resistance spectrum, susceptibility testing of isolates from patients who fail to respond to therapy always should be performed. With effective treatment, ulcers should improve symptomatically within three days and objectively within seven days after starting therapy. Clinical resolution of lymphadenopathy occurs more slowly than that of ulcers. If no clinical improvement becomes evident in seven days, consider the following:

- Is the *H. ducreyi* a resistant strain?
- Is the diagnosis incorrect?
- Is there coinfection with another STD?
- Is the patient also infected with HIV?

Sex partners within the 10 days preceding the onset of symptoms in an infected patient, whether symptomatic or not, should be examined and treated with a recommended regimen. Many centers may not have the specialized media readily available for transport and growth of the organism. In the absence of a proven bacteriologic diagnosis, the patient should be treated if clinical evidence suggests a diagnosis of chancroid.

## Suggested Readings

Chouinard A. Winnipeg suffered second chancroid outbreak: team reports. Can Med Assoc J 1989;140:72–73.

Jessamine PG, Ronald AR. Chancroid and the role of genital ulcer disease in the spread of human retroviruses. Med Clin North Am 1990;74:1417–1431.

Johnson AP, Abeck D, Davies HA. The structure, pathogenicity, and genetics of *Haemophilus ducreyi*. J Infect 1988;17:99–106.

Martin DH, Sargent SJ. Comparison of azithromycin and ceftriaxone for the treatment of chancroid. Clin Infect Dis 1995;21:409–414.

McCarley ME, Cruz PD Jr, Sontheimer RD. Chancroid: clinical variants and other findings from an epidemic in Dallas County, 1986–1987. J Am Acad Dermatol 1988;19(2 Pt 1):330–337.

Morse SA. Chancroid and *Haemophilus ducreyi*. Clin Microbiol Rev 1989;2:137–157.

CHAPTER

# 48

# *Lymphogranuloma Venereum*

*Gael P. Wager*

## Background and Incidence

Lymphogranuloma venereum (LGV) is a systemic disease caused by the L-serotypes of *Chlamydia trachomatis* (L1, L2, and L3). These serovars are often referred to as *C. trachomatis biovar lymphogranuloma* and are identified by means of microimmunofluorescence techniques.

LGV has the potential for systemic dissemination and often persists as a chronic disorder. It is endemic in Africa, India, parts of Southeast Asia, South America, and the Caribbean. It can appear sporadically anywhere in the world, however. Prevalence data are unreliable even in endemic areas.

The lymphadenitis of LGV was recognized by Greek, Roman, and Arab physicians. Durand, Nicolas, and Favre established the infection as a clinical and pathologic entity in 1913. In 1924, Frei developed a specific skin test that permitted more accurate diagnosis.

## Pathophysiology

The infecting organism in LGV is generally transmitted by sexual contact. Once it has gained entry into the host, it incubates at the infection site and induces a primary lesion. It then invades the lymphatic system, causing thrombolymphangitis and perilymphangitis. Eventually, the inflammatory process spreads from infected lymph nodes into the surrounding tissue.

The infected nodes become enlarged and develop areas of necrosis, which then form "stellate abscesses." As the inflammation progresses, the abscesses coalesce and rupture the node, forming loculated abscesses, fistulas, or sinus tracts.

The acute inflammatory process lasts several weeks to months before subsiding. Healing takes place by fibrosis, which destroys the normal structure and function of the lymph nodes and vessels. The resulting chronic edema and fibrotic changes produce induration and enlargement of the affected areas. Fibrosis also compromises the blood supply to the overlying skin and mucous membrane, leading to ulceration.

## Diagnosis

LGV is predominantly an infection of lymphatic tissue. It appears in a variety of acute and late manifestations. Three stages usually characterize the clinical course of the disease:

- A primary stage, extending from the incubation period through formation of the initial lesion
- A secondary stage, with inflammation and swelling of the regional lymph nodes (the inguinal syndrome)
- A tertiary stage, which includes the late sequelae of the infection (anogenital syndrome)

### Primary Stage

The LGV infection is believed to occur primarily during sexual contact. Because chlamydial organisms cannot penetrate intact skin or mucous membranes, they probably enter through minute lacerations or abrasions. The incubation period after exposure has not been definitively identified, but appears to range from 3 to 21 days. After this period, a primary lesion may develop. This lesion may appear as a papule, a small or shallow ulcer or erosion, a small herpetiform ulcer (the most common presentation), or even as nonspecific urethritis. It is generally small, transient, and painless, and therefore often goes unnoticed by the patient.

Healing is spontaneous and without scarring. The most common sites in men are the coronal sulcus, glans, penile shaft, urethra, and scrotum. In women, the lesion is most commonly located on the posterior vaginal wall, the fourchette, the posterior lip of the cervix, or the vulva.

## Secondary Stage (Inguinal Syndrome)

The secondary stage is characterized by painful inflammation and enlargement of the inguinal nodes. This presentation is seen mostly in men, probably because the penis and scrotum are the most common sites of primary infection and because the lymphatic drainage from this area occurs to the inguinal nodes. In women, the vagina and cervix are the primary sites and the principal lymphatic drainage flows to the deep iliac, perirectal, and lumbrosacral nodes. Involvement of the deep iliac and retroperitoneal lymph nodes may be signified by a pelvic mass. Abdominal, pelvic, and lower back pain are frequently seen as well.

When the femoral nodes are concomitantly involved, a characteristic cleft appears between the inguinal and femoral nodes, due to the presence of Poupart's ligament. This finding, which is referred to as the "groove sign," is considered pathognomonic for LGV. At this stage, many patients will manifest systemic symptoms such as fever, headache, malaise, and anorexia in addition to the enlarging femoral nodes.

The lymph nodes may suppurate as a result of inflammatory enlargement. Rupture through the overlying skin may occur, with immediate relief of pain and fever. Numerous sinus tracts are then formed, which continue to drain thick, yellowish pus for long periods.

The organism also may gain access to the bloodstream and cause systemic disease. Manifestations of such a dissemination may include arthritis, pericarditis, pneumonia, hepatitis, erythema nodosum, and erythema multiforme.

## Tertiary Stage (Anogenital Syndrome)

The tertiary stage of LGV is characterized by proctocolitis, rectal stricture, rectovaginal fistulae, esthiomene, and elephantiasis. The vast majority of patients experiencing these late complications are women or homosexual men.

The early symptoms of rectal infection include anal pruritus and a mucous rectal discharge resulting from edema and hyperemia of the anorectal mucosa. The mucosa becomes friable, easily traumatized, and prone to ulceration. Ulcers are replaced by granulation tissue, and the granulomatous process progressively involves all layers of the bowel wall. The muscle layers are replaced by fibrous tissue that contracts over time.

The region 2 to 10 cm above the rectal sphincter is the area most commonly affected. Patients may complain of colicky pain, abdominal distension, constipation, and narrow-caliber stools ("pencil stools"). The rectal mucosa distal to the stricture and the skin around the anus are frequent sites of perirectal abscesses and anal fissures.

The combination of chronic inflammation and lymphatic stasis induces marked changes in the genital structures. Perianal outgrowths of lymphatic tissue that grossly resemble hemorrhoids (lymphorrhoids) may be seen. Women may experience severe edema and enlargement of the vulvar structures. Subsequent compromise of the blood supply to the superficial tissues will lead to development of painful ulcers. This presentation is referred to as esthiomene (Greek for "eating away"). In men, penile, scrotal, or perineal sinuses may develop. Penoscrotal elephantiasis may be seen as well.

## Other Manifestations

Autoinoculation of infectious discharge to the conjunctiva may occur in LGV. In such cases, the maxillary and posterior auricular lymph nodes may become involved.

LGV lesions of the mouth and pharynx may appear when infection is acquired by fellatio or cunnilingus. Cases of supraclavicular lymphadenitis with mediastinal lymphadenopathy and pericarditis have been reported with the presentation of LGV.

The literature also records the recovery of *C. trachomatis* from the gallbladder wall in cases of chronic cholecystitis as well as from fibrous perihepatic abdominal and pelvic adhesions (in cases of Fitz-Hugh–Curtis syndrome).

## Laboratory Confirmation

For decades, the Frei antigen skin test constituted the definitive method for confirming the diagnosis of LGV. The Frei antigen is no longer available in the United States. Instead, the diagnosis is now made on one of three bases:

- A positive serologic test, either complement-fixation (CF) or microimmunofluorescence (MIF)
- Isolation of chlamydial organisms
- Histologic identification of chlamydial elementary and/or inclusion bodies in infected tissue

The CF test, which was introduced in the 1930s, can detect antibodies to either *C. trachomatis* or *C. psittaci.* The CF antigen is common to all members of the *Chlamydia* genus. In patients with LGV, the CF test usually becomes positive within the first two weeks of infection. Titers may remain positive for the remainder of the patient's life. Titers of 1:64 or greater are generally associated with LGV infection; titers in individuals with other *C. trachomatis* infections are generally 1:16 or less.

The MIF test was developed by Wang and Grayson to serotype strains of *C. trachomatis.* It detects type-specific antibodies produced against each chlamydial serotype. The specimen is run against a panel of antigens, with the diagnosis being based on the pattern of reactivity. The disadvantage of the MIF test is that it is available in only a few specialized laboratories.

Chlamydial organisms can be isolated from infected tissue by inoculation into HeLa-229 or McCoy cells. Specimens of pus obtained from a fluctuant lymph node yield the highest rates. Most laboratories do not maintain active cell lines for chlamydial isolation, however. Reported recovery rates range from 24% to 30%.

Histologic identification of chlamydial elementary and inclusion bodies can be made both outside and inside cells in secretions and infected tissues. Fluorescent antibody staining and Giemsa's iodine are used for this purpose. Overall, the diagnosis of LGV by histologic and cytologic methods has not been very successful.

### Differential Diagnosis

Conditions to exclude when findings suggest LGV are genital herpes, donovanosis (granuloma inguinale), chancroid, cat-scratch fever, bacterial lymphadenitis, Hodgkin's disease, and non-Hodgkin's lymphoma. Because other sexually transmitted infections may occur at the same time, the diagnosis must exclude common infections such as syphilis and gonorrhea when LGV is suspected.

## Treatment

A number of antibiotics have been shown to be effective in treating LGV, although no single drug has demonstrated superior efficacy. Antibiotics that have been used in the treatment of LGV have included the tetracyclines, chloramphenicol, erythromycin, sulfadiazine, sulfamethoxazole, and rifampin. Treatment administered in the early stages of the infection achieves a better clinical response than therapy begun at the later, more chronic stages.

The most recent recommendations for LGV from the Centers for Disease Control and Prevention suggest that patients receive treatment for three weeks. The drug of choice is doxycycline, 100 mg orally two times per day. An alternative regimen is erythromycin base, 500 mg orally four times per day. Clinical data on use of azithromycin are lacking, but this agent's activity against *C. trachomatis* suggests that it may be effective in multiple doses given over two to three weeks.

Patients should be followed clinically until their signs and symptoms resolve completely. Pregnant women should be treated with the erythromycin regimen.

### Suggested Readings

Centers for Disease Control and Prevention. 1998 guidelines for treatment of sexually transmitted diseases. MMWR 1998;47 (RR-1):27–28.

Faro S. Lymphogranuloma venereum, chancroid, and granuloma inguinale. Obstet Gynecol Clin N Am 1989;16:517–530.

Hammerschlag MR. Lymphogranuloma venereum. In: Felman YM, ed. Sexually transmitted diseases. New York: Churchill Livingstone, 1986: Ch. 7.

Perine PL, Osoba AO. Lymphogranuloma venereum. In: Holmes KK, Mårdh PA, Sparling PF, et al., eds. Sexually transmitted diseases, 2nd ed. New York: McGraw-Hill, 1990: Ch. 17.

Sweet RL, Gibbs RS. Infectious diseases of the female genital tract. Baltimore: Williams & Wilkins, 1985:34–36.

CHAPTER

# 49

# *Granuloma Inguinale (Donovanosis)*

*Noelle C. Bowdler*
*Rudolph P. Galask*

## BACKGROUND

Granuloma inguinale (donovanosis) is a progressive, ulcerative bacterial infection of the genitalia that occurs most commonly in tropical and subtropical areas. First described by McLeod in 1882, the disease has been identified by several names, including granuloma venereum and donovanosis. The causative agent, which was discovered by Donovan in 1905, is currently known as *Calymmatobacterium granulomatis*. Infection with this organism can lead to significant tissue destruction and scarring, and the condition may be associated with the subsequent development of carcinoma. In addition, granuloma inguinale, like other ulcerative genital infections, is believed to be a cofactor for the transmission of the human immunodeficiency virus (HIV).

Granuloma inguinale occurs primarily in India, Africa, the Caribbean, Brazil, southern China, and Papua New Guinea; it is endemic in the aboriginal population of central Australia. Although it is uncommon in the United States, granuloma inguinale has been found in the southeastern region, particularly in the African American population.

This infection is believed to be transmitted sexually, although it is not highly contagious. Various studies have found that as many as 52% of the sexual partners of affected patients have the disease after repeated unprotected sexual contact. The fact that lesions almost always occur on the external genitalia or uterine cervices of sexually active women supports the hypothesis that the disease is transmitted sexually. The appearance of oral lesions is believed to follow from orogenital contact.

Transmission of granuloma inguinale by nonsexual contact with material from genital lesions is believed to occur as well. One investigator infected himself by inoculating an abrasion on his leg with the contents of a patient's lesion. Others have developed lesions after inoculation with pus from pseudobuboes. Vertical transmission of infection from mother to fetus most likely occurs at the time of delivery. Because the organism requires living tissue to grow in vitro, it has been suggested that a break in the host's skin or mucous membranes is required to allow infection.

## Pathophysiology and Clinical Presentation

After an incubation period, which usually varies from 8 to 80 days but can last even longer, single or multiple subcutaneous nodules appear in the infected person and erode through the skin to produce ulcers. Ulcerated areas are sharply defined but irregular in contour, and the base is often described as "beefy red." The lesions are granulomatous and friable, and they may become secondarily infected. Autoinoculation, with the development of lesions in closely approximated skin ("kissing lesions"), is common. As the primary lesion extends, it produces progressive destruction of affected tissues as well as fibrosis. Lymphedema distal to lesions is common. In as many as 20% of patients, enlargement of the affected genitalia progresses to pseudoelephantiasis.

In women, the lesions of granuloma inguinale are found most often on the inner labia, particularly near the clitoris. The uterine cervix is a primary site for infection as well. In men, lesions generally appear on the glans or prepuce. The inguinal regions are involved in approximately 10% of cases, with formation of pseudobuboes. The perianal tissues are affected in 5% to 10% of cases. Infants typically experience infections of the umbilicus, vulva, or penis, and may develop disseminated disease.

Local extension from the cervix to the endometrium, fallopian tubes, and ovaries, or from the external genitalia to underlying bone, bladder, or bowel, occasionally occurs. Distant sites are involved in approximately 5% of cases. Primary infections of the head (in particular, the mouth and throat), chest, extremities, and buttocks have been reported. Spread of infection from the genitalia to distant sites may occur by autoinoculation or by hematogenous dissemination. Infections of the liver, spleen, lung, and distant bony sites have been described, for example.

Constitutional symptoms are rare when the infection remains confined to the skin. Such symptoms may occur, however, if ulcers become secondarily infected or the infection spreads to certain extragenital sites.

## Diagnosis

A diagnosis of granuloma inguinale may be suggested by the patient's history and physical findings. Confirmation depends on the identification of Donovan bodies in a smear or biopsy specimen taken from the margin of an ulcer. To increase the likelihood of detecting Donovan bodies, prepare biopsy specimens from crushed tissue or by thin section. Donovan bodies are calymmatobacteria located within the cytoplasmic vacuoles of macrophages. The bacteria are pleomorphic rods that turn blue upon Giemsa staining. Leishman's stain, Wright's stain, the Rapidiff stain, and various silver stains can also be used to identify this organism. Donovan bodies have been identified in Papanicolaou-stained cervical smears as well.

*C. granulomatis* can be cultured in the yolk sac of chicken embryos, but has not been isolated using routine microbiological techniques on artificial media. In a preliminary study, researchers amplified *Klebsiella*-like sequences from biopsy specimens of three patients with granuloma inguinale, suggesting that polymerase chain reaction (PCR) tests may have a role in the diagnosis of this disease.

Complement fixation has been studied in patients with granuloma inguinale, as has a serologic test employing indirect immunofluorescence. As yet, no serologic tests are currently in general clinical use.

The differential diagnosis for granuloma inguinale includes infectious diseases that cause genital ulcers, such as chancroid. Early lesions may resemble the syphilitic chancre. Perianal lesions are often verrucous, and can be confused with the condylomata lata of secondary syphilis. Differentiation of granuloma inguinale from other disorders is hampered by the fact that it often coexists with other sexually transmitted diseases.

When lesions are chronic, carcinoma of the vulva must be taken into account in the differential diagnosis. Evaluation for carcinoma is particularly important in this setting because it may occur as a complication of granuloma inguinale.

## Treatment

A number of antibiotic regimens have been reported to be effective treatments for granuloma inguinale. To date, these agents have not been systematically compared. Reports on several of these drugs involve the treatment of only small numbers of patients. In general, it is recommended that treatment continue until all of the patient's lesions have healed. Lesions usually begin to decrease in size within days after the initiation of therapy. In most cases, they are completely healed within two to three weeks, although healing may sometimes take longer. A change in antibiotic regimen is recommended if the lesions do not change within two weeks of beginning treatment. Table 49-1 summarizes the CDC's 1998 recommendations for treating granuloma inguinale.

Tetracycline, 500 mg four times per day, is a commonly used agent. Doxycycline, 100 mg orally twice per day, also is acceptable. Resistance of the infecting organism to tetracycline has been reported.

An alternative oral regimen is trimethoprim/sulfamethoxazole, two tablets twice per day. This regimen can be used during pregnancy, except in the late third trimester.

Erythromycin, 500 mg orally every six hours, is another option for use during pregnancy. It is most effective, however, when combined with agents such as ampicillin or lincomycin.

Another macrolide, azithromycin, has been shown to be an effective treatment in reports on small numbers of patients.

**Table 49-1.** CDC Guidelines for Treating Granuloma Inguinale (Donovanosis)*

**Recommended Regimens**

Trimethoprim/sulfamethoxazole, one double-strength tablet orally twice daily

*or*

Doxycycline, 100 mg orally twice daily

**Alternative Regimens**

Ciprofloxacin, 750 mg orally twice daily

*or*

Erythromycin base, 500 mg orally four times daily

* Minimum treatment duration is three weeks. Consider adding an aminoglycoside such as gentamicin, 1 mg/kg IV every eight hours, if lesions do not respond within the first few days of therapy.

SOURCE: Centers for Disease Control and Prevention. 1998 guidelines for treatment of sexually transmitted diseases. MMWR 1998;47(RR-1):26–27.

Regimens employed include 1 g orally once per week for four weeks; 500 mg orally once per day for seven days; and 1 g orally on day 1, followed by 500 mg a day on days 2 through 5.

Norfloxacin, 400 mg orally twice per day for 7 to 10 days, was shown to be useful for treating granuloma inguinale in a study of 10 patients, as was ciprofloxacin, 500 mg orally twice per day, in a report on three patients. Chloramphenicol, 2 g per day orally in divided doses for 10 to 14 days, is effective as well, but its use is discouraged because of its rare potential to cause profound bone marrow suppression.

Parenteral regimens for granuloma inguinale include gentamicin, 1 mg/kg three times per day, and streptomycin, 1 g intramuscularly twice per day. Ceftriaxone, 1 g intramuscularly once per day, has been used successfully to treat 12 patients with chronic granuloma inguinale, all of whom had failed treatment with other antibiotic regimens.

Vulvectomy is undertaken in cases that are resistant to antibiotic treatment. Surgery also may be necessary if significant residual lymphedema of the vulva persists after antibiotic treatment or if the patient has suffered extensive destruction of vulvar tissues.

Screen patients with granuloma inguinale for other sexually transmitted infections. Also, treat their sexual partners.

Recommend that infected individuals abstain from sexual activity until all lesions heal.

## Sequelae

Long-standing infection with *C. granulomatis* may lead to destruction of the affected tissues and scarring at the site of involvement. Stenosis of the vagina or anus may result. An increased incidence of vulvar carcinoma has been reported in patients with a history of granuloma inguinale, although the strength and nature of this association are unclear.

Ulcerative genital infections are now recognized as cofactors for the sexual transmission of HIV. A program for eradicating granuloma inguinale has been proposed as a means to limit the spread of HIV.

### Suggested Readings

Faro S. Lymphogranuloma venereum, chancroid, and granuloma inguinale. Obstet Gynecol Clin North Am 1989;16:517–530.

Hart G. Donovanosis. In: Mandell GL, Douglas RG Jr, Bennet JE, eds. Principles and practice of infectious diseases, 3rd ed. Edinburgh: Churchill Livingstone, 1990;393.

Hart G. Donovanosis. Clin Infect Dis 1997;25:24–30.

Joseph AK, Rosen TR. Laboratory techniques used in the diagnosis of chancroid, granuloma inguinale, and lymphogranuloma venereum. Dermatol Clin 1994;12:l–8.

Latif AS, Mason PR, Paraiwa E. The treatment of donovanosis (granuloma inguinale). Sex Transm Dis 1988;15:27–29.

Merianos A, Gilles M, Chuah J. Ceftriaxone in the treatment of chronic donovanosis in central Australia. Genitourin Med 1994; 70:84–89.

O'Farrell N. Global eradication of donovanosis: an opportunity for limiting the spread of HIV-1 infection. Genitourin Med 1995; 71:27–31.

Schwarz RH. Chancroid and granuloma inguinale. Clin Obstet Gynecol 1983;26:138–142.

CHAPTER

# 50

# *Pediculosis Pubis*

*Mahmoud A. Ismail*

## Background and Incidence

Lice infestations have been recognized for centuries both as endemic and as epidemic disorders. Conditions of poor personal hygiene and overcrowding have been associated with such epidemics. Recently, a resurgence of skin disease caused by the pubic or crab louse has been recognized, paralleling an increase in the incidence of other sexually transmitted diseases (STDs).

Lice infestations have been observed in virtually every inhabited area of the world. The trend toward greater sexual permissiveness has aided its spread to all strata of society. Pediculosis pubis usually is spread through sexual contact. It is more contagious than any other STD; the chance of contracting the disease during a single sexual encounter is 95%.

After infection, pubic lice can be found on any terminal hair of the body. The organism's transfer from the pubic hair is probably mechanical, being assisted by animated scratching, fingernails, towels, and other similar means rather than by self-propulsion. The perineal and axillary hair often is infected, and the hair of the trunk, beard, scalp, and eyelashes is occasionally contaminated. Pediculosis pubis is most commonly encountered during adolescence and young adulthood.

## Etiology

*Phthirus rubis*, the crab louse, is the organism that causes pediculosis pubis. The organism is 1 to 2 mm long, gray, tough-skinned, and square. It resembles a crab—hence its nickname. It tends to remain in a restricted area in the genital region, where it attaches to the base of a pubic hair and feeds through mouth parts adapted to piercing skin. The sites of feeding nits are sometimes marked by small bluish hemorrhages in the skin.

The life cycle of the crab louse is 25 to 30 days from egg to egg. The female begins to lay eggs within 24 hours after mating, attaching them to a hair near the root. After an incubation time of 7 days, a nymph hatches and proceeds through three molts over the next 13 to 17 days. Once the louse reaches sexual maturity, the adult's life expectancy is 3 to 4 weeks.

## Diagnosis

Pediculosis pubis infestations usually cause pruritus and itching. The intense itching is believed to follow from the body's allergic reaction to foreign material injected by the organism during feeding. Bites often exhibit a hemorrhagic component thought to result from injections of anticoagulant material at the time of feeding. Pubic lice infestations of eyelashes may produce a pruritic and, occasionally, secondary marginal blepharitis.

Visualization of adult lice and their eggs (nits) with a magnifying glass is diagnostic for pediculosis pubis. Confirm the diagnosis by microscopic examination of a crab, its nit, or both. On occasion, the patient may see the crab louse moving over the skin.

## Treatment

The recommended treatment regimen relies on a permethrin (1%) cream rinse that is applied to the affected area and washed off after 10 minutes. Alternatives include pyrethrins and piperonyl butoxide (applied to the affected area and washed off after 10 minutes) or lindane (1%) shampoo (applied for 4 minutes and then thoroughly washed off). Lindane treatment is not recommended for pregnant or lactating women or for children younger than two years of age.

Patients should be reevaluated after one week if symptoms persist. Retreatment may be necessary if lice are found or eggs are observed at the hair–skin junction. The patient's sex partners within the past month should be treated as well.

Therapy for pediculosis of the eyelashes involves the application of occlusive ophthalmic ointment to the eyelid margins two times per day for 10 days to smother lice and nits. Lindane or other drugs should not be applied to the eyes. Clothing or bed linen that may have been contaminated by the patient within the past two days should be washed and dried by machine (hot cycles) or dry-cleaned.

Persons with HIV infection and pediculosis pubis should receive the same treatment as those without HIV infection.

## Suggested Readings

Centers for Disease Control and Prevention. 1998 guidelines for treatment of sexually transmitted diseases. MMWR 1998;47 (RR-1):105–106.

Couch JM, Green WR, Hirst LW, et al. Diagnosing and treating *Phthirus pubis palpebrarum.* Surv Opthalmol 1982;26:219–225.

Felman YM, Nikitas JA. Pediculosis pubis. Cutis 1980;25:482,487–489,559.

Orkin M. Pediculosis today. Minn Med 1974;57:848–852.

CHAPTER

# 51

# *Scabies*

*Mahmoud A. Ismail*

## Background and Incidence

Scabies is a disease of great antiquity and possibly the cause for the "seven-year itch" known to medicine for centuries. Napoleon's troops during the Russian campaign were thought to have had rampant scabies. This infection is common throughout the world, and its prevalence appears to increase in 30-year cycles. In the United States, scabies has been on the rise since 1973.

Although the disease has a worldwide distribution, its actual prevalence is unknown. Epidemics have been associated with world wars. Overcrowding, poor hygiene, malnutrition, and sexual promiscuity probably are contributing factors to its spread.

Scabies is now considered a sexually transmitted disease (STD), but prolonged contact with an infected person is required for transmission. Nonsexual transmission has been reported in hospitals during nursing activities such as sponge-bathing of patients and application of body lotions. Transfer of mites through infested bedding, clothes, or other fomites has also been implicated as a major node of transmission.

## Etiology

Human scabies is caused by the itch mite *Sarcoptes scabiei* var. *hominis*. The full-grown adult female is only about 0.35 mm long and is rounded, with three pairs of short, stubby legs. *S.*

*scabiei* moves briskly across the skin and can travel from neck to waist in a few hours.

Eggs are laid by the fertilized female in burrows several millimeters to several centimeters long, created at the base of the stratum corneum of the epidermis. Approximately 72 to 84 hours later, nymphs emerge and undergo several molts to become adult mites. The adult mites mate 17 days later; shortly afterward the male dies, but the grown female proceeds to burrow and complete the life cycle.

## Diagnosis

Scabies manifests itself by causing intense itching in the host, which usually becomes worse at night. The rash has an insidious onset and a characteristic pattern of involvement that includes the interdigital web spaces, wrists, elbows, anterior axillary folds, periumbilical skin, genitals, buttocks, and sides of the feet. In infants and small children, the palms, soles, face, and scalp may be affected.

The physical findings in scabies include classic linear burrows, particularly in the interdigital spaces and on the penis. The burrows are 5 to 10 mm long, and the organisms may be seen as tiny brown-and-white specks at the inner ends of them. In infants, scabies may sometimes be vesicular or even bullous, and secondary pyoderma may obscure the underlying cause.

Scabies may present as eczematous or urticarial eruptions. Approximately 7% of infected persons exhibit a nodular variant with scattered, pruritic, reddish-brown nodules, particularly on the penis and in the axillae and perineum. These lesions may be a manifestation of strong delayed hypersensitivity to retained mite products and may persist for weeks or even months.

Immunocompromised or debilitated patients may be infested with large numbers of mites found in thickened psoriasis-like skin lesions. This condition, known as Norwegian scabies, is extremely contagious.

The burrow of *S. scabiei* is pathognomonic. In many cases, however, burrows may not be readily apparent. Application of blue or black ink to the skin overlying a suspected burrow can aid diagnosis. By capillary action, the ink will be pulled into the burrow. Removal of the excess external ink with an alcohol swab will leave a line of ink in the burrow to demonstrate its presence. The burrow containing the organism's egg and feces will yield a positive scraping that can be used to confirm the diagnosis on microscopic examination. Fresh lesions should be used for obtaining mites.

Scabies is called the "great imitator," because patients may have a variety of lesions. Dermatologic conditions such as eczema, acute urticaria, impetigo, erythrasma, insect bites, neurodermatitis, and dermatitis herpetiformis must be considered in the differential diagnosis. The history of insidious onset, the presence of nocturnal pruritus and pleomorphic lesions, and the characteristic distribution of lesions are all strongly suggestive of scabies.

## Treatment

Treatment of scabies remains controversial. Success depends on correct application of scabicide to the patient, sexual contacts, and family members.

For adults and older children, the recommended regimen is either permethrin cream (5%), applied to all areas of the body from the neck down and washed off after 8 to 14 hours, or lindane (1%), 1 ounce of lotion or 30 g of cream, applied thinly to all areas of the body from the neck down and washed off thoroughly after 8 hours. Sex partners and close household contacts should receive this treatment as well.

Lindane should not be used following a bath. It is contraindicated in persons with extensive dermatitis, pregnant or lactating women, or children younger than two years of age.

An alternative regimen is crotamiton (10%), applied to the entire body from the neck down nightly for two consecutive nights and washed off thoroughly 24 hours after the second application. Infants, children up to 2 years old, and pregnant and lactating women may be treated with permethrin or crotamiton regimens.

A potential option not yet available in the United States is ivermectin, an anthelmintic agent that has an excellent safety record in the treatment of onchocerciasis (river blindness). A recent study demonstrated that a single oral dose of 200 μg/kg of ivermectin is highly effective in the treatment of scabies in both healthy and immunocompromised patients. No adverse side effects were noted in this study. Although not FDA-approved for use in children younger than age 5 or for the treatment of scabies in humans, ivermectin appears to be the first highly effective, inexpensive, and safe oral agent for the treatment of this common skin infestation. In particular, it is effective in immunocompromised patients in whom very severe skin manifestations of scabies may develop. The oral formulation offers several advantages, including the ability to assure compliance by observing the patient taking the single required dose and avoiding the problems of improper or inadequate application of topical agents. Its use also should facilitate the control of outbreaks in institutions. Furthermore, the oral route of administration appears to offer more rapid resolution of pruritus than does topical treatment.

Pruritus may persist for several weeks, even after adequate therapy with permethrin, lindane, or crotamiton. A single retreatment after one week may be considered if the patient does not show any clinical improvement. Additional weekly treatments are appropriate only if live mites continue to be found. Both sexual and close personal or household contacts within the past month should be examined and treated.

Clothing or bed linen that may have been contaminated by the patient within the past two days should be washed and dried by machine (hot cycles) or dry-cleaned. Fumigation of living areas is not necessary.

Persons with HIV infection and uncomplicated scabies should receive the same treatment as persons without HIV infection. Persons with HIV infection and others who are immunosuppressed are at increased risk for Norwegian scabies, a disseminated dermatologic infection. Such patients should be managed in consultation with an expert.

## Suggested Readings

Centers for Disease Control and Prevention. 1998 guidelines for treatment of sexually transmitted diseases. MMWR 1998;47 (RR-1):106–108.

Cohen HB. Scabies continues. Int J Dermatol 1982;21:134–135.

Meinking TL, Taplin D, Hermida JL, et al. The treatment of scabies with ivermectin. N Engl J Med 1995;333:26–30.

Oriel JD. Ectoparasites. In: Holmes KK, Mårdh PA, eds. International perspectives on neglected sexually transmitted diseases. Washington, DC: Hemisphere Publishing, 1983:131–138.

CHAPTER

# 52

# *Molluscum Contagiosum*

*David E. Soper*

## Background

Molluscum contagiosum is a benign dermatologic infection caused by an unclassified poxvirus. In children, the lesions appear sporadically in a generalized distribution and usually involve the face, trunk, and arms. After puberty, lesions are found typically on or near the genitalia.

## Pathophysiology

Most investigators believe that the molluscum contagiosum virus (MCV) is spread by direct contact. Patient histories and clinical data support the assumption that MCV may be sexually transmitted in some cases. In adults, skin-to-skin contact associated with sexual intercourse is considered the most common method of transmitting the virus. Nonsexual transmission has been reported in patients treated by a surgeon who had hand lesions and in association with wrestling, tattooing, and the use of gymnastic equipment and towels.

Initially, MCV infects the basal keratinocytes. The virus persists in the epidermis in a progressively maturing form similar to that seen in human papillomavirus infections. MCV lesions consist of focal areas of hyperplastic epidermis that surround cystic lobules filled with keratinized debris and degenerating molluscum bodies. The molluscum bodies (Henderson-Paterson bodies) are composed of large masses of maturing virions. The pathologic changes remain limited to the epidermis. In some cases, dermal inflammation may occur as a reaction to viral antigen or keratin infiltration. Resolution usually follows.

The average incubation period for MCV infections is two to three months. Most patients are asymptomatic, with the MCV lesions being incidental to a variety of nonvenereal and nondermatologic conditions. Occasionally, patients complain of pruritus, tenderness, and pain.

The lesions are usually flesh-colored, but can have a gray-white, yellow, or pink color. They begin as tiny, pinpoint papules that grow over several weeks to a diameter of 3 to 5 mm. The papules are smooth, firm, and dome-shaped. They have a highly characteristic central umbilication from which caseous material can be expressed.

One to 20 lesions are commonly found on the skin of the labia majora, mons pubis, buttocks, and inner thighs. They rarely, if ever, cover mucosal surfaces. The linear orientation of some lesions suggests autoinoculation by scratching. Occasionally, multiple lesions become confluent and converge into a "giant molluscum."

Individuals with deficiencies of cell-mediated immunity (for example, AIDS patients) are at risk for extensive outbreaks.

## Diagnosis

The diagnosis of molluscum contagiosum can be made reliably on clinical grounds alone. Excisional biopsy reveals typical enlarged epithelial cells with intracytoplasmic inclusion bodies. Diagnostic confirmation may also be obtained by noting sheets of ovoid, homogenous bodies as large as 25 μm in diameter after crushing the contents of a lesion on a slide and application of Giemsa, Wright's, or Gram's stain. Electron microscopic examination will reveal the typical poxvirus particles.

## Treatment

The natural history of MCV infection is characterized by spontaneous regression of mature lesions, followed by continued emergence of new lesions. Molluscum contagiosum persists from six months to three years in the absence of therapy.

Lesions may be eradicated by mechanical destruction or techniques that induce local epidermal inflammation. Although such treatment may hasten the resolution of individual lesions and reduce the incidence of autoinoculation and transmission to other individuals, recurrence is frequent. The benign and self-limited nature of the infection must therefore be weighed against the potential harm of destructive therapies.

The most widely used method of therapy is excisional curettage. Individual lesions are curetted, and the bases are treated with light electrodesiccation. Cryotherapy and topical treatment with podophyllin or trichloroacetic acid have also been used with favorable results. No currently available therapy appears to be effective in immunocompromised patients, however, probably because of the persistent recurrence of new lesions.

Cryotherapy with a liquid nitrogen spray apparatus is one practical approach to therapy. Such units can be purchased or are available in most dermatologists' offices. The lesions are sprayed until they turn white and are surrounded by a white ring approximately 1 mm in diameter. Large lesions can be sprayed twice with a freeze-thaw-freeze technique.

## Suggested Readings

Brown ST, Nalley JF, Kraus SJ. Molluscum contagiosum. Sex Transm Dis 1981;8:227–234.

Douglas JM. Molluscum contagiosum. In: Holmes KK, Mårdh PA, Sparling PF, et al, eds. Sexually transmitted diseases. New York: McGraw-Hill, 1990.

Wilkin JK. Molluscum contagiosum venereum in a women's outpatient clinic: a venereally transmitted disease. Am J Obstet Gynecol 1977;128:531–535.

CHAPTER

53

# Genital Herpes Simplex Infections

*James H. Harger*

## Background and Incidence

Genital herpes simplex virus (HSV) infections are common in women, although the majority produce no symptoms or result in mild symptoms that may be overlooked. In a recent longitudinal study of 4781 sexually active women attending five family planning clinics in southwestern Pennsylvania, 27.4% had antibodies to glycoprotein (gG-2) of HSV type 2 (HSV-2). Only 4.9% of the women gave a history of genital HSV infections, however. Of the history-positive women, 95.1% tested positive for antibodies to gG-1 or gG-2. In that same population, previous results showed that only 63% of the isolates from the initial case of genital HSV infection were HSV-2. The other isolates (37%) were HSV-1.

The actual prevalence of genital HSV infection is difficult to determine because of the disparity between symptomatic and asymptomatic cases. One study indicated that more than half of all cases of neonatal HSV infection arise in babies born to women with no known history of genital HSV infections. This finding shows that such women harbor the disease and can be considered contagious. Similarly, men may have asymptomatic genital HSV infection.

Serologic surveys using Western blot techniques have shown that antibodies against HSV-2 can be measured in 16% of adults in the United States, in 7% to 28% of various groups in Europe, and in 20% to 45% of men and women in selected

African nations. Because approximately one-third of the isolates from women with initial genital HSV infections involve HSV-1, however, the use of antibody tests that are more or less specific for HSV-2 probably underestimates the actual prevalence of genital HSV infections by a modest proportion. The subtle and highly variable course of this disease can prove vexing to both patients and clinicians.

## Pathophysiology

To plan an effective, appropriate management strategy, the clinician must understand the nature of genital HSV infection. The first episode is as variable as the recurrences.

### Initial Episodes

The classic, severe primary episode occurs in 30% of women who have no preexisting antibodies against HSV-1 or HSV-2. It lasts approximately 20 days. Most initial episodes are less severe, however, and may not produce any symptoms. These initial, mild nonprimary episodes of genital HSV infection may occur because the patient developed anti-HSV antibodies during previous oral HSV infections that confer partial protection.

Both true primary (seronegative) and initial nonprimary (negative history but seropositive) genital HSV infections usually begin with a flu-like syndrome of fatigue, malaise, myalgia, nausea, and fever, which develops three to five days after sexual activity with the source contact. Vulvar burning and pruritus precede the multiple vesicles that occur in two or more anatomic regions of the vulva, the vagina, and (rarely) the cervix. These vesicles may remain intact for 24 to 36 hours before evolving into painful, tender, shallow ulcers. During the first several days of initial infection, crops of vesicles may appear at new sites or near old ones.

Several studies have revealed that the mean duration of pain in primary lesions is 9 to 13 days and the mean time to crusting is 9 to 15 days. Complete healing of the genital lesions requires anywhere from 10 to 22 days, and HSV cultures remain positive (HSV shedding) for a mean of 8 to 14 days. Continuous HSV shedding from the cervix has been observed in some cases for as long as 41 days after the onset of a primary episode, even when vulvar lesions were entirely healed. The ideal duration of drug therapy for such initial episodes, therefore, remains difficult to establish.

## Recurrent Episodes

After the initial episode resolves, the pattern of recurrence varies. Researchers have found a rough correlation between the severity of the first episode and the frequency of recurrences in the first year. After a severe primary episode of genital HSV-2 infection, the patient usually experiences one to six recurrences in the first year. In some women, the recurrences come further apart from the beginning; a few unfortunate patients will have monthly bouts for several years. Patients with HSV-1 genital infection tend to have few to no recurrences.

After a mild or equivocal initial episode, most women develop only sporadic recurrences. These attacks often do not result in lesions but rather produce prodromal lancinating pain, vulvar pruritus, vulvar tenderness, and localized swelling without ulceration. Infrequently, however, women with mild primary episodes will develop frequent recurrences. Whatever the overall pattern, many women will experience stretches of several months in which the recurrence frequency actually increases temporarily. At such times, these patients may seek medical advice for the first time.

The recurrent genital HSV lesions are less severe and last for a shorter period of time than those associated with the primary episodes. Most recurrences produce one or two vesicles, which usually ulcerate within 12 hours. Only one area on the vulva is typically affected, and that site is often the same during recurrences. The mean duration of HSV shedding varies from 3.1 to 7.4 days; crusting of the lesions takes a mean of 2.7 to 5.0 days; and complete healing may require 9.0 to 11.3 days. Patients experience pain in the lesions for a mean of 3.1 to 8.6 days.

Investigators have found that 36% of women having only HSV-1 antibodies developed a culture-positive symptomatic recurrence. In contrast, 66% of women with only HSV-2 antibodies experienced a culture-positive symptomatic recurrence. Women with both HSV-1 and HSV-2 antibodies underwent a culture-documented symptomatic recurrence in 77% of the cases studied. The median number of symptomatic recurrences per year, however, was zero for women with only HSV-1 antibodies but 7.5 for women with only HSV-2 antibodies; this finding confirms the greater tendency toward recurrences caused by HSV-2.

Women who had symptomatic recurrences experienced a mean of 6.5 episodes per year, although the original population was already self-selected for frequent recurrences and probably should not be considered representative of all women with genital HSV infection. Within this group of patients, 57% of the recurrent episodes lasted only one day, 23% lasted two days, 11% lasted three days, and 9% lasted four days or longer. Women who did not experience recurrent symptomatic episodes during the assessment period had a mean of 3.8 asymptomatic culture-positive episodes per year; 75% of those lasted only one day and another 14% lasted only two days. In women with any symptomatic recurrences at all, the mean number of days of viral shedding was 4.7 per year compared with only 5.5 days for those without any symptomatic recurrences.

Asymptomatic HSV shedding from genital sites was found 2.1 times more often in the year following primary occurrence than in the subsequent years. Women experiencing more than 12 recurrences per year were 5.1 times more likely to shed herpes virus than either women with no recurrences or those with fewer than 12 recurrences per year. Asymptomatic HSV genital shedding was 3.3 times more common in women with more than 12 recurrences per year. Frequent recurrences and recent development of genital herpes were the most important markers of a greater risk of asymptomatic shedding. This pattern may lead to unexpected sexual transmission of HSV infection and, perhaps, vertical transmission to a neonate as well. Marked variability in the recurrence pattern makes it difficult to assess the efficacy of therapy for HSV infections.

## Diagnosis

Although a diagnosis of genital HSV ulcers is generally made on clinical grounds, it should be confirmed at least once by laboratory methods before the patient begins pharmacologic therapy. If the patient has an ulcerated or vesicular lesion on cornified squamous epithelium, obtain a Tzanck smear by gently scraping the base of the lesion; transfer the cells to a glass slide, and fix them immediately. The presence of multinucleated giant cells is strongly suggestive of HSV. The Tzanck smear's sensitivity ranges from 85% to 95%, and its specificity exceeds 95%. Papanicolaou smears of moist mucous membranes for HSV shedding also offer better than 95% specificity, but their sensitivity is only 60% to 70% (i.e., 30% to 40% give false-negative results).

The current standard method for detecting HSV shedding consists of tissue culture. Gently, but persistently, rub a swab moistened in Hanks balanced salt solution over the mucous membrane or the base of the lesion. Place the swab into the transport medium, and send it to the laboratory as soon as possible. If the delay in transport exceeds 1 hour, cool the transport tube to 4 °C (refrigerator temperature) or freeze it at –80 °C in a special virology freezer. Freezing the transport medium at –20 °C—the temperature usually maintained in a household freezer—will rapidly reduce the viral titer and might cause a false-negative result.

Once the specimen is inoculated into tissue culture, 95% of HSV can be detected within three days, depending on the size of the inoculum. Typing of HSV may help both the patient and physician. Discerning whether the organism is HSV-1 or HSV-2 can prove beneficial for predicting recurrent disease, for example. Serum antibody levels to HSV usually offer no help because 70% of the adult population is seropositive for HSV-1. Most adults acquire HSV-1 oral infection in childhood.

The greater sensitivity of polymerase chain reaction (PCR) testing for HSV in genital secretions has provided some interesting findings. This technique's high sensitivity can lead to false-positive results because it increases the chance of cross-contamination with previous samples. A potential problem is that PCR detects both intact, infectious HSV particles and

HSV fragments. The latter would give the false impression that the patient's HSV infection remains active.

## Treatment

The goals of treating genital HSV infections depend on the nature and severity of the episode. HSV encephalitis, disseminated HSV infection, and HSV-related hepatitis are rare. Approximately 10% of HSV infections are associated with headache, photophobia, nausea, and meningeal signs.

Almost all women with primary genital HSV infection experience dysuria so severe that many limit their liquid intake to decrease the necessity of voiding frequently. This pain can be overcome by pouring warm water over the vulva while urinating (to dilute the urine) or by urinating while sitting in a tub of warm water. A much smaller proportion of women with primary genital HSV infection, however, develop a true sensory neurogenic bladder and cannot urinate at all. These women will probably require hospitalization, implantation of a suprapubic bladder catheter, and IV antiviral drug therapy. Antibiotics have no place in the treatment of primary genital HSV infections, because they are ineffective against the herpes virus or viruses in general. Likewise, analgesics have little therapeutic value but they may help patients sleep. Topical antiviral agents do not shorten episodes, and topical lidocaine gel provides temporary relief but may lead to allergic reaction.

Recurrent genital HSV infections are rarely frequent or painful enough to warrant pharmacologic treatment. Nevertheless, the loss of self-esteem, the loss of a sense of control over her own body, and the fear of transmitting HSV infections to others usually encourages the patient to seek help in preventing and treating recurrences.

Counseling and education may help patients understand their disease and reduce the risks of HSV transmission. In addition, three effective antiviral agents are currently available in the United States: acyclovir, valacyclovir, and famciclovir. These DNA-polymerase inhibitors are activated only in the nucleus of HSV-infected cells by an HSV-encoded thymidine kinase.

Oral acyclovir has been available since 1984, and its effects and complications are well characterized. When given orally, this agent has poor bioavailability, with only 15% to 20% of the drug being absorbed. On the other hand, this route of administration brings few side effects and is usually well tolerated over prolonged periods. When given intravenously to treat seriously ill patients, acyclovir can be nephrotoxic. Renal function must, therefore, be monitored carefully, and the patient should be kept well hydrated. Long-term effects of acyclovir are not harmful.

In an effort to achieve higher serum concentrations of acyclovir, a new oral prodrug named valacyclovir was introduced in 1995. The 1-valyl ester of acyclovir, valacyclovir is absorbed more completely from the gastrointestinal tract. It is then hydrolyzed in the gut and liver to acyclovir, resulting in bioavailability of about 50% of the oral dose. The steady-state peak plasma concentrations after a 200 mg or 800 mg dose of oral acyclovir are 3.5 and 7.0 μmol/L, respectively, whereas the peak plasma concentration after a 500 mg dose of valacyclovir is 14.4 μmol/L. In this fashion, valacyclovir may be administered twice per day compared with the consistent four-hour doses needed with acyclovir. Future studies may also show that the higher peak plasma concentrations achieved with 1 g oral doses of valacyclovir (24.9 μmol/L) may make it possible to replace parenteral acyclovir therapy with oral valacyclovir in some applications.

Similarly, the antiviral famciclovir is a prodrug with 77% oral bioavailability. Famciclovir is metabolized in the gut and liver to penciclovir, an active agent that inhibits herpes virus replication in cells infected by HSV by the same mechanism as acyclovir (blocking of viral DNA polymerase activity by the penciclovir triphosphate). Because penciclovir has a longer intracellular half-life, somewhat lower doses may suffice.

## Treating Primary Infections

Pharmacologic therapy for the initial episode of genital HSV infection can significantly diminish the duration of symptoms and lesions. Initiate oral acyclovir at a dosage of 200 mg five times per day for 10 days. In studies, this regimen reduced HSV shedding from 9 days in controls to 2 days. Mean time to crusting of lesions was reduced from 10 to 7 days. Duration of lesions declined from 16 days to 12 days and mean duration of local pain diminished from 7 days to 5 days. Acyclovir also decreased the mean duration of constitutional symptoms from 6 days to 3 days.

Antiviral therapy should not be initiated empirically because the onset of the first recurrence—if one occurs at all—cannot be predicted. Therapy should end after the patient completes a course and the signs and symptoms of the infection resolve. Observe the patient to determine the frequency of subsequent recurrences before deciding whether further treatment is warranted.

Although the newer antiviral drugs (valacyclovir and famciclovir) may be as effective in treating the initial genital HSV episodes, no recent studies support the use of these agents for this purpose. Because valacyclovir is converted to acyclovir by hepatic metabolism, it seems likely to be effective, but the necessary dose and the dosing interval remain to be established. Less information is available for famciclovir because the active agent, penciclovir, has not been used in the United States to this point.

Although hospitalization is rarely necessary for initial episodes, some reasonable indications for parenteral acyclovir therapy exist (Table 53-1). In such cases, parenteral acyclovir should be slowly infused IV over 60 minutes to avoid phlebitis (Table 53-2). Maintain the patient in a well-hydrated state to avoid crystallization of acyclovir in renal tubules and obstructive uropathy. Determine serum creatinine levels daily

**Table 53-1.** Indications for Parenteral Acyclovir and Hospitalization

| |
|---|
| Meningeal signs (nuchal rigidity) |
| Photophobia |
| Severe headache |
| Severe nausea |
| Upper-right-quadrant tenderness and/or pain |
| Urinary retention |
| Vomiting |

**Table 53-2.** Dosage of Acyclovir

| |
|---|
| **Mild Disease (Severe Nausea, Vomiting, Urinary Retention)** |
| 5 mg/kg of body weight, administered q8h* |
| **Severe Illness** |
| 10 mg/kg of body weight, administered q8h* |

* Adminster IV over 1 hour.

**Table 53-3.** Side Effects of Acyclovir

| |
|---|
| Acne |
| Arthralgia |
| Confusion |
| Delirium |
| Diarrhea |
| Fatigue |
| Fever |
| Hallucinations |
| Hepatic dysfunction |
| Insomnia |
| Lethargy |
| Lymphadenopathy |
| Menstrual abnormalities |
| Muscle cramps |
| Rash |
| Renal toxicity |
| Seizures |
| Sore throat |
| Tremors |
| Vertigo |

to monitor for nephrotoxicity, a reversible condition that represents the major complication of IV acyclovir (Table 53-3). Uncommon side effects include neutropenia, rash, diaphoresis, and hypotension.

## Therapy for Recurrent Disease

Once a patient develops recurrent genital HSV infections, confirm the diagnosis by culture on one occasion to ensure that the lesions represent recurrent HSV infection. If the signs and symptoms are consistent and typical, further HSV cultures are unnecessary. Obtain a careful history to determine the frequency and duration of the episodes. Three alternative strategies are available to manage recurrent genital HSV infections: education, episodic therapy, and suppression.

### *1. Education*

Pharmacologic therapy may be unnecessary. Because the safety of oral acyclovir, valacyclovir, and famciclovir during pregnancy has not been established, these drugs should not be given to women who are attempting to conceive. In fact, effective contraception should be advised for any reproductive-age woman who is beginning antiviral therapy. In many cases, the frequency of the recurrent infections is so low and the severity so minimal that the patient may be satisfied with the option of using pharmacologic therapy any time she chooses. Simply having this sense of control and an understanding of the disease may allow the patient to reduce the risk of HSV transmission to sexual partners and obviate antiviral drug therapy.

### *2. Intermittent ("Episodic") Oral Antiviral Drug Therapy*

When the recurrences develop at intervals exceeding two months, continuous use of pharmacologic therapy seems wasteful and unnecessary. If the infrequent recurrences last for 5 to 10 days or more, their duration can be reduced by giving acyclovir, 200 mg, five times each day. In a multicenter, randomized, placebo-controlled study of 250 patients, oral acyclovir reduced the mean duration of HSV shedding from 3.4 days to 2.1 days, mean time to crusting of lesions from 3.2 days to 2.4 days, mean duration of pruritus from 3.6 days to 2.8 days, mean duration of pain from 3.4 days to 3.0 days, and mean duration of lesions from 6.5 days in placebo patients to 5.5 days in drug recipients.

In the only published trial of patient-initiated valacyclovir therapy, given as 500 mg b.i.d. for episodic treatment of recurrent HSV, the median time required for lesion healing was reduced from 6.0 days in 259 controls to 4.1 days in 360 cases.

The median duration of pain declined from 4 and 3 days in controls to 3 and 2 days in treated women and men, respectively; the median duration of HSV shedding decreased from 4 days in controls to 2 days in treated cases of both sexes. No further improvement in these outcome variables was observed when a dose of 1 g b.i.d. was given. In the only published study of three different doses of patient-initiated famciclovir therapy for genital HSV recurrences, no significant differences were found between b.i.d. doses of 125 ($n$ = 117), 250 ($n$ = 128), and 500 mg ($n$ = 121). All three dose levels, however, reduced the median time to lesion healing from 3.8 days in 101 controls to 3.7 to 4.1 days in cases. The median time to complete resolution of all symptoms decreased from 3.7 days in controls to 3.0 to 3.2 days in treated patients.

Although such differences may seem subtle, all were statistically significant. Because the gains are relatively small with any of the three available antiviral agents, however, therapy will achieve virtually no appreciable improvement in recurrences that last fewer than four days. Some patients may benefit more from the knowledge that they have some measure of control over the recurrences than from actual use of the drug.

The multicenter study demonstrated a better effect from oral acyclovir when it was begun very early in the course of the recurrence. Similar findings arose with valacyclovir and famciclovir when physician-initiated therapy was compared with patient-initiated drug treatment. For that reason, the patient should not wait to see the clinician for confirmation of each recurrence. Rather, she should purchase the antiviral drug to keep on hand until prodromal symptoms are perceived and then commence therapy immediately after symptoms appear.

No clear choice of antiviral agent has emerged, because the efficacy of the three available drugs seems similar, although they have not been tested against one another. Given that each reduces symptoms and lesion healing by 30% to 50%, convenience and cost may determine the preferred agent. Because acyclovir must be taken five times daily compared with twice daily for valacyclovir and famciclovir, the latter two would seem easier to use. The current retail cost for the three agents given over a five-day course for HSV recurrences is approximately \$33 for acyclovir (25 capsules at \$1.32 per capsule), \$30 for valacyclovir (10 caplets at $3.03 per caplet), and $25 for famciclovir (10 tablets at $2.53 per tablet). Note, however, that prices may change in the future.

### *3. Suppression*

The third strategy for recurrent genital HSV infection is prophylactic therapy. In patients whose recurrences develop more than six to eight times per year, continuous administration of oral acyclovir can usually reduce the frequency of recurrences in a dramatic fashion. Two large studies (of 950 and 261 patients, respectively) in which subjects received one year of oral acyclovir at a dose of 400 mg twice daily showed that 44% and 46% of patients had no recurrences at all, whereas only 2% and 5% of placebo-treated controls remained free of recurrences. In other words, acyclovir-treated patients developed a mean of 1.8 recurrences per year in the two studies compared with mean recurrence rates in controls of 11.4 and 8.7 per year in the studies.

These and other studies of smaller populations and shorter therapy demonstrate that suppressive therapy with acyclovir can be effective and safe. Athough studies of suppression with various doses of valacyclovir and famciclovir are under way, the results of these trials have not yet been published. No hepatic or renal toxicity of oral acyclovir has been observed in any study. Determination of long-term safety, of course, must await 15 to 25 years of postmarketing evaluation. Finally, suppression therapy with acyclovir in immunocompetent patients has not yielded any clinically significant HSV isolates that are resistant to the drug. A 1994 report by members of the Acyclovir Study Group found 4 of 113 (3.5%) isolates of resistant HSV strains cultured from 239 immunocompetent adults treated with continuous acyclovir suppression for six years.

When administering acyclovir for suppression of frequent genital HSV recurrences, it is reasonable to begin with the proven dose of 400 mg twice daily and then reduce the dose gradually as long as no recurrence develops. Alternatively, the potential hazards and cost of acyclovir may be minimized by beginning at a level of 200 mg twice daily and then raising the dose if this lower level proves insufficient to prevent recurrences. Furthermore, suppressive doses of acyclovir have been continued beyond one year to two years or more without any adverse effects. Although many physicians refuse to extend prescriptions for acyclovir suppression beyond the 12 months approved by the Food and Drug Administration, the FDA does not actually limit the physician's clinical use of this agent.

Acyclovir suppression does not alter the natural history of genital HSV recurrences. In some cases, however, the frequency of recurrences may diminish spontaneously. The long-term study revealed that 205 (85.8%) of the 239 adults had at least one HSV recurrence in year 7 after receiving six years of suppressive therapy; 75% had two recurrences. By the Kaplan-Meier method, the median time to the first recurrence after stopping acyclovir was found to be 68 days (range 1 to 363 days) and the median time to the second recurrence was 180 days (range 18 to 364 days). Patients taking long courses of acyclovir should occasionally interrupt their therapy to assess any changes in the frequency of recurrence that would render further suppression unnecessary.

## Suggested Readings

Baker DA, Blythe JG, Kaufman R, et al. One-year suppression of frequent recurrences of genital herpes with oral acyclovir. Obstet Gynecol 1989;73:84–87.

Deardourff SL, Deture FA, Drylie DM, et al. Association between herpes hominis type 2 and the male genitourinary tract. J Urol 1974;112:126–127.

Fife KH, Crumpacker CS, Mertz GJ, et al. Recurrence and resistance patterns of herpes simplex virus following cessation of ≥6 years of chronic suppression with acyclovir. J Infect Dis 1994;169: 1338–1341.

Goldberg LH, Kaufman R, Kurtz TO, et al. Long-term suppression of recurrent genital herpes with acyclovir. Arch Dermatol 1993;129:582–587.

Harger JH, Pazin GJ, Breinig MC, et al. Current understanding of the natural history of genital herpes simplex infections. J Reprod Med 1986;31:365–373.

Johnson RE, Nahmias AJ, Magder LS, et al. A seroepidemiological survey of the prevalence of herpes simplex virus type 2 in the United States. N Engl J Med 1989;321:7–12.

Koutsky LA, Steven CE, Holmes KK, et al. Underdiagnosis of genital herpes by current clinical and viral-isolation procedures. N Engl J Med 1992;326:1533–1539.

Kurtz TO, Boone GS, Acyclovir Study Group. Safety and efficacy of long-term suppressive Zovirax treatment of frequently recurrent genital herpes: year 5 results. Abstract 1107. 30th Interscience Conference on Antimicrobial Agents and Chemotherapy, Atlanta, Oct. 21–24, 1990.

Mertz GJ, Critchlow CW, Benedetti J, et al. Double-blind placebo-controlled trial of oral acyclovir in first-episode genital herpes simplex virus infection. JAMA 1984;252:1147–1151.

Mertz GJ, Jones CC, Mills J, et al. Long-term acyclovir suppression of frequently recurring genital herpes simplex virus infections: a multicenter double-blind trial. JAMA 1988;260:201–206.

Nahmias AJ, Lee FK, Beckman-Nahmias S. Sero-epidemiological and sociological patterns of herpes simplex virus infections in the world. Scand J Infect Dis 1990;69:19–36.

Pazin GJ, Harger JH, Armstrong JA, et al. Leukocyte interferon in the treatment of initial episodes of genital herpes. J Infect Dis 1987;156:891–898.

Reichman RC, Badger GJ, Mertz GJ, et al. Treatment of recurrent genital herpes simplex infections with oral acyclovir. JAMA 1984;251:2103–2107.

Sacks SL, Aoki FY, Diaz-Mitoma F, et al. Patient-initiated, twice-daily oral famciclovir for early recurrent genital herpes: a randomized, double-blind multicenter trial. JAMA 1996;276:44–49.

Saltzman R, Jurewicz R, Boon R. Safety of famciclovir in patients with herpes zoster and genital herpes. Antimicrob Agents Chemother 1994;38:2454–2457.

Spruance SL, Tying SK, DeGregorio B, et al. A large-scale, placebo-controlled, dose-ranging trial of peroral valacyclovir for episode treatment of recurrent herpes genitalis. Arch Internal Med 1996; 156:1729–1735.

Straus SE, Croen KD, Sawyer MH, et al. Acyclovir suppression of frequently recurrent genital herpes: efficacy and diminishing need during successive years of treatment. JAMA 1988;260:2227–2230.

Wald A, Zeh J, Selke S, et al. Virologic characteristics of subclinical and symptomatic genital herpes infections. N Engl J Med 1995; 333:770–775.

Whitley RJ, Nahmias AJ, Visintine AM, et al. The natural history of herpes simplex virus infection in mother and newborn. Pediatrics 1980;66:489–494.

CHAPTER

# 54

# *Human Papillomavirus Infection*

*Stanley A. Gall*

## Background and Incidence

Genital warts have been recognized for centuries, although their infectious nature was not described until 1894. A virus was implicated as an etiologic agent in 1907, but the human papillomavirus (HPV) particle was not seen with electron microscopy until 1949. To this day, no effective method for culturing HPV in tissue has been developed.

The spectrum of disease linked to this condition includes clinical (genital warts) and subclinical HPV infection of the cervix, vagina, vulva, perineal body, and anus; an association of HPV with intraepithelial neoplasia of the vulva, vagina, cervix, and penis; and juvenile laryngeal papillomatosis. More recently, researchers have demonstrated that HPV DNA is present in practically every squamous malignancy of the female and male genital tracts. Because of this association with malignant disease, the diagnosis and therapy of HPV infection has taken on greater significance.

An increase of more than 1000% in the HPV-related case load has been noted in sexually transmitted disease (STD) clinics and private office consultations over the past decade. The prevalence of HPV infection correlates with sexual activity. Peak occurrence is between ages 15 and 35. HPV infection also is associated with other STDs. Between 50% and 70% of sexual partners of women with HPV infection have or will develop genital warts.

Human papillomavirus produces an overt infection in 30% of cases and subclinical infection in 70%. The virus can also persist in a latent state. During this latency period, it can be identified only by recombinant DNA technology.

In studies using cervical cytology to estimate the prevalence of genital HPV infection, 2% to 3% of unselected Pap smears were positive. When HPV DNA sequencing was applied to these Pap smears, an additional 20% tested positive for HPV infection.

Human papillomavirus can occupy multiple sites in the female genital tract. In 77% of women with an infected cervix, vaginal lesions are present. Similarly, 36% of women who have vulvar infection will also have an infected cervix. These facts suggest that HPV satisfies the criteria for an infectious etiology as a multicentric source of carcinoma of the vulva and vagina. Although most investigators do not believe that HPV is the primary etiologic agent of genital squamous tract malignancies, most believe that it represents a strong cocarcinogen. Finding HPV in any area of the genital tract suggests the virus will be present in the remainder of the genital tract.

## Pathophysiology

One hypothesis suggests that microtrauma allows the virus to enter the skin or mucosa of the genital tract. The virus enters the cells at the basal layer and matures as it passes through the parabasal, spinous, and granular layers of the epithelium. At the granular cell level, viral DNA replication, late protein synthesis, and viral particle assembly take place. Integration of the viral DNA into the host genome does not occur until the cervical intraepithelial neoplasia (CIN) III/carcinoma in situ (CIS) stage of development.

HPV DNA has been found in as many as 90% of cervical cancers examined; the remaining 10% may represent HPV DNA types not yet characterized. HPV DNA type 16 (found in 50% of cancers), HPV 18 (14%), HPV 45 (8%), and HPV 31 (5%) are the most prevalent types on a worldwide basis. Thus far, 16 genital HPV types have been detected in cervical cancer, including HPV 6, 11, 26, 33, 35, 51, 52, 55, 56, 58, 64, and 68 in addition to the four just named. These types belong to a group of viruses prevailing in high-grade squamous intraepithelial lesions of the cervix. HPV 18 appears to be the predominant type in adenocarcinomas and adenosquamous tumors, which account for approximately 5% of cervical tumors.

No general agreement has been reached on the prognostic meaning of the HPV type in carcinomas of the cervix. Although some reports have implicated HPV types 16 and 18 as risk factors influencing the frequency of nodal metastases and relapse, other reports have failed to show any correlation between HPV type and prognosis.

## Clinical Findings

Overt condyloma acuminatum may be seen in the perianal area, perineal body, vulva, vagina, or cervix. Subclinical HPV infection may be seen in the same areas.

Vulvar condylomas appear as pinkish, whitish, or pigmented sessile tumors with lobulated or pointed finger-like projections on their surfaces. They are found most commonly in the vulvar area and less commonly in the vagina and the cervix. When HPV infection manifests as a flat lesion with minimal elevation or as a pink papular plaque with a smooth surface, it may be missed during routine examination.

Subclinical HPV infection is more common than overt infection. The most common lesion is an elongated vaginal papilla with clustered epithelial projections in a central capillary. Aceto-white epithelium, another common manifestation, may be detected by a colposcopic examination of the vulva after application of 5% acetic acid, which causes the individual cells to swell, giving a white color to the wart or neoplastic epithelium. The lesions are usually multifocal and appear more commonly in the upper third of the vagina.

Human papillomavirus may be detected with great frequency if the clinician pays special attention to the vagina. Vaginal condylomas can be detected in as many as one-third of patients who have vulvar condylomas. In general, condylomas in the upper third of the vagina are considered to confer a high risk of cancer, as the HPV DNA types found here tend to be those associated with malignant potential (types 16, 18, and 31).

Condylomas in the lower third of the vagina tend to carry a low risk and tend to be associated with HPV DNA type 6 or 11. Most patients have multiple condylomas in the vagina that appear as white elevations. Frequently, a vaginal discharge accompanies the infection. The presence of HPV should be investigated in patients with recurrent episodes of bacterial vaginosis or *Candida albicans* infection, as mild immunosuppression allows both HPV and *C. albicans* to flourish.

In the past, condyloma acuminatum of the cervix was a rare lesion. Today, however, it is seen with increased frequency. Subclinical papillomavirus infection is generally accepted as the most common manifestation of HPV disease in the cervix.

## Diagnosis

Techniques for detecting HPV infection include physical examination, cytology, colposcopy, histologic studies, HPV antigen detection studies, and HPV DNA molecular hybridization.

Physical examination of the genital tract is simple and noninvasive. When used alone, however, this method misses only 10% of HPV infections. Other diagnoses that may be confused with genital warts include fibroepithelial polyps, introital papillosis, molluscum contagiosum, melanocytic nevi, condyloma latum, and vulvar intraepithelial neoplasia (VIN). On occasion, even normal anatomy may be mistaken for condyloma.

Cytologic studies are a relatively inexpensive approach to diagnosing HPV infection. Positive findings include koilocytosis, dyskaryosis, atypical parabasal cells, and multinucleation. Nevertheless, HPV is underdiagnosed in routine cytologic examinations. Colposcopic examination after soaking with 5% acetic acid allows detection of 70% of subclinical papillomavirus infections. The colposcope is also helpful in selecting areas to be biopsied.

The histologic findings of genital warts are basal cell hyperplasia, papillomatosis, koilocytosis, and parakeratosis. Koilocytosis is the most commonly used marker for HPV infection. The specific koilocytotic atypia seen in lesions, however, is caused by high-grade HPV DNA types such as 16 and 18, especially in advanced-grade CIN.

Antigens to HPV can be detected in cytologic and histologic specimens by using immunostaining techniques with antiserum from rabbits immunized to bovine papillomavirus. The cells carrying the virus are well differentiated. As dysplasia progresses, it becomes increasingly difficult to detect HPV antigen; at the CIN III/CIS stage, for example, it is not detectable.

Cloning techniques have now given us the ability to obtain typing of HPV DNA. As noted earlier, HPV DNA types 6 and 11 are thought to have low malignant potential and generally are found in the vulva and lower third of the vagina. HPV DNA types 16, 18, 31, and other high-number types are found in the upper third of the vagina and the cervix; they are more frequently associated with malignant conditions. Because the physician will treat the clinical or histologic condition rather than the HPV DNA type, the use of routine HPV DNA typing may not be indicated. In questionable situations, HPV DNA typing can be useful—for example, when lesions might be confused with those of HPV and in cases involving koilocytosis with atypia in patients who desire to know their HPV type.

## TREATMENT

Human papillomavirus infection must be regarded as having the potential for infecting the entire genital tract, as only very early disease tends to be localized. The therapeutic objective is to remove all overt and subclinical HPV infections detected during the diagnostic evaluation. All currently available treatment methods have been associated with a high degree of recurrence. Therapy options that attack the HPV locally will prove helpful only for conditions in which the virus remains localized.

The recurrence of HPV infection after therapy is difficult to assess. Recurrences indicate a failure of therapy, failure to treat all areas involved, resistant virus, or reinfection. Most recurrences are seen within three to six months of therapy. If the disease persists after six months despite repeated attempts at therapy, it is called resistant and persistent HPV disease.

Treatment options include keratolytic agents, physical agents, and immunotherapy. Because of the variety of presentations, the volume of disease, the areas infected, and possibly the DNA type of the papillomavirus, no single agent has yet emerged as a standard treatment. When a patient presents with a small amount of localized disease, a simple approach is best. When the patient has more extensive disease, more intensive therapy may be needed.

Podophyllin resin is one keratolytic agent that has been widely used for this indication. It acts by poisoning the mitotic spindle of the virus. The resin is applied directly to the surface of the wart and washed off after six hours; it is then reapplied on a weekly basis.

Podophyllin resin varies from lot to lot, and it produces unpredictable side effects. It is contraindicated during pregnancy because of the possibility of teratogenesis and even carcinogenesis. Its use should be severely limited when applied to mucosal surfaces. The best course of action may be to reserve it for use in patients with minimal vulvar or perianal lesions.

Trichloroacetic acid (TCA), another keratolytic agent, acts by precipitating surface proteins. It should be used at a strength of 85% and applied directly to the vulvar, anal, or vaginal lesions with a small cotton-tipped applicator. It produces a white slough that peels in several days, leaving a small ulcer. Application of 85% TCA can be repeated every two to three weeks. Again, recurrences are frequent with this agent.

5-Fluorouracil (5-FU) is a pyrimidine antimetabolite that causes sloughing of growing tissue. At 5% concentration, 5-FU may prove helpful in the treatment of multiple, small, nonkeratinized vaginal lesions; it may also be used for lesions of the vulva. This agent is more effective for small HPV lesions involving the vestibule and inside labia minora. It is usually applied on a once-weekly basis into the vagina and/or the vestibule of the vulva for 12 weeks. It is important to instruct the patient in use of 5-FU and to obtain informed consent.

Cryotherapy for HPV disease may be applied either as a single cycle or as repetitive 2-minute freeze-and-thaw cycles to destroy infected wart tissue. It may be performed either by probe or by application of liquid nitrogen. Patients frequently require more than one application to clear the overt or subclinical papillomavirus infection. Comparative studies have shown that cryotherapy is more effective than podophyllin and as effective as electrical cautery or laser therapy. Treatment of the vulvar area should be preceded by application of a local anesthetic agent.

The use of laser therapy is widespread and has the theoretic advantage of precise control of depth, margins, and hemostasis. On the other hand, laser ablation has the disadvantages of requiring operator control and expertise and of treating only visible disease. The vulva and vestibule are the most convenient areas for laser therapy. Laser therapy of the vagina may be complicated by difficulty in application and by scarring. Studies have shown that recurrences occur in 25% to 100% of cases treated by this method. Some researchers have recommended extending the field of laser therapy in an attempt to destroy latent virus at the margins; studies have shown that this approach is of little value, however, and increases morbidity excessively. The use of 5-FU immediately following laser therapy in the vagina or vulva has been advocated, but success and morbidity rates need to be confirmed.

The laser plume, which contains carbon, water vapor, cells, and—in some cases—viral DNA, represents a potential hazard to the surgeon, operating room staff, and patient. Smoke evacuation units equipped with high-efficiency filters (0.1 μm) should be used to remove as much plume as possible. Suction tubing held within 1 cm of the tissue impact site can trap approximately 98% of the plume; if the tubing is held at a distance of 2 cm, approximately 50% of the plume will escape. Although intact viral particles have been found in laser plume, viral transmission via airborne debris has not been demonstrated to date. Masks with finer filtering ability are available, but no evidence has been gathered to show that these masks significantly reduce the number of particles inhaled by the laser surgeon. Thus careful plume evacuation should be the mainstay of inhalation safety.

The use of electrocautery to destroy small volumes of condyloma acuminatum appears to be effective. This method is particularly convenient for office use. Although surgical ablation has also been widely used to treat condyloma, it offers less precision than laser therapy and has the disadvantage of increasing scarring in the vulvar area. A number of investigators have focused on vaccine therapy, but this option has been found to be no better than placebo in controlled trials.

Interferons—a family of proteins with antiviral, antiprolific, and immunomodulatory properties—are also being used to treat

HPV infection. Three preparations are currently available: α-interferon II-A, α-interferon II-B, and α-interferon N-1. These agents may be given by intramuscular injection at a dosage of 2.5 to 3 million U three times per week for a minimum of eight weeks, or 3 million U/$m^2$ to a maximum of 4.5 million U three times per week for at least eight weeks. The duration of this therapy can be extended two to four weeks if the patient experiences at least a partial response.

A second route of interferon therapy is intralesional injection at a dosage of 250,000 to 1 million U for each wart, as many as five warts at one time, three times per week for three weeks. Because this mode of therapy is regional, the therapy duration may need to be extended beyond three weeks. Also, because the doses are somewhat lower for the α-interferon N-1 preparation, the prescribing information should be reviewed.

Side effects are dose-related and almost absent with the regimen of 3 million U three times per week. The most frequent side effect of interferon is transient fever for 8 to 12 hours following injection. Other potential side effects include fatigue, myalgia, and headache; a transient decrease in the white blood cell (WBC) count and elevation of liver function tests appear in fewer than 10% of individuals.

Interferons may be used for either small or large volumes of HPV disease. They are effective for both intravaginal and vulvar warts. Recent unpublished data suggest that superior results are obtained by using interferon as initial therapy followed by cryotherapy, laser therapy, or 5-FU. It has also been suggested that this approach permits use of a lower dosage (1 million U) of interferon.

A newer product, imiquimod, is an interferon and cytokine inducer. It is available as a cream that is rubbed into external genital warts three times per week. The complete clearance rate in females is 72%, as reported in the initial marketing literature.

Still another chemotherapeutic option is dinitrochlorobenzene (DNCB) therapy. This treatment is unique in that the patient is sensitized to the agent first. The sensitization procedure involves application of a topical solution of DNCB (1000 μg/0.1 mL) to the volar surface of the forearm. A challenge dose of 50 μg of DNCB is applied to the same forearm two weeks after the sensitizing dose. Induration of greater than 0.5 cm indicates a positive reaction.

After this sensitization procedure, the DNCB is placed in a cream and applied to the lesion. The patient develops a delayed hypersensitivity reaction that destroys the wart. Disadvantages of this therapy include (1) the inability to sensitize all patients to DNCB, (2) the reluctance of patients to have a hypersensitivity reaction occur in the perineal area, and (3) varied sensitivity to DNCB, with a potential for severe reaction.

## Treatment During Pregnancy

In general, overt condylomas will enlarge during pregnancy. This growth probably results from high progesterone levels in the mother. In some cases, the lesions may become large enough to cause hemorrhage. Podophyllin therapy is contraindicated because of its toxicity and risk of teratogenesis. Likewise, agents such as bleomycin and 5-FU are contraindicated because of their antimitotic and cytotoxic actions. Trichloroacetic acid solution may prove useful in pregnant patients, however. Cryotherapy and use of the $CO_2$ laser have also been helpful in reducing the number and volume of warts. Imiquimod has a category B rating, but no clinical data on its use during pregnancy are available. In almost every case, HPV disease will diminish after delivery.

Extensive condylomas may develop during pregnancy. If multiple lesions are present in and on the genitalia, cesarean section may become necessary to prevent transmission of HPV infection to the infant. A strong association between clinical maternal genital condylomas and the subsequent development of laryngeal papillomatosis in infants delivered vaginally has been documented epidemiologically and corroborated by detection of HPV DNA sequences in both genital and laryngeal papilloma tissues. In one study, 78% of children with laryngeal papilloma had mothers with genital condylomas. Possible modes of transmission include contact between the fetus and the mother's infected genital tract during delivery, transplacental transmission of maternal infection, and postnatal contact. Despite the high prevalence of genital HPV infection, juvenile laryngeal papillomatosis remains a rare disease, implying that transmission of maternal infection is uncommon. Because the method of transmission is not known and the risk is ill defined, currently no consensus exists regarding whether cesarean delivery offers a protective benefit for the neonate.

## Treatment of Choice

For localized warts, TCA offers the best combination of effectiveness, low morbidity, and expense. When the disease affects the labia and vulva, the use of TCA or 5-FU is recommended. For extensive vulvar disease, laser therapy is best used for the labia, perineal body, or perianal areas. Alternatively, intralesional and/or intramuscular interferon, either alone or in combination with laser therapy or 5-FU, may offer the best hope of controlling the virus.

### Suggested Readings

American College of Obstetrics and Gynecology. Genital human papillomavirus infections. ACOG Technical Bulletin No. 105, 1987.

Bosch FX, Manos MM, Munoz N, et al. Prevalence of human papillomavirus in cervical cancer: a worldwide perspective. J Natl Cancer Inst 1995;87:796–802.

Gall SA, Constantine L, Koukol D. Therapy of persistent human papillomavirus disease with two different interferon species. Am J Obstet Gynecol 1991;164:130–134.

Gall SA, Hughes CE, Mounts P, et al. Efficacy of human lymphoblastoid interferon on the therapy of resistant condyloma acuminatum. Obstet Gynecol 1986;67:643–651.

Krebs H. Treatment of vaginal condylomata acuminata by weekly topical application of 5-fluorouracil. Obstet Gynecol 1987;70:68–71.

Krebs H, Helmkamp F. Chronic ulcerations following topical therapy with 5-fluorouracil for vaginal human papillomavirus-associated lesions. Obstet Gynecol 1991;78:205–208.

Shah K, Kashima H, Polk BF, et al. Rarity of cesarean delivery in cases of juvenile-onset respiratory papillomatosis. Obstet Gynecol 1986;68:795–799.

Stoler M, Rhodes CR, Whitbeck A, et al. Human papillomavirus type 16 and 18 gene expression in cervical neoplasias. Hum Pathol 1992;23:117–128.

CHAPTER

55

# Genital Mycoplasmas

*William M. McCormack*

## Background and Incidence

Mycoplasmas are microorganisms that differ from viruses in that they can grow on cell-free media. They differ from bacteria in that they lack a cell wall. Only three species of mycoplasmas have been isolated with any frequency from human genital mucosal surfaces. One, *Mycoplasma genitalium*, is a newly recognized species of uncertain significance. The other two, *Mycoplasma hominis* and *Ureaplasma urealyticum*, are common isolates that have been extensively studied.

The genital mucosa of infants may be colonized during passage through the birth canal. Ureaplasmas can be recovered from vaginal cultures from about one-third of infant girls. *M. hominis*, in contrast, is isolated less often from girls. Boys are less likely than girls to be colonized by either species.

Neonatal colonization tends not to persist. Ureaplasmas can be isolated from approximately 10% of 1-year-old girls. Colonization continues at this low level until puberty.

Following puberty, colonization is influenced primarily by sexual experience. Sexually inexperienced adolescents have low rates of mycoplasmal and ureaplasmal colonization, similar to those seen in prepubertal children. After the initiation of sexual intercourse, colonization rates increase in relation to the number of sex partners.

Infection rates are higher among socially disadvantaged groups. *M. hominis* has been isolated from approximately 50% of patients attending public clinics and from about 20% of patients visiting private physicians' offices. Ureaplasmas have been recovered from 80% of patients seen in public clinics and from 50% of private patients.

Thus both *M. hominis* and *U. urealyticum* are common inhabitants of the genital mucosa of normal sexually experienced adult men and women. It is against this background that we must assess their role in human disease.

## Pathophysiology

Both *M. hominis* and *U. urealyticum* are prominent components of the abnormal flora of bacterial vaginosis (BV). Both species also have been isolated from women who have intra-amniotic infection, postpartum endometritis, and pelvic inflammatory disease.

In each of these conditions, mycoplasmas and ureaplasmas have rarely been isolated in pure culture; rather, they have been isolated along with other organisms, which are often components of the abnormal flora of BV. These data suggest that organisms found in BV may be responsible for the aforementioned infections of the upper genital tract in women and that the isolation of *M. hominis* or *U. urealyticum* may be a marker for BV or a BV-related infection.

In addition, ureaplasmas have been associated with disorders of reproduction such as habitual spontaneous abortion, unexplained involuntary infertility, and low birthweight. More data, especially from placebo-controlled, double-blind treatment studies, are needed to establish a role for *U. urealyticum* in these disorders.

## Diagnosis

As noted earlier, both *M. hominis* and *U. urealyticum* can be isolated from the vaginal mucosa of a significant proportion of normal sexually experienced women. Also mentioned previously was the infrequency with which either of these species is isolated in pure culture from women who have upper genital tract infection and the lack of conclusive evidence of a role for these organisms in disorders of reproduction.

It follows that cultures for *M. hominis* or *U. urealyticum* have no place in clinical practice. Examination of vaginal or other specimens for mycoplasmas or ureaplasmas is justified only in the context of a research protocol. Specimens from the vaginal mucosa are more likely to yield an isolate than are specimens from the endocervical canal or periurethral area.

## Treatment

Although most isolates of *U. urealyticum* are susceptible to tetracyclines and erythromycins, it is difficult to eradicate these organisms from the vagina. *M. hominis* is susceptible to tetracyclines but not to erythromycins. Because the prevalence of tetracycline-resistant isolates of *M. hominis* is increasing, clindamycin may be more effective against this agent.

As noted earlier, examining cultures for genital mycoplasmas is seldom justifiable in clinical practice. Nevertheless, any treatment regimen for the upper genital tract syndromes with which *M. hominis* and *U. urealyticum* have been associated should contain an antimicrobial agent that shows in vitro activity against these organisms.

## Prevention

Regular use of barrier contraceptives retards genital colonization by mycoplasmas. These organisms are so widespread, however, that it is difficult to imagine any approach that would prevent a significant portion of sexually experienced adults from eventually becoming colonized.

### Suggested Readings

Glatt AE, McCormack WM, Taylor-Robinson D. Genital mycoplasma. In: Holmes KK, Mårdh P-A, Sparling PF, eds. Sexually transmitted disease, 2nd ed. New York: McGraw Hill, 1989:279–293.

Taylor-Robinson D. Infections due to species of *Mycoplasma* and *Ureaplasma:* an update. Clin Infect Dis 1996;23:671–682.

Taylor-Robinson D. *Ureaplasma urealyticum* (T-strain Mycoplasma) and *Mycoplasma hominis*. In: Mandell GL, Bennett JE, Dolin R, eds. Principles and practice of infectious diseases, 4th ed. New York: Churchill Livingstone, 1995:1713–1718.

CHAPTER

56

# *Pelvic Inflammatory Disease: Incidence and Diagnosis*

*Pål Wölner-Hanssen*

## Background and Incidence

Pelvic inflammatory disease (PID) describes infection ascending from the cervix through the uterus into the fallopian tubes and peritoneal cavity. Acute salpingitis is an infection of the fallopian tubes only, although the terms are often used interchangeably. For women with suspected but unconfirmed acute salpingitis, acute PID is a more appropriate term and diagnosis.

More than 1 million cases of PID occur annually in the United States, with 250,000 to 300,000 of them requiring hospitalization. In 1988, 11% of U.S. women of reproductive age reported that they had received treatment for PID. These figures may actually either overestimate or underestimate the incidence of women actually having PID, for two reasons:

- Many cases diagnosed as PID are not confirmed laparoscopically.
- The number of cases of PID never recognized by the patient or the physician (known as "silent" or "atypical" PID) is unknown.

As a result, the true overall incidence remains to be determined. Nevertheless, reports from around the world suggest that the incidence of PID has been declining in recent years. In Amsterdam, for example, the estimated incidence declined from 50 per 10,000 women to 24 per 10,000 between 1986 and 1990. This decline was limited to non-teenaged women.

The persistent incidence of PID among teenagers in the Dutch study underscores the well-known fact that young age is a risk factor for PID among sexually active women. The risk of acquiring a sexually transmitted disease (STD), and hence acute STD-related salpingitis, is highly correlated with the number of sex partners. Youth is a risk factor for PID in part because young sexually active women tend to have less stable sexual relationships than somewhat older women and therefore may expose themselves to genital infections more often. For example, women with 10 or more lifetime partners are more than three times as likely to report a history of PID as women with only one male partner. Another possible explanation for the increased incidence of PID noted among young women is that these women may have less immunity against STD agents than older women, in part because the columnar epithelium of the endocervix is more exposed in adolescents and younger women.

Other risk factors for PID include ethnicity, postmarital status, and contraceptive practices:

- In 1988, the cumulative incidence of self-reported PID among African American women was almost twice that among white women (17% versus 10%).
- Formerly married women have a cumulative incidence of self-reported PID three times that of never-married women.
- Many consider the use of an IUD to be a risk factor for PID among women with multiple sex partners. In contrast, oral contraceptives and barrier methods may reduce this risk.

In recent studies, vaginal douching has emerged as one of the few preventable risk factors for PID. Vaginal douching is a hygienic practice particularly common among less educated women in the southeastern United States. The association between douching and PID is stronger among white women (50% increased risk of PID) than among African American women, probably because of the high prevalence of douching among the latter.

An association between bacterial vaginosis with both adnexal tenderness and a clinical diagnosis of PID has been reported. In addition, cigarette smoking has been statistically associated with PID, although no causal relationship has been proven.

## Diagnosis

Abdominal pain is the principal symptom of acute salpingitis, although it is not always present. Women with acute PID may experience severe pain (common in women with perihepatitis) or no pain at all ("silent" PID). The character of the pain (aching, burning, cramping, or stabbing), and location (unilateral versus bilateral) is nonspecific. The pain usually is bilateral, but it may be unilateral and indistinguishable from that caused by appendicitis.

Patients with acute PID may report both genital and extragenital symptoms. These include symptoms related to the gastrointestinal tract (vomiting, diarrhea, constipation, tenesmus), the urinary tract (dysuria, frequency, urgency), and the genital tract (increased discharge, abnormal odor from the vagina, abnormal bleeding). Adnexal, uterine, and cervical motion tenderness are also nonspecific signs of acute PID. Purulent cervical discharge is another sign that suggests acute PID in a woman with acute abdominal pain, although lack of mucopus does not rule out acute salpingitis. Some clinicians evaluate vaginal "wet smears" for the presence of leukocytes, using leukocyte dominance as a criterion for upper genital tract infection, although no published data support this approach. Fever is a sign often believed to be required for a diagnosis of PID. In studies using intentionally loose criteria for enrollment but stringent criteria for the final diagnosis, however, fever was an uncommon sign of PID. Among women with acute chlamydial salpingitis, only 20% developed fever.

Few laboratory tests are useful for evaluating women with suspected PID. A sensitive pregnancy test is important for sexually active women with abdominal pain because ectopic pregnancy and acute PID often have similar manifestations. An elevated erythrocyte sedimentation rate (ESR), white blood cell (WBC) count, or serum C-reactive protein level suggests inflammation of some sort, but none of these tests is specific for acute PID. In one study, for example, 25% of women with acute PID had a normal ESR and 53% of those without confirmed PID had an elevated ESR. In another study, 70% of women with acute chlamydial salpingitis had normal WBC counts.

**Table 56-1.** Clinical Criteria for Diagnosis of PID

| |
|---|
| **Necessary for Diagnosis** |
| Abdominal direct tenderness, with or without rebound tenderness |
| Tenderness with motion of cervix and uterus |
| Adnexal tenderness |
| **One or More Necessary for Diagnosis** |
| Gram's stain of endocervix positive for gram-negative intracellular diplococci |
| Temperature > 38 °C |
| Leukocytosis (WBC > 10,000) |
| Purulent material (WBC present) from peritoneal cavity obtained by culdocentesis or laparoscopy |
| Pelvic abscess or inflammatory complex on bimanual exam or by sonography |

SOURCE: Hager WD, Eschenbach DA, Spence MR, et al. Criteria for diagnosis and grading of salpingitis. Obstet Gynecol 1983;61:113–114.

In their classic work, Jacobson and Weström could not confirm acute PID in one-third of women with clinical symptoms and signs suggesting the infection. Later investigators have encountered the same difficulty in making a diagnosis. Although laparoscopic examination has become the "gold standard" for making a definitive diagnosis, most studies continue to base the diagnosis of PID on clinical criteria for several reasons. Laparoscopy is not generally performed for women with suspected PID because it requires hospitalization and anesthesia. Moreover, certainty of diagnosis may be mandatory for research but less important for routine clinical care. Nevertheless, laparoscopy remains the best technique for distinguishing causes of acute lower abdominal pain. Usually, one can readily visualize the appendix and the genital tract through the laparoscope. Clinical criteria for diagnosis have been described by Hager and coworkers and endorsed by the Infectious Diseases Society for Obstetrics and Gynecology (Tables 56-1 and 56-2). These authors have also outlined a severity staging system based on laparoscopic findings.

Endometrial biopsy is a newly developed method for confirming acute PID. Among women with acute pelvic pain and

**Table 56-2.** Grading of PID by Clinical Examination

I. Uncomplicated (limited to fallopian tubes and/or ovaries)
   A. Without pelvic peritonitis
   B. With pelvic peritonitis

II. Complicated (inflammatory mass or abscess involving fallopian tubes and/or ovaries)
   A. Without pelvic peritonitis
   B. With pelvic peritonitis

III. Spread to structures beyond pelvis (ruptured tubo-ovarian abscess)

SOURCE: Hager WD, Eschenbach DA, Spence MR, et al. Criteria for diagnosis and grading of salpingitis. Obstet Gynecol 1983;61:113–114.

adnexal tenderness, the presence of one or more plasma cells per 120× field of endometrial stroma is associated with PID. This method suffers a disadvantage in that results are not available for several days. The technique may therefore have greater utility in research than in routine care.

Transvaginal ultrasound examination might be useful in evaluating women with clinical evidence of PID. In one study, for example, in women with acute pelvic pain, observation of thickened, fluid-filled fallopian tubes on transvaginal ultrasound examination was 100% specific for plasma cell endometritis. Ultrasonography may also help in monitoring drainage of tubo-ovarian abscesses and for assessing the effectiveness of therapy in patients who are difficult to examine—obese women, for example.

## Microbiologic Evaluation

*Neisseria gonorrhoeae* and *Chlamydia trachomatis* cause most cases of acute PID. Consequently, cervical specimens for detection of *N. gonorrhoeae* and *C. trachomatis* should be obtained in all cases of suspected PID. Antigen-detection techniques such as Microtrak (Syva Company, Palo Alto, California), Chlamydiazyme (Abbott Laboratories, Abbott Park, Illinois), or polymerase chain reaction (PCR) tests are adequate alternatives to chlamydial cultures. It makes no sense to take culture specimens from the cervix for anaerobic or facultative (other than *N. gonorrhoeae*) microorganisms, because these organisms are part of the normal flora.

With women undergoing laparoscopy, the clinician has an opportunity to collect specimens from the fallopian tubes and the cul-de-sac fluid directly without contaminating the specimens with vaginal flora. Organisms isolated from the fallopian tubes probably cause the acute inflammation. Regrettably, most women with obvious acute PID have no detectable microorganisms in the tubes.

Culdocentesis includes aspiration of cul-de-sac fluid via needle puncture of the posterior vaginal fornix. Purulent cul-de-sac fluid suggests intra-abdominal infection (PID, appendicitis, or diverticulitis). Clear fluid, however, does not rule out infection. Culture of culdocentesis material has little value, because vaginal microorganisms may have contaminated the fluid.

## Summary

To possibly decrease the sequelae of PID, we must improve the efficiency of our clinical criteria for diagnosis in evaluating women with abdominal pain. We must maintain a high index of suspicion in young, sexually active women with abdominal pain. In addition, we must consider the use of laparoscopy whenever the diagnosis is uncertain.

### Suggested Readings

Aral SO, Mosher WD, Cates W Jr. Self-reported pelvic inflammatory disease in the United States, 1988. JAMA 1991;266:2570–2573.

Coutinho RA, Rijsdijk AJ, van den Hoek JA, et al. Decreasing incidence of PID in Amsterdam. Genitourin Med 1992;69:353–355.

Hager WD, Eschenbach DA, Spence MR, et al. Criteria for diagnosis and grading of salpingitis. Obstet Gynecol 1983;61:113–114.

Jacobson L, Weström L. Objectivized diagnosis of acute pelvic inflammatory disease. Am J Obstet Gynecol 1969;105:1088–1098.

Washington AE, Cates W Jr, Wasserheit JN. Preventing pelvic inflammatory disease. JAMA 1991;266:2574–2582.

Wölner-Hanssen P, Eschenbach DA, Paavonen J, et al. Association between vaginal douching and acute pelvic inflammatory disease. JAMA 1990;263:1936–1941.

CHAPTER

# 57

# *Pelvic Inflammatory Disease: Treatment*

*Richard L. Sweet*

## Background and Incidence

Pelvic inflammatory disease (PID), or acute salpingitis, continues to be a major medical, economic, and public health problem for reproductive-aged women in the United States. Among young women, PID is the most common serious complication of sexually transmitted disease (STD). It is also the most common gynecologic disorder leading to hospitalization for women of reproductive age in the United States. More than 1 million cases of clinically apparent PID are estimated to occur each year in the United States, associated with annual costs of more than $7 billion. Unrecognized or atypical PID is believed to occur as frequently as apparent disease.

Involuntary (predominantly tubal factor) infertility affects 20% of PID patients—a sevenfold increase relative to women without this disease—and ectopic pregnancy is increased six- to tenfold in women with PID. Chronic pelvic pain, dyspareunia, pelvic adhesions, and other inflammatory residua, which often require surgical intervention, occur in 15% to 20% of cases. In addition, tubo-ovarian abscess—the major early complication associated with acute PID—occurs in 5% to 10% of hospitalized acute PID patients.

## Etiology

At one time, *Neisseria gonorrhoeae* was considered the primary etiologic agent for acute PID in the Western world. Thus, based on cervical culture results, PID was designated as either gonococcal or nongonococcal disease. More recently, advances in the technology for obtaining microbiologic specimens directly from the fallopian tubes, endometrial cavity, or peritoneal fluid, combined with advances in microbiologic isolation techniques, have resulted in the recovery of nongonococcal organisms such as *Chlamydia trachomatis* and anaerobic and facultative bacteria from both the cervix and upper genital tracts of women with acute PID.

Thorough microbiologic assessment of the upper genital tract indicates that PID is polymicrobial. Studies report recovery of *N. gonorrhoeae*, *C. trachomatis*, or both, in two-thirds of women with acute PID. Among the one-third with nongonococcal/nonchlamydial microorganisms isolated from the upper genital tract, mixed anaerobic organisms (*Prevotella* sp. and peptostreptococci) and facultative bacteria (*Gardnerella vaginalis*, streptococci, *Escherichia coli*, and *Haemophilus influenzae*) are the most common findings. Several studies have demonstrated an important association between organisms causing bacterial vaginosis (BV) and PID. Although genital tract mycoplasmas, such as *Mycoplasma hominis* and *Ureaplasma urealyticum*, have also been recovered from women with PID, their role in etiology remains uncertain.

## Treatment

The goals of management in PID are to preserve fertility, prevent ectopic pregnancy, and reduce long-term inflammatory sequelae. Optimal treatment requires early diagnosis and prompt institution of antimicrobial agents effective against major pathogens known to be involved in the disease process. Recently, treatment within 48 hours of the onset of symptoms has been shown to be crucial in preventing PID sequelae.

Initially, single-agent antimicrobial therapy focused on eradication of *N. gonorrhoeae*. Most often, however, these

**Table 57-1.** Oral and IM Treatment Guidelines for Acute PID

**Regimen A**
Ofloxacin, 400 mg orally twice a day for 14 days
*plus*
Metronidazole, 500 mg orally twice a day for 14 days

**Regimen B**
Ceftriaxone, 250 mg IM once
*or*
Cefoxitin, 2 g IM, plus probenecid, 1 g orally in a single dose concurrently once
*or*
Other parenteral third-generation cephalosporins (e.g., ceftizoxime or cefotaxime)
*plus*
Doxycycline, 100 mg orally twice a day for 14 days (include with one of the preceding Regimen B options)

SOURCE: Centers for Disease Control and Prevention. 1998 guidelines for treatment of sexually transmitted diseases. MMWR 1998;47(RR-1):84.

drugs failed to eradicate *C. trachomatis* and mixed aerobic–anaerobic bacteria and therefore produced largely unsatisfactory results.

In the early 1980s, broad-spectrum antibiotic treatment with single agents such as cefoxitin, cefotetan, and third-generation cephalosporins addressed the issue of coverage for mixed anaerobic–aerobic bacteria. Unfortunately, this approach failed to provide adequate coverage against *C. trachomatis* and led to persistent chlamydial infection of the upper genital tract despite supposed clinical cure. Subsequently, the Centers for Disease Control and Prevention (CDC) established guidelines for inpatient and outpatient treatment of acute PID using antibiotic combinations that provide coverage for *C. trachomatis* and anaerobic–aerobic bacteria as well as *N. gonorrhoeae*. Tables 57-1 and 57-2 provide the current CDC guidelines for oral and parenteral treatment of acute PID, respectively.

Alternative parenteral regimens include the following:

- Ofloxacin, 400 mg IV every 12 hours, plus metronidazole, 500 mg IV every 8 hours
- Ampicillin–sulbactam, 3 g IV every 6 hours, plus doxycycline, 100 mg IV or orally every 12 hours

**Table 57-2.** Parenteral Inpatient/Outpatient Treatment Guidelines for Acute PID

**Regimen A**
Cefotetan, 2 g IV every 12 hours
*or*
Cefoxitin, 2 g IV every 6 hours
*plus*
Doxycycline, 100 mg IV or orally every 12 hours

**Regimen B**
Clindamycin, 900 mg IV every 8 hours
*plus*
Gentamicin, loading dose IV or IM (2 mg/kg of body weight), followed by a maintenance dose (1.5 mg/kg) every 8 hours. Single daily dosing may be substituted.

For both Regimen A and Regimen B, parenteral therapy may be discontinued 24 hours after clinical improvement. Continue oral doxycycline, 100 mg twice daily, for 14 days.

SOURCE: Centers for Disease Control and Prevention. 1998 guidelines for treatment of sexually transmitted diseases. MMWR 1998;47(RR-1):82–83.

- Ciprofloxacin, 200 mg IV every 12 hours, plus doxycycline, 100 mg IV or orally every 12 hours, plus metronidazole, 500 mg IV or orally every 8 hours

An alternative oral regimen is amoxicillin–clavulanic acid plus doxycycline, 100 mg orally every 12 hours for 14 days. In order to cover anaerobes and bacterial vaginosis, many experts recommend adding metronidazole 500 mg orally twice a day for 7 days to oral regimen B.

It is unclear whether oral treatment or parenteral antibiotic therapy offers greater effectiveness in preventing complications and long-term sequelae. Economic and logistic considerations dictate that the majority of PID patients be treated on an outpatient basis. Since 1982, a number of studies have compared the outcomes obtained with various inpatient regimens. In general, combination regimens with either clindamycin plus an aminoglycoside or an extended-spectrum cephalosporin plus doxycycline have produced excellent initial beneficial clinical responses. On the other hand, single-agent fluoroquinolone treatment has been followed by a high rate of post-treatment persistence of anaerobic bacteria in the endometrial cavity despite apparent clinical response—a situation similar to the persistent chlamydial infection in supposed clinical cures when *C. trachomatis* is not covered. Unmet needs in this field include randomized, prospective studies with meticulous clinical or laparoscopic grading, microbiologic analysis, and long-term follow-up to assess these regimens' effectiveness in preventing subsequent episodes of PID, as well as adverse reproductive sequelae such as infertility, ectopic pregnancy, and chronic pelvic pain.

Hospitalization is recommended for pregnant patients and for patients for whom the diagnosis cannot exclude surgical emergencies such as appendicitis. Parenteral treatment (inpatient or outpatient) is recommended in the following settings:

- Failure to respond clinically to oral therapy
- Inability to follow or tolerate an oral regimen
- Severe illness, with high fever, nausea, and vomiting
- Tubo-ovarian abscess
- Current immunodeficiency (including HIV infection with a low CD4 count)

The decision of whether to hospitalize the patient or undertake ambulatory parenteral therapy in these situations should be based on the provider's judgment and discretion.

To minimize the likelihood of reinfection, we recommend that all partners of women with PID be screened for *N. gonorrhoeae* and *C. trachomatis*. Those found positive for these pathogens should be treated with a regimen effective against both *N. gonorrhoeae* and *C. trachomatis*—most commonly, a single 125 mg IM dose of ceftriaxone plus 100 mg of doxycycline orally twice daily for seven days, or a single 1 g oral dose of azithromycin.

It is crucial to institute treatment as soon as possible to maximize future reproductive potential. Scandinavian studies suggest that the critical period of time is the initial 48 hours after the onset of symptoms. Whether inpatient therapy is preferable remains unclear. Likewise, it remains to be seen whether concomitant anti-inflammatory agents will prevent long-term sequelae of infertility or ectopic pregnancy.

## Suggested Readings

Centers for Disease Control and Prevention. 1998 guidelines for treatment of sexually transmitted diseases. MMWR 1998;47 (RR-1):79–86.

Eschenbach DA, Buchanan TM, Pollock HM, et al. Polymicrobial etiology of acute pelvic inflammatory disease. N Engl J Med 1975;293:166–171.

Joessens MO, Schachter J, Sweet RL. Risk factors associated with pelvic inflammatory disease of differing microbial etiologies. Obstet Gyncecol 1994;83:989–997.

Paavonen J, Teisala K, Heinonen PK, et al. Microbiological and histopathological findings in acute pelvic inflammatory disease. Br J Obstet Gynaecol 1987;94:454–460.

Sweet RL. Role of bacterial vaginosis in pelvic inflammatory disease. Clin Infect Dis 1995;20(suppl 2):S271–S275.

Sweet RL, Draper DL, Schachter J, et al. Microbiology and pathogenesis of acute salpingitis as determined by laparoscopy: what is the appropriate site to sample? Am J Obstet Gynecol 1980;138: 985–989.

Sweet RL, Schachter J, Robbie MO. Failure of ß-lactam antibiotics to eradicate *Chlamydia trachomatis* in the endometrium despite apparent clinical cure of acute salpingitis. JAMA 1983;250: 2641–2645.

Thompson SE, Brooks C, Eschenbach DA, et al. High failure rates in outpatient treatment of salpingitis with either tetracycline alone or penicillin/ampicillin combination. Am J Obstet Gynecol 1985;152:635–641.

Walker CK, Kahn JG, Washington AE, et al. Pelvic inflammatory disease: meta-analysis of antimicrobial regimen efficacy. J Infect Dis 1993;168:969–978.

Washington AE, Katz P. Cost of and payment source for pelvic inflammatory disease. Trends and projections, 1983 through 2000. JAMA 1991;266:2565–2569.

Wölner-Hanssen PW, Kiviat NB, Holmes KK, et al. Atypical pelvic inflammatory disease: subacute, chronic, or subclinical upper genital tract infection in women. In: Holmes KK, Mårdh P-A, Sparling PF, et al., eds. Sexually transmitted diseases, ed 2. New York: McGraw-Hill, 1990:615–620.

CHAPTER

# 58

# *Chronic Sequelae of Salpingitis*

*Mark Gibson*

## Background and Incidence

For most victims of salpingitis, the most important consequences occur only after the pain, fever, and limitation of normal activity of acute illness subside. For these patients, chronic sequelae of adnexal inflammation—in the form of tubal inflammatory damage (TID)—exact the greatest cost by causing both symptoms and reproductive dysfunction.

TID-related infertility, which appears in approximately 20% of TID cases, affects an estimated 1% to 2% of all women. Peritubal and periovarian adhesions may interfere with normal tubo-ovarian relationships and by themselves produce infertility. The most sensitive targets of salpingitis are the tube's ampulla and fimbria, where minor postinflammatory changes include phimosis of the tubal orifice and subtle degrees of fimbrial agglutination. More severe damage to the distal tube results in the classic retort-shaped sactosalpinx, most typically drawn posterolaterally beneath the ovary and bound there by webs or bands of adhesions.

In tubes that are totally occluded at the fimbriated end, abnormal mucosa and muscularis are the rule. In addition, the tube's isthmic portion may become occluded by fibrosis, plugged by amorphous inspissations, or distorted by fibrosis and diverticula in a configuration known as salpingitis isthmica nodosa. These proximal tubal abnormalities are assumed to result from salpingitis, as they are frequently associated with typical residua of salpingitis on the adnexa.

Salpingitis clearly can cause infertility because of TID. Data from Weström's group in Sweden suggest that approximately 6% of aggressively treated cases of gonococcal salpingitis and 17% of cases of nongonococcal salpingitis lead to infertility. The laparoscopic severity of the acute infection predicts long-term success at live birth, ranging from 90% to 57% for patients with mild and severe disease, respectively. Association of instrumentation—from intrauterine devices or pregnancy termination—with the infection or recurrence of infection increases the likelihood that TID will eventually produce infertility. Nevertheless, even advanced salpingitis, manifesting as an inflammatory tubo-ovarian complex, is associated with successful pregnancy in 33% of women who attempt childbearing after medical treatment. This fact encourages aggressive medical treatment of advanced pelvic infection when the patient hopes to have children at some later date.

The relationship between salpingitis, defined as an acute, symptomatic illness, and TID leading to infertility is therefore not as clear as it might first appear. Most women experiencing a bout of salpingitis remain fertile, and only a minority with TID-associated infertility (ranging from 25% to 50% in several series) have a history of salpingitis. Consequently, given the estimate that 2% of all women are infertile because of TID, one or both of the following propositions must be true:

1. An important incidence of asymptomatic pelvic infection irreversibly damages the adnexa, distinct from the incidence that is commonly clinically termed pelvic inflammatory disease (PID).
2. Salpingitis is frequently undiagnosed because of mild symptoms, lack of patient sensitivity to symptoms' possible significance, or both.

The resolution of this conundrum is important, as it will allow progress to be made in preventing TID. Fertility in patients who have TID is not restored by surgery in most cases, and in vitro fertilization remains an expensive and frequently unsuccessful last resort.

## Diagnosis

Complementary information derived by hysterosalpingography (HSG) and laparoscopy is needed to diagnose TID. The HSG results will reveal isthmic or interstitial obstruction, although a finding of proximal tubal obstruction in a single HSG is frequently spurious. Findings of salpingitis isthmica nodosa are highly characteristic and reliable. Phimosis of the ampullary tubal ostium is difficult to detect on HSG, but complete obstruction with sactosalpinx is shown readily and reliably. By revealing the presence or absence of rugal folds in the ampulla, the HSG demonstrates the degree of mucosal preservation in cases of distal occlusion—a finding predictive of the success of subsequent attempts at repair.

Laparoscopy with chromopertubation confirms HSG findings and may invalidate false-positive findings, such as those frequently produced by unilateral proximal tubal occlusion. In addition, laparoscopy can identify abnormalities that usually escape detection on the HSG, such as periadnexal adhesions and tubal phimosis.

## Treatment for Tubal Damage

When TID is the culprit in infertility, surgical correction represents merely one therapeutic option in an array that includes in vitro fertilization and adoption. Even with the most meticulous and expert surgical reconstruction, the outlook for pregnancy is often poor, and the anguish of failure or repeated ectopic gestations serve the couple poorly and consume valuable time in their quest for a family. Frank and expert preoperative counseling is important.

Correcting isolated occlusion of the proximal tube in an otherwise normal pelvis often proves successful. Microsurgical anastomosis after resection of the occluded segment yields pregnancy rates between 50% and 75%. Recently, hysteroscopically or fluoroscopically guided cannulation of such obstruction has produced favorable outcomes. The use of this cannulation technique sometimes affords good results with less surgical invasiveness, morbidity, and cost.

Likewise, the prognosis often is excellent when adhesiolysis alone is all that is required to restore normal adnexal relationships. Although the likelihood of pregnancy depends on the extent and character of the adhesions, pregnancy generally can be anticipated in 50% to 70% of patients in this category.

By contrast, repair of distal occlusion is associated with much poorer outcomes. Advances in microsurgical technique have not improved results as dramatically in this group as in others. The best outcomes are associated with occlusions amenable to simple fimbrial dissection. Sactosalpinx dimensions are inversely correlated with success, as is the extent of mucosal destruction and of associated pelvic adhesion formation. Overall, pregnancy rates of 25% to 50% are seen after surgical correction of distal tubal obstruction.

The surgical reconstruction data do not compare favorably with contemporary success rates for in vitro fertilization. Despite the fact that in vitro fertilization offers the best hope of pregnancy for women with severe TID, mounting evidence suggests that the presence of hydrosalpinx decreases implantation rates and increases pregnancy loss rates in women undergoing such treatment. The idea that this trend may reflect a toxic influence of hydrosalpinx fluid and therefore may be ameliorated by salpingostomy or salpingectomy has not been evaluated.

## SEQUELAE
## Ectopic Pregnancy

A frequent outcome after any surgical correction of post-inflammatory adnexal damage, ectopic pregnancy accounts for one-third of resulting pregnancies. Both preoperative and post-operative counseling should clearly address this possibility. Early, close biochemical and ultrasonographic monitoring of pregnancies after reconstructive surgery is mandatory for patient safety and permits earlier, more conservative intervention in the event of tubal gestation.

Ectopic pregnancy occurs more often in women with a history of salpingitis. The reported increase in the incidence of ectopic pregnancy has been attributed to salpingitis, and histologic evidence of past salpingitis often appears in fallopian tubes removed because of ectopic pregnancy. Women with a history of salpingitis should be monitored closely during early pregnancy for evidence of ectopic gestation so as to reduce the risk of hemorrhage and to facilitate less invasive and more conservative management in the event of an ectopic pregnancy.

## Pelvic Pain

The incidence of chronic pelvic pain is higher in women who have experienced PID. Many clinicians suspect pelvic pain arises as a result of TID, but the entity has not been systematically described or characterized by appropriate studies.

Pelvic pain in women with a history of PID may result from reinfection or exacerbation of chronic infection or from causes unrelated to pelvic infection. Some patients have portions of one or both adnexa trapped by TID and presumably experience pain because of this condition. Symptoms in these patients typically include sharp or nagging unilateral discomfort, as well as abrupt periovulatory or luteal exacerbation. The latter feature may reflect effects of follicular rupture, corpus luteum formation, luteal enlargement from intraluteal hemorrhage on the adhesions with resulting traction, pressure on the adjacent peritoneum or on the ovary itself, or all these occurrences. A decrease in symptoms during a trial of gonadal quiescence induced by oral contraceptives may assist in the diagnosis.

Lysing adhesions and restoring normal relationships and mobility of the tubes and ovaries may afford relief to the patient. These steps are often possible at the time of diagnostic laparoscopy. A study designed to (1) confirm the existence of a pain syndrome arising specifically from TID, (2) evaluate the reliability of its diagnosis through a trial of gonadal quiescence, and (3) show the effectiveness of adhesiolysis remains an unmet need in this disease.

## Suggested Readings

Brumsted JR, Clifford PM, Nakajima ST, et al. Reproductive outcome after medical management of complicated pelvic inflammatory disease. Fertil Steril 1988;50:667–669.

Deaton JL, Gibson M, Riddick DH, et al. Diagnosis and treatment of cornual obstruction using a flexible tip guidewire. Fertil Steril 1990;53:232–236.

Dinsmoor M, Gibson M. Early recognition of ectopic pregnancy in an infertility population. Obstet Gynecol 1986;68:859–862.

Jacobs LA, Thie J, Patton PE, et al. Primary microsurgery for postinflammatory tubal infertility. Fertil Steril 1988;50:855–859.

Lepine LA, Hillis SD, Marchbanks PA, et al. Severity of the pelvic inflammatory disease as a predictor of the probability of live birth. Am J Obstet Gynecol 1998;178:977–981.

Mäkinen JI, Erkkola RU, Laippala PJ. Causes of the increase in the incidence of ectopic pregnancy: a study on 1,017 patients from 1966 to 1985 in Turku, Finland. Am J Obstet Gynecol 1989;160:642–646.

Pauerstein CJ, Coxatto HB, Eddy CA, et al. Anatomy and pathology of tubal pregnancy. Obstet Gynecol 1986;67:301–308.

Rosenfeld DL, Seidman SM, Bronson RA, et al. Unsuspected chronic pelvic inflammatory disease in the infertile female. Fertil Steril 1983;39:44–48.

Weström L. Effect of acute pelvic inflammatory disease on fertility. Am J Obstet Gynecol 1975;121:707–713.

Zeyneloglu HB, Arici A, Olive DL. Adverse effects of hydrosalpinx on pregnancy rates after in vitro fertilization—embryo transfer. Fertil Steril 1998;70:492–499.

CHAPTER

# 59

# *Tubo-ovarian Abscess*

*Charles H. Livengood III*

## Background

Abscess formation represents an important host defense mechanism for controlling a progressive infection. An abscess has one of two fates: either the containment holds and the infection is eventually sterilized (a process that may include spontaneous drainage into a hollow viscus), or the containment fails and the infection spreads rapidly. Either course can occur even if the patient receives antimicrobial therapy. Abscess formation is one of the last lines of host defense, and an infection that reaches this stage is by definition severe and dangerous. Accordingly, pelvic inflammatory disease (PID) with tubo-ovarian abscess (TOA) formation is regarded as the most severe form of the disease. TOA may also arise in infections following pelvic surgery, uterine perforation, bowel perforation, appendicitis, and diverticulitis, as well as in pelvic malignancy. Regardless of the origin of the abscess, the pathogenesis and management of TOA are similar. Approximately 50,000 to 100,000 TOAs are treated annually in the United States, representing 5% to 10% of all patients with PID.

## Pathogenesis

Pelvic inflammatory disease results when the barrier function of the endocervical canal becomes compromised by a sexually transmitted agent (*Neisseria gonorrhoeae, Chlamydia trachomatis* serotypes D–K, and possibly others); the breach allows pathogenic bacteria to gain access to the upper genital epithelium. If these organisms are not checked by host immunity or medical treatment, they proliferate and damage host tissue. Denuded surfaces of the fallopian tubes coapt and agglutinate, and an abscess forms in that closed space as bacteria, white cells, and fluids accumulate within it. The ovary may adhere to the fimbria of the infected oviduct (pyosalpinx) and become the distal wall of the abscess, or primary ovarian infection originating in a cortical defect may initiate the abscess. The bowel, parietal peritoneum, uterus, and omentum are usually involved secondarily and may host a loculation that forms to control pus leaked from the TOA; such loculations may evolve into a cul-de-sac abscess. Vascular perfusion of the inner wall of the abscess becomes compromised as well. An anaerobic environment evolves, with redox potential falling as low as –400 mV.

Tubo-ovarian abscess always should be considered a mixed (facultative and anaerobic) polymicrobial infection. Aerobic and anaerobic *Streptococcus* species including enterococci, Enterobacteriaceae (most often *Escherichia coli* and *Proteus* species), *Peptostreptococcus, Bacteroides, Prevotella*, and *Porphyromonas* species are commonly found in this disease. Highly resistant facultative gram-negative rods such as *Pseudomonas* species remain rare in TOA. Cultures are reported as negative in as many as one-third of TOAs. Although some of these cases may represent a successful host immunologic effort, most probably comprise technical culture failures.

## Diagnosis

Any patient suspected of having PID is at risk for developing a TOA. Patients with TOA tend to be somewhat older than the general PID population, most commonly in the third and fourth decades of life. A history of PID and use of IUD contraception are no longer considered to be indicators of a greater probability of TOA.

More severe pain is the rule with TOA, but exceptions occur. Findings of ileus—nausea, vomiting, and abdominal distension—are not uncommon.

The literature provides little information about the proportion of abscesses that are palpable on bimanual examination. While most are palpable, an unsuspected TOA is often discovered in a patient undergoing laparotomy for failure of medical therapy for PID. Most patients with acute TOA present with fever and leukocytosis; those with chronic TOAs usually do not have these findings. The differential diagnosis is extensive—ectopic pregnancy, all of the pelvic neoplasms, ovarian cyst or hematoma, appendiceal and diverticular abscesses, and degenerating uterine myomas all must be considered. Without surgery, it remains virtually impossible to distinguish between TOA and torsion of an adnexal mass.

Use ultrasonography or computed tomography when you suspect a pelvic mass in a patient with PID, when you cannot perform a pelvic examination because of pain, or when a PID patient fails to respond to antibiotic therapy. TOA causes more than 80% of medical therapy failures in PID and may progress rapidly to sepsis and death with or without rupture. Furthermore, if sonography reveals the presence of TOA, a search for metastatic abscesses (most often found in the right subphrenic space) should be undertaken.

Equally important, ultrasound is the best means for differentiating between a TOA and a tubo-ovarian complex (TOC); this important distinction has become fully appreciated only in the past 15 years. TOC is an inflammatory pelvic mass representing edematous, adherent, infected pelvic structures in PID; although sinus tracts containing pus are often present, no devitalized abscess wall or accumulation of pus within a cavity occurs. The TOC is perfused, living tissue. Although it may be large, it responds to medical therapy in more than 95% of cases. TOC and TOA cannot be differentiated by palpation. Sonographically, TOA will appear as one or more (usually contiguous) relatively homogeneous, somewhat symmetrical, cystic, thin-walled mass(es); TOC is a markedly heterogeneous, thick-walled mass with vague margins and no dominant cystic component or symmetry.

Imaging techniques such as magnetic resonance imaging, $^{111}$I-labeled leukocyte scanning, and others may offer an advantage over modern ultrasound only in certain special circumstances, and they are certainly more expensive. A decrease in the uterine artery pulsatility index has been reported in TOA and may predict a poor response to medical therapy.

## TREATMENT

The introduction of potent new antibiotics, the trend toward earlier presentation for medical care, the advent of invasive imaging capabilities, and greater understanding of the difference between TOA and TOC have been the apparent sources of recent changes in management of TOA. From 1950 to 1970, leaders in the field made a strong case for early hysterectomy with bilateral adnexectomy and pelvic drainage in all cases of TOA, citing a decline in mortality of up to sevenfold with this approach. During the early 1980s, when the distinction between TOA and TOC was elucidated, publications by Hager and by Ginsburg and coworkers provided further strong support for surgical treatment of TOA, although these authors did suggest selective resection of devitalized tissues. At the same time, Landers and Sweet reported successful medical management of TOA in two-thirds of the women in their large series when clindamycin was included in the regimen and in one-third when it was not; they concluded that conservative medical therapy including a strong anti-anaerobe drug is appropriate for initial management of TOA.

In the subsequent decade, the literature on TOA has focused on the success of minimally invasive drainage with medical therapy. A number of small series have shown initial responses in approximately 90% of patients and very good long-term responses as well. Interestingly, these good results are obtained regardless of whether the drainage is done preemptively or after failure of medical therapy alone; whether the approach is transcutaneous, transvaginal, or through the laparoscope; and whether a one-time needle drainage is performed or a catheter is placed for several days.

At present, no indisputable standard of care exists for TOA. A physician should not be criticized for undertaking immediate extirpative pelvic laparotomy for a patient with TOA (particularly if her condition is unstable or she has completed childbearing) or for attempting medical management alone with potent broad-spectrum antibiotics and careful monitoring (particularly if the patient is young and in stable condition). Some boundaries have been established, however. Initial outpatient management of TOA is unsafe; rupture and sepsis syndrome may occur unexpectedly and still carry mortality approaching 25%. Oral antibiotic regimens and those lacking broad-spectrum facultative and anaerobic coverage are inadequate. TOC should first be treated medically.

Furthermore, treatment of the patient with TOA depends on whether the abscess remains intact. The patient with an intact TOA usually will have pelvic peritonitis, but the upper abdomen will remain unaffected. Bowel sounds are hypoactive but not totally absent. A flat plate and upright X ray of the abdomen usually do not reveal air fluid levels or thickening of the bowel wall. Women with intact TOAs and thin-walled abscesses usually have good blood flow to the masses and therefore should respond to antibiotic therapy. On the other hand, patients with thick-walled abscesses will likely have poor blood flow; if the abscess is multiloculated, it probably will not be well perfused. If antibiotic therapy is administered, allow for a trial of 72 to 96 hours (as long as the patient's condition does not worsen) before declaring failure. When you suspect a ruptured TOA or find evidence of septic shock in a patient with TOA, immediately perform an exploratory laparotomy. To adequately examine the pelvis, the entire bowel, and subhepatic and subdiaphragmatic spaces, use a vertical abdominal wall incision.

The following protocol is offered as a general guideline, which aims to make the safest and most effective use of our current resources. When TOA is diagnosed:

1. Begin intravenous fluids.
2. Begin broad-spectrum antibiotics, choosing:
    a. ampicillin *plus* gentamicin *plus* metronidazole;
    b. ofloxacin *plus* metronidazole; or
    c. single-agent therapy with one of the following: ticarcillin/clavulanate, piperacillin/tazobactam, trovafloxacin, or imipenem.

    The antibiotic regimen employed has three functions: (1) to treat the abscess; (2) to be effective in preventing and treating the potential bacteremia that may occur; and (3) to be effective in treating intra-abdominal sepsis. Therefore, the antibiotic regimen must show efficacy against gram-positive and gram-negative facultative, and anaerobic bacteria. Some authorities feel strongly that coverage of enterococci is an essential component of antibiotic selection in TOA.

3. Survey for sepsis syndrome, including:
   a. vital signs and physical examination (including mental status);
   b. blood cell counts and chemistries;
   c. coagulation studies;
   d. chest X ray and electrocardiography; and
   e. urine ouput.
4. Place a nasogastric tube to suction if ileus has developed.
5. Strongly consider guided drainage of TOA within 24 to 48 hours.
   a. A transvaginal approach using an endovaginal probe with needle guide should be considered first; if this technique is not possible, proceed to a transcutaneous or laparoscopic approach.
   b. Place an indwelling catheter if the contents are too viscous to aspirate.
   c. Use colpotomy drainage only if the abscess is fixed and distends the low rectovaginal septum in the midline.
   d. Send the aspirate for microbiologic evaluation (and cytologic analysis if the fluid is serous or cloudy).
6. Correct any underlying medical derangements, such as anemia, hyperglycemia, hypoproteinemia, or hypoxia.

When treated with this regimen, patients should show a clear clinical response within approximately four days. For those who do not, consider reviewing the microbiology and sensitivities of the abscess contents, imaging the abscess for reaccumulation, performing water-soluble contrast bowel studies, blood cultures and echocardiography, and analyzing the patient for concomitant disease. Nevertheless, almost all of these patients will require surgery.

If the pelvic infection is not resolved by the preceding protocol or if the patient shows evidence of sepsis syndrome (hypotension and dysfunction of two or more organ systems) at *any* time during the course of treatment, laparotomy should be performed immediately for resection of all infected tissues in the pelvis. Closed suction drainage through the vagina may be a useful addition to this surgery. A mass closure of peritoneum, muscle, and fascia with monofilament suture and retention stitches is advised. Closure of the skin and subcutaneous layer primarily is appropriate only for women with no free pus in the abdomen. Postoperative management in an intensive care unit should be considered for those with septic shock, particularly if the clinician suspects adult respiratory distress syndrome.

For patients showing a good response to this conservative protocol, comprehensive antibiotic treatment should be continued for at least 10 days (in compliant patients, this course may be completed with oral outpatient therapy after resolution of clinical signs of infection), and they should be checked weekly with bimanual examination for two to three weeks after initial resolution. The mass associated with the TOA may not fully resolve for several months. Any increase in its size should spur careful evaluation and consideration of additional treatment. Sexually transmissible disease counseling should be reinforced. Patients should be advised that pregnancy remains possible, and that they should be promptly evaluated for any episode of amenorrhea or abdominal pain because of the risk for ectopic pregnancy.

## Suggested Readings

Ginsburg DS, Stern JL, Hamod KA, et al. Tubo-ovarian abscess: a retrospective review. Am J Obstet Gynecol 1980;138:1055–1058.

Hager WD. Follow-up of patients with tubo-ovarian abscess(es) in association with salpingitis. Obstet Gynecol 1983;61:680–684.

Landers DV, Sweet RL. Current trends in the diagnosis and treatment of tubo-ovarian abscess. Am J Obstet Gynecol 1985;151:1098–1110.

Landers DV, Sweet RL. Tubo-ovarian abscess: contemporary approach to management. Rev Infect Dis 1983;5:876–884.

Nelson AL, Sinow RM, Renslo R, et al. Endovaginal ultrasonographically guided transvaginal drainage for treatment of pelvic abscesses. Am J Obstet Gynecol 1995;172:1926–1932.

Shulman A, Maymon R, Shapiro A, et al. Percutaneous catheter drainage of tubo-ovarian abscess. Obstet Gynecol 1992;80:555–557.

CHAPTER

# 60

# *Perihepatitis*

*Stephen J. Fortunato*

## Background and Incidence

The clinical syndrome of perihepatitis complicating active or previously treated salpingitis is known in the United States as Fitz-Hugh–Curtis syndrome. This syndrome originally was described by Carlos Stajano in a presentation to the Society of Obstetricians and Gynecologists of Montevideo, Uruguay, in 1919. In the 1930s, Thomas Fitz-Hugh and Arthur Curtis independently described perihepatic inflammation with stringy adhesions between the peritoneum and hepatic capsule as a complication of acute gonococcal salpingitis.

The diagnosis of salpingitis-associated perihepatitis has been made on the basis of typical symptoms in as many as 20% of patients with salpingitis. The same diagnosis has been made on the basis of laparoscopic findings in 5% to 15% of patients with salpingitis.

## Etiology

Initially, *Neisseria gonorrhoeae* was believed to be the only organism responsible for salpingitis-associated perihepatitis. In earlier reports, however, fewer than half of patients with clinical symptoms consistent with salpingitis-associated perihepatitis had cervical cultures positive for *N. gonorrhoeae*. For several reasons, positive cultures have been obtained much less frequently from the surface of the liver.

In the 1970s, growing recognition of the importance of *Chlamydia trachomatis* in salpingitis, along with improvements in the ability to culture this organism, spurred interest in *C. trachomatis* as an etiologic agent in salpingitis-associated perihepatitis. As it became increasingly evident that *C. trachomatis* was present in a large percentage of salpingitis cases, the tubal pathology associated with this organism was likened to that seen in perihepatitis. In 1978, Muller-Schoop and coworkers reported an association between laparoscopically documented peritonitis and perihepatitis with serologic evidence of recent *C. trachomatis* infection. Subsequently, Wölner-Hanssen and coworkers reported three cases of acute genital chlamydial infection, confirmed by culture and serology, in which they obtained laparoscopic evidence of both salpingitis and perihepatitis. None of the patients in these cases showed evidence of acute gonococcal infection.

Additional reports have strengthened the etiologic association of *C. trachomatis* with salpingitis-associated perihepatitis. In fact, sufficient evidence has accumulated to suggest that *C. trachomatis* may be the etiologic agent of perihepatitis, with *N. gonorrhoeae* representing a frequently accompanying, but ultimately innocent, bystander. Recently published studies by Eschenbach and Wölner-Hanssen indicated that *N. gonorrhoeae* was isolated in only 10% of cervical cultures from women with perihepatitis and *C. trachomatis* in 50% of these women; in addition, serologic evidence of acute chlamydial infection was present in 81% of cases. To date, no evidence has indicated that other organisms play a role in the pathogenesis of this syndrome.

## Pathophysiology

Only a small percentage of women with salpingitis will develop perihepatitis. Host factors and microbiologic virulence factors remain undefined.

Investigators have proposed three mechanisms of spread from the pelvis to the liver: (1) direct intraperitoneal, (2) lymphatic, and (3) hematogenous. In direct intraperitoneal spread, purulent exudate from the fallopian tubes travels up to the paracolic gutter and collects in the subhepatic space, the most dependent portion of the abdominal cavity when a woman is supine.

This process results in an inflammatory reaction involving a liver capsule. The gross pathology observed during the early phase of this disease includes areas of purulent and fibrinous peritonitis on the liver capsule and hemorrhagic areas on the parietal peritoneum. Characteristic "violin string" adhesions do not appear until later in the course of the syndrome; these avascular bands between the liver capsule and the anterior abdominal wall are usually found after resolution of the acute inflammatory process.

The contribution of lymphatic and hematogenous spread of microorganisms to the pathogenesis of the perihepatitis syndrome remains unclear, but the occurrence of the condition in men necessitates an alternative explanation for direct intraperitoneal spread. Intraparenchymal liver damage has not been reported as a histologic feature of this syndrome.

## Diagnosis

Acute salpingitis-associated perihepatitis should be suspected when right-upper-quadrant pain accompanies the clinical diagnosis of pelvic inflammatory disease (PID). The diagnosis can be confirmed by direct laparoscopic inspection that reveals both salpingitis and perihepatic adhesions. The right-upper-quadrant pain associated with this condition often takes a sudden and intense form. It occasionally radiates to the shoulder and is commonly exacerbated by breathing or coughing. In the majority of cases, it occurs simultaneously with the pelvic pain associated with salpingitis, although it may arise days to weeks after the onset of pelvic pain. In cases of salpingitis that is incompletely treated or mistakenly diagnosed, where *C. trachomatis* has not been considered as an offending organism, the patient may present with chronic right-upper-quadrant pain of long duration. Focused questioning may reveal a history of onset commensurate with an intra-abdominal process that resolved after oral or intravenous antibiotic treatment, leaving behind right-upper-quadrant pain resistant to both diagnosis and treatment by the patient's primary-care provider.

The differential diagnosis of this condition is extensive and is not limited to those conditions associated only with right-upper-quadrant pain. Acute cholecystitis, hepatitis, and pancreatitis are among the most common conditions confused with salpingitis-associated perihepatitis; conditions such as pneumonia, hepatic and subdiaphragmatic abscess, pleuritis, pleurodynia, perforated abdominal viscus, appendicitis, and even pyelonephritis have been mistaken for this condition as well.

Liver enzymes are frequently elevated to a mild degree (25% to 50%) but rarely prove helpful in making the differential diagnosis. Patients with pronounced enzyme elevations should undergo serologic testing for viral hepatitis (including hepatitis A, B, C, and E) as well as cytomegalovirus and Epstein-Barr virus.

Ultrasound and chest X rays may also aid in making the correct diagnosis. Ultrasound images of the gallbladder, bile ducts, and liver parenchyma should appear normal, although thin, stringy adhesions between the liver capsule and the anterior abdomen have been described in the presence of ascites. The chest X ray will occasionally show a small amount of pleural fluid; a larger pleural effusion or pulmonary infiltrate is not seen in salpingitis-associated perihepatitis and should suggest another diagnosis.

## TREATMENT

Parenteral regimens currently recommended for the treatment of acute PID are adequate for treating salpingitis-associated perihepatitis. In addition, azithromycin has been approved for the treatment of chlamydial infections as a single oral 1 g dose. If perihepatitis proves to have a chlamydial origin rather than being a gonococcal infection, this single-dose therapy should adequately treat perihepatitis. In that event, single-dose azithromycin should be able to replace doxycycline in the following regimens and improve patient compliance. Interestingly, in the Centers for Disease Control and Prevention's (CDC's) 1998 guidelines for treating sexually transmitted diseases, azithromycin is recommended for chlamydial coverage for uncomplicated gonococcal infection but not for PID. This recommendation is most likely an oversight.

Approved regimens for salpingitis-associated perihepatitis include the following:

1. cefotetan, 2 g IV every 12 hours, plus doxycycline, 100 mg every 12 hours orally or IV
2. clindamycin, 900 mg IV every 8 hours, plus gentamicin, loading dose (2 mg/kg) IV or IM followed by a maintenance dose (1.5 mg/kg) every 8 hours plus doxycycline
3. ampicillin/sulbactam, 3 g IV every 6 hours, plus doxycycline as above

The patient should receive intravenous antibiotic therapy for at least 48 hours after she improves clinically. Continuation of doxycycline at 100 mg orally two times per day for a total of 10 to 14 days is recommended. Usually acute upper abdominal pain resolves rapidly after IV therapy begins. Sometimes, however, chronic right-upper-quadrant pain may persist even after adequate therapy.

## Suggested Readings


Centers for Disease Control and Prevention. 1998 guidelines for treatment of sexually transmitted diseases. MMWR 1998;47 (RR-1):49–69,79–86.

Darougar S, Forsey T, Wood JJ, et al. *Chlamydia* and the Curtis–Fitz-Hugh syndrome. Br J Vener Dis 1981;57:391–394.

Eschenbach DA, Wolner-Hansen PA. Fitz-Hugh–Curtis syndrome. In: Holmes KK, ed. Sexually transmitted disease, 2nd ed. New York: McGraw-Hill, 1990:612–626.

Gjonnaess H, Dalaker K, Anestad G, et al. Pelvic inflammatory disease: etiologic studies with emphasis on chlamydial infection. Obstet Gynecol 1982;50:550–555.

Muller-Schoop JW, Wang SP, Munzinger J, et al. *Chlamydia trachomatis* as possible cause of peritonitis and perihepatitis in young women. Br Med J 1978;1:1022–1024.

Owens S, Yeka TR, Bloy R, et al. Laparoscopic treatment of painful perihepatic adhesions in Fitz-Hugh–Curtis syndrome. Obstet Gynecol 1991;78:542–543.

Paavonen J, Saikku P, von Knorring J, et al. Association of infection with *Chlamydia trachomatis* with Fitz-Hugh–Curtis syndrome. J Infect Dis 1981;144:176.

Wang SP, Eschenbach DA, Holmes KK, et al. *Chlamydia trachomatis* infection in Fitz-Hugh–Curtis syndrome. Am J Obstet Gynecol 1980;138:1034–1038.

CHAPTER

# 61

# *Pelvic Tuberculosis*

*Walter Chaim*
*Eli Maymon*

## BACKGROUND

Tuberculosis again has become a serious threat to public health in the United States. A recent report from the Centers for Disease Control and Prevention (CDC) indicated an increase of 20% in the total incidence of tuberculosis during the last decade, with 44% of the increase occurring among persons aged 25 to 44 years and 27% among children younger than 15 years of age.

Tuberculosis remains endemic in some parts of the world, especially in less developed countries. The demographic characteristics of what appears to be a new "tuberculosis epidemic" both worldwide and in the United States reflect the medical and social problems of poverty in urban populations, with increasing prevalence of risk factors such as homelessness, drug addiction, and HIV infection. In homeless persons in the United States, the prevalence rate of active tuberculosis is 1.6% to 6.8%, and estimates of latent infection range as high as 18% to 51%.

The resurgence of this disease worldwide, and in the United States in particular, has been strongly linked to the increasing incidence of HIV infection. Indeed, the occurrence of tuberculosis has increased 500-fold in patients with AIDS during the last decade. In the United States, the rate of HIV seropositivity among those attending tuberculosis clinics is as high as 45%. The increasing number of women with HIV infection and the potential for spread of primary pulmonary infection to the pelvis has increased the risk of pelvic tuberculosis infection among women in the United States.

Currently, pelvic tuberculosis is frequently observed in India, the Far East, the Caribbean region, and South America. Increasing immigration from these areas, added to the increased risk posed by the rise in HIV infection among U.S. women, underscores the need to remain alert for the possibility of pelvic tuberculosis. Approximately 10% of patients with pulmonary tuberculosis also develop genital tuberculosis, although less than 1% of salpingitis infection can be attributed to *Mycobacterium tuberculosis*.

## Pathophysiology

Genital tuberculosis usually results from hematogenic spread of a primary pulmonary tuberculous infection. It generally occurs during the first one or two years after the primary infection, presenting with a long and indolent course. The fallopian tubes are the first pelvic target of hematogenic spread in 90% to 100% of cases. The ampulla is invariably involved, whereas the isthmus is affected in only 80% of cases and the interstitial portions are never involved. This pattern of infection probably reflects the distribution of the blood supply to the fallopian tubes.

The tubal involvement in pelvic tuberculosis means that mechanical infertility is the most common symptom. From the tubes, spread follows by direct extension to the endometrium in 50% to 60% of cases, to the ovaries in 20% to 30% of cases, to the cervix in 5% to 15% of cases, and less frequently to the peritoneum. An ascending infection from the lower genital tract by sexual contamination of epididymal origin is very rare.

## Diagnosis

In the majority of cases, genital tuberculosis is associated with infertility and pelvic pain. It is therefore more often diagnosed during the premenopausal period. Nevertheless, 10%

of cases may be diagnosed only after menopause, with presenting symptoms such as vaginal bleeding or pain. In 20% of the cases of genital tuberculosis, a family history of tuberculosis may be present. Simultaneous active pulmonary infection is uncommon.

Pelvic tuberculosis may present in three clinical forms: latent genital tuberculosis, tuberculous salpingitis, and tuberculous peritonitis. The diagnosis of latent genital tuberculosis most frequently results from an infertility workup or endometrial biopsy. The latency period may extend to as long as 30 years after primary infection. Signs and symptoms of salpingitis presenting in a virgin should arouse strong suspicion of pelvic tuberculosis.

Diagnostic laparoscopy for pelvic inflammatory disease that does not respond to prolonged antibiotic treatment may reveal gross enlargement of the tubes caused by an inflammatory reaction to tuberculosis. Biopsy of a lesion and histologic examination may reveal the presence of tuberculous salpingitis. In such cases, the patient should receive antibiotic therapy.

Tuberculous peritonitis has a much different laparoscopic appearance. In this manifestation, infection may extend over all of the peritoneal surfaces, with typical tubercles taking the form of small nodules accompanied by ascites and adhesions. This clinical form of pelvic tuberculosis does not necessarily imply occluded tubes and is the product of hematogenous or lymphatic spread.

A negative tubercular skin test (purified protein derivative [PPD] or Mantoux test) virtually rules out the possibility of tuberculosis. The diagnosis of pelvic tuberculosis is established by isolating *M. tuberculosis* from an endometrial biopsy specimen obtained during the week preceding menstruation for histologic examination and culture. Repeated cultures of menstrual flow may serve as a diagnostic alternative. If these test results are negative, endometrial curettage is indicated. If none of these tests verifies the diagnosis, perform a laparotomy or an open laparoscopy, taking care not to perforate possibly adherent intestinal loops.

Performance of hysterosalpingography is not recommended when pelvic tuberculosis is suspected, to avoid a possible exacerbation of the disease.

**Table 61-1.** Antituberculous Therapy

| | | |
|---|---|---|
| **First-Line Regimens** | | |
| Isoniazid | 5 mg/kg/day to a total of 300 mg/day | Oral or IM |
| Rifampin | 10 mg/kg/day to a total of 600 mg/day | Oral |
| Ethambutol | 5–25 mg/kg/day to a total of 2.5 g/day | Oral |
| Pyrazinamide | 15–30 mg/kg/day to a total of 2 g/day | Oral |
| **Additional Regimens** | | |
| Capreomycin | 15–30 mg/kg/day to a total of 0.75–1 g/day | IM |
| Cycloserine | 10–15 mg/kg/day to a total of 250–1000 mg/day | Oral |
| Ethionamide | 15–20 mg/kg/day to a total of 1 g/day | Oral |
| Kanamycin | 15–30 mg/kg/day to a total of 0.75–1 g/day | IM |
| *Para*-amino-salicylic acid | 150 mg/kg/day to a total of 10–12 g/day | Oral |
| Streptomycin | 15 mg/kg/day to a total of 1.5 g/day | IM |
| Viomycin | 15–30 mg/kg/day to a total of 0.75–1 g/day | IM |

SOURCE: Bass JB Jr, Farer LS, Hopewell PC, et al. Treatment of tuberculosis and tuberculosis infection in adults and children. American Thoracic Society and Centers for Disease and Prevention. Am J Respir Crit Care Med 1994;149:1359–1374.

## TREATMENT

The principles and duration of the treatment of pelvic tuberculosis are similar to those of pulmonary tuberculosis. Treatment should be administered in consultation with an infectious disease specialist. Current regimens vary from six to nine months in length and typically include two to four drugs, depending on the suspicion of drug-resistant disease and the patient's response to therapy.

Isoniazid, rifampin, ethambutol, and pyrazinamide are the first-line choices among the drugs commonly used to treat tuberculosis (Table 61-1). Isoniazid is an inexpensive drug that can penetrate all body fluids and cavities and effectively kill *M. tuberculosis* organisms in caseous material. Its most common side effect is hepatitis. Rifampin also may cause hepatitis and perhaps interact with and degrade the activity of other drugs, including oral contraceptives (OCs). Women taking OCs should therefore switch to an alternative contraceptive method while receiving rifampin therapy. Use of ethambutol may cause a dose- and time-related retrobulbar neuritis with blurred vision, central scotomata, and red-green color blindness. Use of pyrazinamide inhibits renal tubular excretion of uric acid, increasing serum uric acid level. This side effect may spur the development of a nongouty polyarthralgia, but it need not require discontinuation of the drug. The American Thoracic Society and CDC recommend pyrazinamide as part of the initial treatment of tuberculosis. Other drugs available to treat tuberculosis are effective but poorly tolerated by women because of their frequent side effects.

The initial phase of a six-month regimen of therapy for pelvic tuberculosis requires at least two months of daily isoniazid, rifampin, and pyrazinamide; ethambutol or streptomycin are added if isoniazid resistance emerges or the patient develops life-threatening disease. The second phase of treatment, lasting four months, includes isoniazid and rifampin on a daily or twice-weekly basis.

The nine-month treatment protocol is similar to the six-month protocol, with the same drugs used for longer periods of time.

Surgery is necessary for pelvic tuberculosis only in circumstances such as the presence of an adnexal mass. In older women, total abdominal hysterectomy with bilateral salpingo-oophorectomy is the operation of choice. Surgical intervention also should be considered when the patient suffers from persistent or recurrent infection or pelvic pain.

Development of drug resistance may be the result of unsupervised treatment, which can lead to inadequate and inappropriate dosing with probable poor drug absorption. It also may follow from mutations in the tubercle bacillus.

## Suggested Readings

Centers for Disease Control and Prevention. Initial therapy for tuberculosis in the era of multidrug resistance. Recommendations of the Advisory Council for the Elimination of Tuberculosis. MMWR 1993;42:1–8.

Eschenbach DA. Genital tuberculosis. In: Scott JR, DiSaia PJ, Hammond CB, et al., eds. Danforth's obstetrics and gynecology, 7th ed. Philadelphia: J. B. Lippincott Company, 1994:661–664.

Gull I, Peyser MR, Yaron Y, et al. The effect of an in-vitro fertilization pregnancy on a woman with genital tuberculosis. Human Reprod 1995;10:3052–3054.

Miller KS, Miller JM Jr. Tuberculosis in pregnancy: interactions, diagnosis, and management. Clin Obstet Gynecol 1996;39:120–142.

Nogales-Ortiz F, Tarancon I, Nogales FF Jr. The pathology of female genital tuberculosis. A 31-year study of 1436 cases. Obstet Gynecol 1979;53:422–428.

Robinson CA, Rose NC. Tuberculosis: current implications and management in obstetrics. Obstet Gynecol Surv 1996;51:115–124.

CHAPTER

# 62

# *IUD-Associated Infections*

*Richard H. Schwarz*

## Background and Incidence

Although an association between the use of an intrauterine contraceptive device (IUD) and increased risk of pelvic inflammatory disease (PID) has been documented for many years, recent studies suggest that this association may have been overestimated. In fact, postinsertion PID has become a relatively uncommon clinical entity given the decreased use of IUDs, the relatively low incidence of problems with currently available devices, careful insertion techniques with or without antibiotic prophylaxis, and proper selection of patients. Methodologic flaws in older studies—such as comparison with inappropriate control groups, overdiagnosis of PID among IUD users, and failure to adjust for confounding variables—artificially increased the apparent risk of IUDs. In addition, the risk of PID with the Dalkon Shield was higher than that observed with other IUDs, and failure to exclude cases involving that particular device may have led to an overestimation of the risk associated with currently available devices.

In 1991, a controversial review by Kronmal and coworkers even questioned the previously reported strong association between PID and the Dalkon Shield. In 1993, a meta-analysis by Sivin specifically confirmed that the Dalkon Shield was associated with significantly higher rates of serious complications than were other devices used in the 1970s as well as those in contemporary use. These complications include higher rates of expulsion, pregnancy, hospitalization for PID, septic abortion, and deaths. Following the cessation of distribution and use of the Dalkon Shield in 1975 and a recommendation by the Food and Drug Administration (FDA) that IUDs be removed in the case of pregnancy, no deaths were reported in pregnant women with IUDs in place in the United States for the subsequent 15 years.

Methodologically sound studies published since the mid-1980s have clarified the association between IUDs and PID. They indicate a relative risk of contracting PID of 1.0 to 2.6 for women using IUDs compared with the risk of women using no contraceptive method.

## Pathophysiology

Contamination of the endometrial cavity at insertion is suspected to be responsible for most cases of IUD-related PID. Risk appears limited to the first four months of use and is probably caused by organisms other than those responsible for sexually transmitted disease (STD). Infections occurring four months or more after insertion are believed to result from acquired sexually transmitted pathogens rather than the IUD itself.

Previously, it was believed that IUD infections spread through lymphatics to produce a perisalpingitis similar to that of postabortal or postpartum infections. Today, however, direct spread of microorganisms from the infected or colonized uterine cavity to the fallopian tubes is suspected to constitute the major pathogenic mechanism. In addition, it was previously hypothesized that unilateral tubo-ovarian abscesses were uniquely associated with IUD infections; this view has subsequently been disproved. Although the multifilamented tail of the Dalkon Shield was purported to act as a "wick" for endometrial contamination, the monofilament tails of currently available IUDs do not appear to have etiologic importance in PID.

Recent pathomorphologic studies of fallopian tubes excised during sterilization of asymptomatic IUD users reveal a sterile foreign-body reaction. A relationship of this sterile reaction to infectious salpingitis has not been established, however.

Spontaneous midtrimester septic abortions were rare until the introduction of the Dalkon Shield in 1970. According to Tatum, the Dalkon Shield appeared to predispose to this serious condition when the 200 to 400 separate fibers forming its sheathed multifilament tail retracted into the endometrial cavity early in the second trimester. In addition, microorganisms lodged between the sheathed fibers of the tail were not exposed to the bacteriocidal and bacteriostatic endocervical mucus, as they are with the unsheathed single or double fibers of conventional modern IUD tails.

## ETIOLOGY

The microorganisms associated with non-STD-related IUD PID are those linked to the endogenous cervicovaginal flora. These infections are always polymicrobial, with anaerobes predominating. Infections occurring more than four months after insertion are probably caused by both sexually transmitted and endogenous organisms that cause non-IUD-related PID (see Chapter 56).

A unique role for *Actinomyces* organisms in IUD PID has been suggested, although this relationship has not yet been fully elucidated. In a review of Pap smears in 1520 IUD users, *Actinomyces*-like organisms were identified in 11.2%, and the rate seemed to increase with duration of use. The presence of the organisms on Pap smears, however, has not been equated with active pelvic actinomycosis, nor has the risk of subsequent pelvic infection been quantified. A literature survey by Fiorino in 1996 revealed 96 recorded cases of actinomycotic pelvic abscess associated with the presence of an IUD. Because the physical findings in these patients frequently suggest pelvic malignancy, these cases often are treated surgically with hysterectomy and salpingo-oophorectomy. If *Actinomyces* infection is suspected, surgery should be delayed because medical therapy with high-dose penicillin may provide complete resolution.

IUD use may increase a woman's susceptibility to bacterial vaginosis (BV), a condition that may itself increase her risk of developing PID. To date, no studies have addressed the risk of postinsertion PID in IUD users with BV.

## Diagnosis

The classic syndrome of IUD-related progressive endometritis, first described by Burnhill, consists of persistent foul-smelling vaginal discharge, intermenstrual spotting, premenstrual bloating, and dull backache during menstruation. Initially, the uterine corpus is tender on bimanual palpation, but adnexal tenderness and cervical motion tenderness are late findings. This syndrome has virtually disappeared with the discontinuance of older devices such as the Dalkon Shield, Birnberg bow, and Majzlin spring; Burnhill feels it is largely of historical interest.

Postinsertion and STD-related IUD PID can be asymptomatic or they may present with the same signs and symptoms as non–IUD-related PID. The diagnosis is established in the same way as in the latter condition, and laparoscopy should be employed if the diagnosis is uncertain.

The syndrome of midtrimester septic abortion also has essentially disappeared with the abandonment of the Dalkon Shield. In this syndrome, patients often progressed to severe infection with minimal signs and symptoms, and septic shock and adult respiratory distress syndrome (ARDS) were frequent and early complications.

## Treatment

### Progressive Endometritis

Progressive endometritis is rarely seen today. In the past, patients diagnosed before adnexal involvement occurred were found to respond to a 7- to 10-day course of oral tetracycline, with removal of the IUD after 24 hours of antibiotic therapy.

### Postinsertion and STD-Related IUD PID

Antibiotic management of postinsertion and STD-related IUD PID generally is the same as that for any acute salpingitis. We prefer parenteral therapy (clindamycin plus gentamicin, cefotetan plus doxycycline, or ampicillin/sulbactam plus doxycycline) on an inpatient basis for IUD users with salpingitis. The IUD should be removed as soon as systemic antimicrobial levels are established. Failure to respond to therapy, including treatment for tubo-ovarian abscess, is managed exactly as with other acute PID conditions (see Chapter 57).

## *Actinomyces* Colonization/Infection

When *Actinomyces* is identified in an asymptomatic IUD user (almost always on a Pap smear), removal of the device will result in clearing of the organism (see Chapter 63). Removal should be followed by another Pap smear after one or two menstrual cycles to confirm the result. After the finding of a negative smear, a new device may be reinserted.

Symptomatic patients should be treated with parenteral antimicrobial therapy and the IUD removed. The exact role of the *Actinomyces* organism in abscess formation remains unclear, as does the mechanism of its apparent relationship to the IUD. Whether *Actinomyces* is a sole pathogen or merely a marker for mixed aerobic–anaerobic infection is an unresolved question. We consider mixed infection more likely and therefore prefer to prescribe broad-spectrum antibiotic coverage. If *Actinomyces* infection appears in association with a tubo-ovarian abscess, antibiotic therapy for one to three months must follow surgical extirpation of the infected tissue. Penicillin is the drug of choice; cephalosporins, clindamycin, and chloramphenicol are alternative agents. Metronidazole, although extremely active against most anaerobes, is not effective against *Actinomyces*.

## IUDs and Pregnancy

If a patient conceives with an IUD in place and wishes to continue the pregnancy, the device should be removed if the string is visible. If it cannot be removed, the patient must be advised of the potential problems and carefully monitored throughout the pregnancy. In the rare event of septic midtrimester abortion, management includes aggressive evacuation of the uterus by the most expeditious means, broad-spectrum parenteral antibiotic therapy, and intensive cardiovascular and respiratory monitoring. Failure to recognize the problem and to treat it aggressively can lead to a high mortality rate.

### IUDs and BV

Bacterial vaginosis should be treated in an IUD user (metronidazole, 500 mg orally twice daily for seven days). The IUD does not need to be removed unless the patient shows signs or symptoms of PID (see Chapter 39).

## Sequelae

The greatest concern following IUD-related PID focuses on tubal damage. Two case-control studies of tubal infertility showed the risk highest with the Dalkon Shield and the lowest risk with copper devices. In a study by Cramer and coworkers, the increased relative risk of primary tubal infertility was statistically significant for users of the Dalkon Shield (*RR* = 3.3), Lippes Loop or Saf-T-Coil (*RR* = 2.9), and copper IUDs (*RR* = 1.6). The higher relative risk of tubal infertility with the Dalkon Shield was confirmed in Sivin's meta-analysis. For secondary tubal infertility, the risk associated with copper devices was not statistically significant. Importantly, women with only one sexual partner had no increased risk of primary tubal infertility associated with IUD use.

In a study by Daling and coworkers, the relative risk of primary tubal infertility was 6.8 for users of the Dalkon Shield, 3.2 for users of the Lippes Loop or Saf-T-Coil, and 1.9 for users of copper devices. The risk associated with the use of a copper device was not statistically significant. As with PID, the risk of infertility appears to be largely related to the likelihood of exposure to STDs.

## Prevention

The IUD, unlike barrier methods of contraception and birth control pills, offers no protection against STDs. This fact is a critical issue in contraceptive choice for a woman who desires fertility in the future. Careful selection of candidates for IUDs appears to offer the greatest opportunity for infection prevention. Only women at low risk for acquiring an STD should receive an IUD. The ideal candidate would be in a stable, mutually monogamous relationship, have no evidence of acute cervicitis, and have no history of ectopic pregnancy, salpingitis, or any STD. Mishell has suggested that IUDs should not be used by any nulliparous woman who may want to conceive in the future, because of the slight possibility of postinsertion PID and its associated tubal infertility risk.

Optimally, the physician should confirm the absence of cervical infection with *Neisseria gonorrhoeae* and/or *Chlamydia trachomatis* before insertion. Frequently, however, this testing is not feasible. If a mucopurulent discharge from the cervix is noted, insertion should be deferred until the cause has been investigated and treated. The presence of the typical BV syndrome, confirmed microscopically, should also lead to delay of insertion until treatment ends.

Aseptic technique must be maintained during the insertion process. The vagina and cervix are routinely cleansed with an antiseptic.

In the 1998 edition of the *Physicians' Desk Reference*, the manufacturer of the Paragard T device states, "Data do not confirm the utility of prophylactic administration of antibiotics in reducing the incidence of PID, and their use in nursing women is not recommended." Although this statement might imply that prophylactic antibiotics might be used for insertion prophylaxis in nonpregnant women, a recent randomized, controlled trial of prophylactic antibiotics administered before IUD insertion showed that prophylaxis with azithromycin did not affect the likelihood that a woman would retain her IUD at 90 days or the frequency of postinsertion medical attention. These authors concluded that routine antibiotic prophylaxis at IUD insertion seems unwarranted in appropriate candidates for intrauterine contraception, in whom infection of the upper genital tract is rare, with or without antibiotic prophylaxis.

The most recent guidelines of the American Heart Association for prevention of bacterial endocarditis do not recommend endocarditis prophylaxis for insertion or removal of intrauterine devices in uninfected tissue.

## Suggested Readings

Burnhill MS. Syndrome of progressive endometritis associated with intrauterine contraceptive devices. Adv Planned Parent 1973;8:144.

Chatwani A, Amin-Hanjani S. Incidence of actinomycosis associated with intrauterine devices. J Reprod Med 1994;39:585–587.

Chi IC. A bill of health for the IUD: where do we go from here? Adv Contracept 1994;10:121–131.

Cramer DW, Schiff I, Schoenbaum SC, et al. Tubal infertility and the intrauterine device. N Engl J Med 1985;312:941–947.

Dajani AS, Taubert KA, Wilson W, et al. Prevention of bacterial endocarditis. Recommendations by the American Heart Association. JAMA 1997;277:1794–1801.

Daling JR, Weiss NS, Metch BJ, et al. Primary tubal infertility in relation to the use of an intrauterine device. N Engl J Med 1985;312:937–941.

Fiorino AS. Intrauterine contraceptive device-associated actinomycotic abscess and *Actinomyces* detection on cervical smear. Obstet Gynecol 1996;87:142–149.

Grimes DA. Intrauterine devices and pelvic inflammatory disease: recent developments. Contraception 1987;36:97–109.

Hager WD, Douglas B, Majmudar B, et al. Pelvic colonization with *Actinomyces* in women using intrauterine contraceptive devices. Am J Obstet Gynecol 1979;135:680–684.

Jossens MO, Schachter J, Sweet RL. Risk factors associated with pelvic inflammatory disease of differing microbial etiologies. Obstet Gynecol 1994;83:989–997.

Kessel E. Pelvic inflammatory disease with intrauterine device use: a reassessment. Fertil Steril 1989;51:1–11.

Kronmal RA, Whitney CW, Mumford SD. The intrauterine device and pelvic inflammatory disease: the Women's Health Study reanalyzed. J Clin Epidemiol 1991;44:109–122.

Lee NC, Rubin GL, Borucki R. The intrauterine device and pelvic inflammatory disease revisited: new results from the Women's Health Study. Obstet Gynecol 1988;72:1–6.

Lee NC, Rubin GL, Ory HW, et al. Type of intrauterine device and the risk of pelvic inflammatory disease. Obstet Gynecol 1983;62:1–6.

Sinei SK, Schulz KF, Lamptey PR, et al. Preventing IUCD-related pelvic infection: the efficacy of prophylactic doxycycline at insertion. Br J Obstet Gynaecol 1990;97:412–419.

Sivin I. Another look at the Dalkon Shield: meta-analysis underscores its problems. Contracept 1993;48:1–12. (Published erratum appears in Contracept 1993;48:192.)

Walsh T, Grimes D, Frezieres R, et al. Randomised controlled trial of prophylactic antibiotics before insertion of intrauterine devices. Lancet 1998;351:1005–1008.

Zorlu CG, Aral K, Cobanoglu O, et al. Pelvic inflammatory disease and intrauterine devices: prophylactic antibodies to reduce febrile complications. Adv Contracept 1993;9:299–302.

CHAPTER

# 63

# *Pelvic Actinomycosis*

*W. David Hager*

## Background

Infection of the female genital tract with *Actinomyces israelii* is not frequent, although colonization with this organism is not uncommon, especially among IUD users. Most of the published data relating to this condition have come from case reports. A 1996 review collected 92 reported cases of pelvic abscesses caused by *Actinomyces* and associated with IUD use. Despite this relative paucity of data, health care professionals often have questions regarding the management of situations involving *Actinomyces* in an IUD user when a cervical cytologic report indicates a possible actinomycotic infection.

## Pathophysiology

*Actinomyces israelii* is one of several species of the genus *Actinomycetes*. This filamentous, gram-positive bacillus has the characteristics of being aerobic or microaerophilic and non-acid-fast. A hyphal organism, it fragments into coccoid or bacillary forms. Unlike fungi, *A. israelii* does not form conidia. It has erroneously been classified as a fungus and as a strict anaerobe in previous reports.

Because this bacterium is not a mucosal invader, it requires tissue injury or a foreign body to establish infection, which explains its association with IUDs and with pelvic infections. Bacteria present in the lower genital tract can migrate up the filamentous IUD string and create an infection at the site of cavitation created by the device. When recovered from patients with a pelvic abscess, *Actinomyces* species usually are found in association with anerobic bacteria.

*Actinomyces israelii* is considered to be part of the normal flora in the oral cavity and the upper intestinal tract. It is from these sites that the organism is transmitted to the pelvis in women who present with genital tract infection.

## Clinical Findings

*Actinomyces israelii* has been isolated from infections in various body systems, including meningitis, brain abscess, endocarditis, chest wall abscess, cervicofacial infection, peritonitis, and rectal abscess, as well as endometritis and pelvic abscess. Characteristically, infection results in sinus tract formation, fistulas, or abscesses. By the time a diagnosis is made, most patients have developed a significant abscess and are severely ill.

The most common presenting symptoms in infected women are abdominal pain, abnormal vaginal discharge, fever, and weight loss. The most frequent findings on examination are abdominal and pelvic tenderness along with a pelvic mass. Women who have *Actinomyces* infection diagnosed on Pap smear usually are completely asymptomatic and have no clinical findings on examination.

Most women who have clinical infection will be diagnosed as having pelvic inflammatory disease (PID) with or without a tubo-ovarian abscess. Patients may also present with a rectal abscess with or without peritonitis. In the five years from 1993 through 1997, 15 case reports cited pelvic abscesses with *A. israelii* as the principal isolate. Thirteen of those 15 cases were associated with the presence of an IUD. In his review of 92 cases from 63 case reports of pelvic actinomycosis resulting in pelvic abscesses and associated with IUD use, Fiorino reported the mean age of the patients to be 37 years and the mean duration of IUD use to be 8 years. The author's group obtained similar results in a prospective study of IUD users who underwent endometrial biopsy and Pap smear. This study revealed that 8% of asymptomatic IUD users had *A. israelii* in the endometrium, as confirmed by biopsy.

## Diagnosis

*Actinomyces* is most commonly recognized when a cervical cytologic specimen returns with a reading of sulfur granules consistent with *A. israelii.* This result indicates that the patient is colonized, but does not necessarily mean that she has an infection. If she also has clinical findings consistent with PID, the diagnosis must be pursued aggressively. The author's group reported seven cases of PID and concurrent isolation of *A. israelii;* in two of those patients, the organism was not apparent on Pap smear, even after a second careful evaluation.

Although culture has been considered the definitive means of diagnosis, tissue diagnosis from an endometrial biopsy, a needle biopsy, or a specimen obtained at surgery offers a better diagnostic yield. The pathology is characterized by a nonspecific acute and chronic inflammatory response consisting of polymorphonuclear leukocytes, lymphocytes, and plasma cells within which the classic "sulfur granules" (a dense, central basophilic mass of tangled filamentous rods) may be identified. An acute, purulent exudate around the organisms is necessary to indicate that it is a pathogen. Special stains such as Gomori's methenamine silver, Ziehl-Neelsen, and Gram's stains may be used to confirm the presence of the organism.

## Treatment

The most frequent question about treatment of pelvic actinomycosis centers on the issue of whether to remove or leave in situ the IUD in a woman whose Pap smear indicates the possible presence of *Actinomyces* organisms. The consensus is that removal is necessary to eradicate the bacteria. In the author's prospective study, all patients had resolution of their colonization after IUD removal. Some have questioned whether a patient for whom the IUD is the only possible method of contraception can keep the device in place and be treated with antibiotics. No controlled trials appear to address this issue. The risk is that subtle infection with *A. israelii* may occur and that the patient may not present until she is extremely ill with PID and a pelvic abscess. If the IUD is left in place, and antibiotic therapy initiated, careful follow-up is essential.

If the IUD is removed in an asymptomatic patient, she should have a follow-up Pap smear in six to eight weeks to check whether the organisms have disappeared. If they have been eliminated, the patient needs no further treatment. If the organisms persist, a pelvic ultrasound scan should be performed to rule out a pelvic abscess. A complete blood count and an erythrocyte sedimentation rate should be obtained as well. If no abscess is present, the patient may be treated with 30 days of oral penicillin, 500 mg four times daily; tetracycline HCl, 500 mg four times daily; or doxycycline, 100 mg twice daily. Amoxicillan/clavulanate, 500 mg twice daily, may also be used. If the patient has an abscess, the recommended treatment would include ampicillin or penicillin, plus an aminoglycoside and clindamycin or metronidazole in standard protocols for the treatment of a pelvic abscess. If surgery is indicated for extirpation of the abscess, antibiotics must be administered before initiating the procedure.

Surgery in a patient with actinomycosis and a pelvic abscess will almost always require removal of the uterus, tubes, and ovaries plus aggressive parenteral antibiotic therapy, because it is difficult to drain all of the abscessed tissue as well as the sinus tracts that have formed.

## SEQUELAE

The consequences of pelvic actinomycosis are those related to PID: tubal damage resulting in tubal occlusion and infertility, ectopic pregnancy, and chronic pelvic pain. When a woman develops PID and *A. israelii* is involved, one or more pelvic abscesses will likely develop with or without sinus tract formation. If allowed to go untreated for several days, the outcome can be lethal, as has been demonstrated by case reports.

Recurrence of pelvic actinomycosis has not been reported in women who had IUDs in place but had them removed when *A. israelii* was identified on a Pap smear. There are no known long-term sequelae in this group of patients.

## Suggested Readings

Cintron JR, Del Pino A, Duarte B, et al. Abdominal actinomycosis. Dis Colon Rectum 1996;39:105–108.

Fiorino AS. Intrauterine contraceptive device-associated actinomycotic abscess and *Actinomyces* detection on cervical smear. Obstet Gynecol 1996;87:142–149.

Garland SM, Rawling D. Pelvic actinomycosis in association with an intrauterine device. Aust N Z J Obstet Gynaecol 1993;33:96–98.

Hager WD, Douglas B, Majmudar B. Pelvic colonization with *Actinomyces* in women using intrauterine contraceptive devices. Am J Obstet Gynecol 1979;135:680–684.

Laurent T, de Grandi P, Schnyder P. Abdominal actinomycosis associated with intrauterine device: CT features. Eur Radiol 1996;6:670–673.

CHAPTER

# 64

# *Cystitis*

*Mark G. Martens*

## Background and Incidence

Cystitis, or lower urinary tract infection (UTI), is a common malady, estimated to occur at least once in 20% of all women in their lifetime. The incidence of bacteriuria varies between 4% and 6% in the reproductive-aged group. It increases 1% to 2% per decade of life, bringing the rate to approximately 10% by the early postmenopausal years.

## Pathophysiology

Colonization of the vaginal introitus and periurethral region by Enterobacteriaceae or gram-positive organisms from the bowel is thought to be the initial step in the pathogenesis of UTIs in women. Progression to cystitis appears to reflect the action of several factors, including intercourse, personal hygiene, and diaphragm use.

## Etiology

The most common cause of simple cystitis is *Escherichia coli* (found in 80% to 85% of cases), with other gram-negative bacteria such as *Klebsiella*, *Proteus*, *Enterobacter*, and *Pseudomonas* species also contributing. The most common gram-positive bacteria recovered are *Staphylococcus saprophyticus* (11%). *Staphylococcus epidermidis*, the enterococci, and group B ß-hemolytic streptococci are also possible pathogens.

## Diagnosis

Asymptomatic bacteriuria is defined as two consecutive urine samples of 100,000 colony-forming units (cfu) per milliliter of urine collected by the clean-catch method from a patient with no complaints. Unless the patient is pregnant and undergoes prenatal urine analysis, asymptomatic bacteriuria usually goes undetected unless she is screened for other reasons, has a voiding difficulty, or experiences suprapubic pain. Examination of the urine in an infected patient reveals evidence of pyuria and hematuria approximately 50% of the time.

Initially, UTI is diagnosed in a patient with clinical symptoms by demonstrating large numbers of bacteria and white blood cells (WBC) in the urine. The bacteria should become visible upon microscopic examination of an unspun specimen, and more than 50 WBC should be seen per high-power field in a spun specimen. Samples can then be sent for Gram staining and culture, and treatment can be initiated.

Urine containing more than $10^5$ bacteria/mL in a woman with clinical symptoms is considered to be diagnostic of cystitis. Nevertheless, 30% to 50% of women with acute lower-tract infections will harbor fewer than $10^5$ bacteria/mL. Stamm and coworkers, using suprapubic aspiration, found $10^2$ or more bacteria/mL to be the best diagnostic criterion, having a sensitivity of 95%.

## Treatment

Cost analyses have demonstrated that 90% of cystitis cases are uncomplicated and respond readily to the empiric antimicrobials chosen, without the use of a culture. Nevertheless, cultures are indicated and helpful in several circumstances:

- Complicated UTI or uncertain diagnosis
- Recent previous UTI (less than three weeks)

**Table 64-1.** Recommended Oral Medications for Cystitis

| Drug | Regimen |
|---|---|
| **First-Line Agents** | |
| Nitrofurantoin macrocrystals | 100 mg twice daily for 7 days |
| Fosfomycin tromethamine | 3 g in 4 oz water in a single dose |
| Trimethoprim/sulfamethoxazole | 80/400 mg four times daily for 7 days |
| Trimethoprim/sulfamethoxazole (double strength) | 160/800 mg twice daily for 3 to 7 days |
| Sulfamethoxasole/sulfisoxazole | 2 g initially; then 500–1,000 mg four times daily for 7 days |
| **For Resistance to First-Line Agents** | |
| Ofloxacin | 200 mg twice daily for 3 days |
| Ciprofloxacin | 100 mg twice daily for 3 days |
| Trovafloxacin | 100 mg once daily for 3 days |
| Amoxicillin/clavulanate | 250 mg three times daily for 7 days |
| Cefixime | 200 mg twice daily for 7 days |
| Cefpodoxime | 100 mg twice daily for 7 days |
| Cefuroxime | 250 mg twice daily for 7 days |

- Symptoms lasting more than seven days
- Recent catheterization
- Genitourinary surgery
- Pregnancy
- Diabetes

Gram's stain of the urine sample can help direct the choice of initial therapy. Penicillin and ampicillin, although inexpensive and effective, are not considered to be first-line UTI agents given the increasing resistance to these agents of several gram-negative organisms (particularly *E. coli*). Initial therapy can be effectively carried out with one of several relatively inexpensive oral agents, such as nitrofurantoin macrocrystals, 50 to 100 mg every 6 to 12 hours; trimethoprim/sulfamethoxazole, one to two tablets every 12 hours; or sulfamethoxazole or sulfisoxazole, 2 g initially, then 500 mg to 1 g every 6 to 8 hours (Table 64-1). These agents provide excellent activity against the most common gram-positive and gram-negative uropathogens. An agent commonly used in

Europe and now available in the United States is fosfomycin tromethamine. It is available as a single 3 g oral dose for the specific treatment of women with uncomplicated UTI.

Quinolone antibiotics (such as ciprofloxacin, ofloxacin, and trovofloxacin), the ß-lactamase-inhibiting combination of amoxicillin and clavulanate, and the extended-spectrum agents cefuroxime, cefixime, and cefpodoxime should be reserved for resistant or complicated UTI, because of their higher costs.

Approximately 20% of women treated for simple cystitis will experience a recurrence of their disease. In these cases, the newer agents can be administered if culture documents the presence of resistance to first-line agents (see Table 64-1). Three-day treatment regimens appear to be as effective as a seven-day treatment course for initial UTI. Several recent reports demonstrate that single-dose therapy can offer adequate efficacy. Given the morbidity associated with recurrences and retreatment, further evaluation of this abbreviated regimen is warranted. Individuals who remain symptomatic following treatment when the infecting organism has not been isolated by culture should be evaluated for conditions such as trichomoniasis, urethritis, and interstitial cystitis.

Reinfections usually occur more than two to three weeks after cessation of previous therapy, and in 95% of cases they reflect the presence of a different organism. In evaluating these patients, radiographic and endoscopic examinations of the urinary tract are rarely beneficial. Instead, the most significant diagnostic aids are culture of the organism and antibiotic sensitivity determinations. Strategies for managing frequent reinfections include prophylaxis, intermittent self-start therapy, and postcoital prophylaxis.

Relapse or persistence with the same pathogen occurs in approximately 5% of all cystitis cases. These episodes usually occur within one to two weeks of cessation of antimicrobial therapy and are often associated with structural abnormalities of the urinary tract. Strategies for managing relapse include radiologic and endoscopic evaluation of the urinary tract and continuation of pharmacologic therapy for two to six weeks or longer. The Food and Drug Administration has approved prophylaxis with cinoxacin, 250 mg orally daily for as long as five months; this regimen has been demonstrated to be safe and more than 90% effective in reducing frequent recurrences in both younger and perimenopausal women.

## Suggested Readings

Carey JC, Wilkerson RG. Urinary tract infections in women. In: Pastorek J, ed. Obstetric and gynecologic infectious disease. New York: Raven Press, 1994:85–88.

Martens MG, Finkelstein LH. Daily cinoxacin as prophylaxis for urinary tract infections in mature women: a prospective trial. Adv Ther 1995;12:207–211.

Stamm WE. Dysuria: establishing a diagnostic protocol. Contemp OB/GYN 1988;32(Oct):81–93.

CHAPTER

# 65

# *Acute Urethral Syndrome*

*Michael G. Gravett*

## Background

Symptoms associated with lower urinary tract infection (UTI) are among the most common reasons that young women visit a physician. In the United States, more than 5 million women seek health care for such infections annually. Although frequency and dysuria are usually attributed to cystitis, these symptoms also can be associated with urethritis or vaginitis. The term "acute urethral syndrome" has been used to refer to acute dysuria or frequency of less than two weeks' duration without significant bacteriuria (defined as $10^5$ or more bacteria/mL of urine).

Acute urethral syndrome should not be confused with the more general "urethral syndrome." The latter phrase denotes lower urinary tract symptoms that are usually of extended duration and without recognized infectious etiologies. Possible etiologies for urethral syndrome include hypoestrogenism, mechanical or functional urethral obstruction, traumatic insult, and neurologic or psychiatric disturbances.

## Pathophysiology

The urethra normally plays an important role in preventing the ascension of UTI. In addition to a midurethral high-pressure zone that acts as a mechanical barrier preventing the ascent of genital microorganisms, mucus-secreting periurethral glands in the posterior portion of the urethra may aid in trapping bacteria and secreting immunoglobulin A. Although an average of six to eight species of microorganisms can usually be recovered from the distal urethras of women, the proximal 1 cm of the urethra normally is sterile.

Acute urethral syndrome may represent the earliest stages of an ascending lower UTI after periurethral colonization by coliform bacteria or other uropathogens. This hypothesis is supported by the observation of O'Grady and coworkers, who found that more than 50% of women with the syndrome prospectively develop significant bacteriuria. The bacteria recovered from urine cultures of these women are identical with those recovered from women with acute cystitis. The reasons why periurethral colonization progresses to acute cystitis in some women remain speculative, but may reflect an arbitrary clinical distinction between the two conditions rather than true differences in pathophysiology.

Clinicians have adopted $10^5$ or more bacteria/mL of urine as the major criterion for the diagnosis of cystitis. This value is based on early work by Kass. Kass, however, used this criterion to distinguish bacteriuria in women with acute pyelonephritis from asymptomatic women or contaminated urine specimens; he did not study women with lower urinary tract symptoms only.

More recent data suggest that among women with dysuria, the demonstration of $10^2$ or more uropathogens/mL of urine is the most sensitive and specific criterion for the diagnosis of cystitis. Thus, a continuum exists for the same disease process. The condition is arbitrarily designated as cystitis when associated with $10^5$ or more bacteria/mL and as acute urethral syndrome when associated with less than $10^5$ bacteria/mL.

## Etiology

Studies using either suprapubic bladder aspiration or sterile urethral catheterization have demonstrated microorganisms from the bladder urine of many patients with acute urethral syndrome. Stamm, Wagner, and coworkers recovered uropathogens from bladder urine of 27 (46%) of 59 women, including *Escherichia coli* in 24 (41%) and *Staphylococcus saprophyticus* in 3 subjects (5%), all in concentrations of $10^4$ or less per mL. Pyuria (defined as 8 or more leukocytes/$mm^3$ of uncentrifuged midstream urine) is strongly correlated with the recovery of uropathogens from the bladder. It was found in 26 (96%) of 27 of those patients from whom a bacterial uropathogen was recovered and in only 7 (20%) of 34 asymptomatic patients.

Sexually transmitted organisms may also cause the disorder. Both *Neisseria gonorrhoeae* and *Chlamydia trachomatis* are common causes of urethritis in men, in whom infection is usually associated with frank urethral discharge. Similarly, both may cause acute urethral syndrome in females, although frank urethral discharge is infrequent in infected women.

Dysuria and frequency are commonly observed among women visiting sexually transmitted disease clinics who have genital infection with *N. gonorrhoeae* and *C. trachomatis*. Particularly intriguing is the role of *C. trachomatis*. Stamm, Counts, and coworkers found evidence of chlamydial infection in 11 of 32 women with acute urethral syndrome and sterile bladder urine. Pyuria, as previously defined, was noted in 10 of these 11 patients. The correlation between *C. trachomatis* infection and sterile pyuria is important. Among 16 patients with sterile bladder cultures and pyuria, evidence of chlamydial infection was found in 10 (62.5%) in contrast with only 1 (6%) of 16 patients with sterile cultures and no evidence of pyuria. Thus infection with *C. trachomatis* must be considered in a patient with acute urethral syndrome, sterile urine, and pyuria.

The role of other potentially pathogenic microorganisms remains controversial. Currently, insufficient evidence exists to suggest that *Lactobacillus* sp. or the genital mycoplasms, including *Mycoplasma hominis* and *Ureaplasma urealyticum*, cause acute urethral syndrome.

## DIAGNOSIS

Dysuria or frequency may be associated with acute urethral syndrome, cystitis, vaginitis, or primary herpetic genital infection. All patients should be carefully evaluated by appropriate physical examination, microscopic examination of the midstream urine, and appropriate urine, urethral, or genital cultures.

Approximately 10% of women with dysuria have vaginitis or genital herpes. Vaginitis-associated dysuria usually is described as external and is characterized as a burning sensation when urine comes into contact with the inflamed genitalia. Vaginitis or primary genital herpes can be excluded on the basis of careful physical examination and microscopic examination of vaginal discharge. The cervix also should be inspected for mucopurulent cervicitis, which may indicate the presence of chlamydial infection, and a Gram's stain from the cervix should be examined for gram-negative intracellular diplococci, which indicates a gonococcal infection. Urethral discharge expressed by gentle pressure on the urethra suggests infection with *N. gonorrhoeae* or *C. trachomatis.*

In the absence of vaginitis, carefully collected midstream or catheterized urine should be cultured for usual uropathogens and examined microscopically. Cystitis, associated with $10^5$ or more bacteria/mL of urine, occurs in approximately 50% of women with dysuria, and acute urethral syndrome affects the remaining 40% of patients.

Initially, uncentrifuged urine should be examined microscopically. When analyzing uncentrifuged urine, the presence of one bacterium per oil immersion field correlates well with the $10^5$ or more bacteria/mL criterion, allowing the diagnosis of acute cystitis to be made. The absence of bacteria in several oil immersion fields suggests a bacterial colony count of $10^4$/mL or less. Urine should also be centrifuged and the sediment examined microscopically under the high dry objective field (400×).

Pyuria, defined as 8 or more leukocytes/mm$^3$ of midstream urine, approximates to 5 to 10 leukocytes per high-dry microscopic field when 10 mL of urine has been centrifuged and the sediment resuspended in 1 mL of urine. Midstream urine should also be cultured. Patients in whom a pure culture of between $10^2$ and $10^4$ uropathogens/mL is recovered and who also have pyuria or dysuria should be considered to have acute urethral syndrome and treated as such.

If the patient has pyuria without bacteriuria and is considered to be at risk for sexually transmitted disease or if a speculum examination reveals that the patient has cervicitis, specimens should be taken from both the cervix and urethra for detection of *N. gonorrhoeae* and *C. trachomatis* by culture, DNA probe, polymerase chain reaction (PCR), or ligase chain reaction (LCR). Recently, LCR testing on first-void urine specimens has been demonstrated to offer sensitivity and specificity of more than 90% in the detection of *C. trachomatis;* this technique offers the advantage of noninvasive self-collection by the patient.

Several biochemical tests for detecting bacteriuria (nitrite tests) or pyuria (leukocyte esterase tests) may prove helpful in diagnosing cystitis. Their role in detecting acute urethral syndrome has not been established as yet, but these tests may aid in screening women with dysuria.

## Treatment

Uncomplicated cystitis may be effectively treated with a three-day regimen (trimethoprim/sulfamethoxazole, one double-strength tablet twice daily; amoxicillin/clavulanic acid, 250 mg three times daily; norfloxacin, 400 mg twice daily; or ciprofloxacin, 500 mg twice daily). Single-dose therapy is no longer recommended. Sulfonamides, ampicillin, and amoxicillin can no longer be primarily recommended for the treatment of UTI because of a high frequency of *E. coli* resistance to these agents.

These shorter therapeutic regimens offer cure rates comparable with those obtained with conventional 7- to 10-day antibiotic regimens for uncomplicated cystitis. As yet, however, clinical trials comparing three-day regimens with longer conventional therapy for acute urethral syndrome have not been reported. It is likely that women with acute urethral syndrome associated with *E. coli* or *S. saprophyticus* can be treated with these shorter regimens. Women in whom either *N. gonorrhoeae* or *C. trachomatis* infection is suspected on epidemiologic grounds or urinalysis (pyuria without bacteriuria) should be treated in accordance with current CDC guidelines.

Current therapeutic recommendations for chlamydial infections include tetracycline, 500 mg orally four times daily for seven days; doxycycline, 100 mg orally twice daily for seven days; ofloxacin, 300 mg orally twice daily for seven days; erythromycin stearate, 500 mg orally four times daily; or azithromycin, a single oral dose of 1 g. In addition, patients with suspected gonococcal infections should receive ceftriaxone, 125 mg IM; ofloxacin, 400 mg orally once; or cefixime, 400 mg orally once.

Patients with acute dysuria without bacteriuria or pyuria do not benefit from antibiotic therapy. These women may be symptomatically treated with phenazopyridine HCl and reevaluated if their symptoms persist. Women with recurrent UTIs or with chronic dysuria not associated with infection should be referred for urologic evaluation.

## Suggested Readings

Centers for Disease Control and Prevention. 1998 guidelines for treatment of sexually transmitted diseases. MMWR 1998;47 (RR-1):49–69.

Fihn SD, Stamm WE. The urethral syndrome. Semin Urol 1983; 1:121–129.

Hamilton-Miller JM. The urethral syndrome and its management. J Antimicrob Chemother 1994;33(suppl A):63–73.

Kass EH. Asymptomatic infections of the urinary tract. Trans Assoc Am Physicians 1956;69:56–63.

Latham RH, Stamm WE. Urethral syndrome in women. Urol Clin North Am 1984;11:95–101.

O'Grady FW, Richards B, McSherry MA, et al. Introital enterobacteria, urinary infection, and the urethral syndrome. Lancet 1970;2:1208–1210.

Stamm WE, Counts GW, Running KR, et al. Diagnosis of coliform infection in acutely dysuric women. N Engl J Med 1982; 307:463–468.

Stamm WE, Wagner KF, Amsel R, et al. Causes of acute urethral syndrome in women. N Engl J Med 1980;303:409–415.

Wong ES, Stamm WE. Urethral infection in men and women. Ann Rev Med 1983;34:337–358.

CHAPTER

66

# *Techniques for Isolating Pelvic Bacterial Pathogens*

*Gale B. Hill*

## Background

Knowledge of the likely etiologic agents in various female pelvic infections can guide the proper collection and transport of patient specimens for microbiologic culture and the choice of appropriate empiric therapy. This information is also helpful in anticipating patterns of antibiotic resistance.

Most obstetric and gynecologic infections, with the exception of uncomplicated endocervical gonococcal or chlamydial infection, involve anaerobic and aerobic bacteria. These mixed infections include chorioamnionitis, endometritis, postabortal sepsis, bacterial vulvovaginal infections, salpingitis, pelvic peritonitis, tubo-ovarian and pelvic abscesses, postoperative wound infections, pelvic cellulitis, and pelvic thrombophlebitis. Septicemia usually involves only one species, but also can be polymicrobic in origin.

## Source of Infections

In general, the source of mixed infections in the female pelvis is the endogenous microflora of the lower genital tract (endocervix and vagina). The external genitalia and urethra also contain a resident aerobic/anaerobic microflora. The types present in the microflora may vary considerably from one individual to another, and not all organisms have the same potential to cause infection.

In reproductive-age women, the physiologic pattern associated with normal vaginal findings consists of a predominance of aerobic lactobacilli, often with diphtheroids, coagulase-negative staphylococci, and other aerobes and anaerobes being present in lower counts. These women have a lowered risk of infection compared with women who have altered microflora.

Among women who have bacterial vaginosis, for instance, the resident flora includes high counts of potentially pathogenic microorganisms among anaerobic gram-negative rods, anaerobic gram-positive cocci, *Gardnerella vaginalis*, and genital mycoplasmas. Aerobic lactobacilli, when present, are in the minority.

Nevertheless, some women may have an altered microflora other than these two patterns. Endogenous or exogenous influences, such as antibiotics or surgery, can cause marked changes in species type and in relative concentrations of resident flora.

## Settings for Infection

Opportunistic pathogens among the endogenous flora can produce infection in tissue when local host defense mechanisms become interrupted or diminished by natural causes or medical intervention. Lowered oxygen tension and oxidation–reduction (redox) potential in tissue are critical factors permitting invasion by anaerobic organisms. Settings that predispose to infection usually involve tissue necrosis or impaired blood supply; they include trauma, surgery, malignancy, foreign bodies, vascular disease, irradiation, shock, edema, and vasoconstrictive agents. Under these circumstances, aerobes and anaerobes in the vagina and endocervix may directly invade contiguous tissue structures in the normally sterile upper genital tract or spread by hematogenous, lymphatic, or other routes.

## Etiologic Agents

Certain species of microorganisms are prevalent in female pelvic infections and are typically present in various mixtures of aerobes and anaerobes. Others are unusual or to be expected only in particular—and perhaps rare—settings.

## Aerobic

Among aerobic (including facultatively anaerobic species) gram-negative rods, *Escherichia coli* is the most common culprit found in female pelvic infections; species of *Klebsiella*, *Enterobacter*, and *Proteus* are less commonly observed. Highly antibiotic-resistant species such as *Pseudomonas* are infrequently isolated, except in occasional cancer patients.

Among the aerobic cocci, α- and nonhemolytic species of *Streptococcus* are particularly common. Group B ß-hemolytic streptococci colonize the vagina of 10% to 30% of pregnant women and represent important pathogens in upper tract gynecologic infections as well as in maternal and neonatal disease. Group A ß-hemolytic streptococci are rarely isolated and are exogenously acquired.

Enterococci are more common in postoperative infections after prophylactic use of certain antimicrobials. *Staphylococcus aureus* is infrequently isolated, except in occasional abdominal wound infections, where it likely derives from an exogenous source. It is the causative agent in toxic shock syndrome, which, although rare, is a risk for the low percentage of women who carry the organism vaginally. *Gardnerella vaginalis* (previously called *Haemophilus vaginalis*) is common in the genital microflora of sexually active women and can be isolated from upper genital tract infections.

## Anaerobic

Among the anaerobic gram-negative rods, species of *Prevotella* and *Porphyromonas* (genera that were previously included in *Bacteroides*)—especially *Prevotella bivia*, *Prevotella disiens*, and black-pigmenting species—are most frequently isolated. The *Bacteroides fragilis* group is occasionally etiologic.

Among the anaerobic gram-positive cocci, *Peptostreptococcus anaerobius*, *Peptostreptococcus asaccharolyticus*,

*Peptostreptococcus magnus*, *Peptostreptococcus prevotii*, and *Peptostreptococcus tetradius* are the most common species in pelvic infections. *Actinomyces* species and *Eubacterium nodatum* are both gram-positive rods that are isolated usually only when a foreign body—particularly an IUD—is present.

*Clostridium perfringens* is common in the gastrointestinal tract and ubiquitous in the environment. The significance of its presumptive detection or actual isolation from a pelvic source must be carefully but speedily weighed in the context of the clinical setting. Careful evaluation of the patient's condition can help to distinguish cellulitis or myonecrosis from simple wound contamination.

### Other Organisms

Some types of bacteria mentioned earlier are the usual agents in conditions such as postoperative infectious complications and endometritis. The etiology of salpingitis, in particular, is more complex. Sexually transmissible agents such as *Neisseria gonorrhoeae* and *Chlamydia trachomatis* may be present with or without the endogenous organisms already discussed (see Chapters 11, 12, 13, 43, 44, and 45). Genital mycoplasmas also are correlated with sexual activity, yet are so commonly present in women that they conveniently can be considered part of the mixed endogenous microflora. *Mycoplasma hominis* and *Ureaplasma urealyticum* are etiologic in perhaps 5% to 10% of cases of salpingitis and may be present in other settings, such as intra-amniotic infection, postpartum endometritis, and bacteremia (see Chapters 2, 7, and 79).

## Collecting Specimens for Culture

Gleaning useful information from microbial culture initially depends upon careful site preparation and collection of an appropriate specimen, followed by protected and timely transport of the specimen to the laboratory. Whenever feasible, procure specimens for microbiologic culture before initiating antimicrobial therapy.

Avoid contaminating specimens with the anaerobic and aerobic endogenous flora of the endocervix and vagina. Certain members of the lower genital tract flora may cause the upper genital tract infection, but the *infected site* alone must be sampled to identify the specific etiologic agent or agents and avoid contamination of the specimen with extraneous microorganisms. Otherwise, culture reports will be impossible to interpret and may be misleading. As a result, the vagina and endocervix would not be acceptable sites for unrestricted culture of aerobes and anaerobes. Culture should be limited to seeking specific infectious agents, such as gonococci or chlamydiae from the cervix, in appropriate clinical settings. With some specific exceptions, then, appropriate specimens for culture generally are taken from normally sterile body sites.

Communicate with laboratory personnel before you collect specimens and culture for unusual organisms. Also, not all laboratories have the facilities or trained personnel to perform all types of culture, such as those for mycoplasmas, *C. trachomatis*, and occasionally anaerobes.

## Specimen Types

The most productive types of specimens for microbiologic culture and diagnosis are tissue samples and aspirated fluid. Samples collected on swabs are less desirable for three reasons:

1. Often they do not provide sufficient material for inoculation of cultures for all likely etiologic agents.
2. They may promote loss of viability of microorganisms prior to culture because of drying and exposure of anaerobes to the toxic effects of oxygen.
3. They are prone to contamination by extraneous bacteria if the infected site is near normally colonized sites in the vagina and endocervix or on the skin.

You can avoid many of these problems by using a swab transport device that provides for a moist, anaerobic environment in transit to the laboratory and by ensuring that the swab is well saturated with infected material. Extraneous contamination generally does not pose a problem with swabs collected in an operating room setting; in this instance, however, the more appropriate tissue or aspirated sample usually should be available. The advancing edge of a soft-tissue infection and the wall of an abscess are examples of tissue samples. Aspirated specimens can be obtained if a collection of fluid or loculation is present; otherwise, it may be necessary to inject a small volume of sterile, nonbacteriostatic saline to aspirate fluid back from infected tissue. Obtain 1 to 3 mL of aspirated fluid, if available.

The remainder of this section describes guidelines for collection of specimens from particular sources.

### *Body Fluids*

Collect body fluids by aspiration whenever possible. Amniotic fluid can be collected by transabdominal amniocentesis, by aspiration at the time of cesarean section, by needle amniotomy of intact membranes after povidone-iodine disinfection, or through a pressure catheter (discard the first 5 to 7 mL drawn) as clinically appropriate. Specimens obtained through a pressure catheter should be cultured and screened only for unusual or predominant organisms or for specific agents such as group B ß-hemolytic streptococci, because the insertion of the catheter will introduce microorganisms from the lower genital tract into the amniotic sac.

### *Blood Culture*

Carefully prepare the venipuncture site with antiseptic to prevent skin organisms from contaminating the culture. Collect at least two blood cultures, preferably at least one hour apart, in the setting of pelvic infection and clinical signs of possible septicemia. The yield with this technique is higher for intra- and postpartum infections and septic abortion than for salpingitis.

### *Decidua, Membranes, or Placenta*

These tissues may be cultured directly at the time of cesarean section. After vaginal delivery, the surface of the placenta should be decontaminated and a wedge of tissue procured. For chorioamnionic membranes, take a sample from between the placental amnion and chorion after peeling membranes apart 4 cm or more back from the torn membrane edge. Avoid the contaminated outer membrane surfaces.

### *Endometrial Culture*

Sample the decidua beyond the endocervix after first cleansing the cervical area. Protected (double- or triple-lumen) endometrial collection devices are highly desirable to prevent contamination by vaginal or cervical secretions. Protected devices designed for aspirating, brushing, or swabbing the endometrium can be prepared in-house or obtained commercially. The Endometrial Pipelle suction curette (Unimar, Inc., Wilton, Connecticut) provides for more specimen volume (tissue and fluid) and offers greater protection against contamination than is obtainable with an unprotected swab. A brush sampling device sheathed within a plastic cannula is available as well (Uterine Sampling Device; Medi-Tech, Watertown, Massachusetts).

### *Culdocentesis*

For aspiration, cleanse the vaginal wall with antiseptic, leaving it in contact for 1 minute. Wipe the area with a sterile gauze pad before inserting the needle. Be careful that aspiration occurs only in the cul-de-sac and not in the vagina (or bowel).

### *Abscesses*

Where applicable, decontaminate unbroken skin or mucosal surface and aspirate pus with a needle and syringe. In an operaing room setting, obtain abscess wall tissue as well as fluid content.

### *Wound Cultures*

Collect the specimen by deep aspiration or tissue biopsy. As appropriate, first cleanse contaminated and exposed surfaces at the collection site with povidone-iodine and then dry the area. Swabs are not preferred because of contamination by extraneous surface microorganisms. If used, the swab must be carefully collected from *deep* within the wound after decontamination of the wound surface.

### *Vaginal Cuff Infection*

If a loculation is present, aspirate it directly after decontamination of the mucosal surface. Otherwise, it may prove difficult to avoid vaginal secretions when procuring drainage from the peritoneal cavity through an opening in the cuff. Because of the probability of vaginal contamination, this type of specimen should be considered only in instances where empiric therapy proved unsuccessful, and the culture should be screened only for an unusual or predominant organism (suggestive only).

## SPECIMEN TRANSPORT

Deliver specimens for culture to the laboratory as soon as possible to avoid degradation of the sample and loss of viability of pathogens. Over time, important pathogens may be overgrown by other organisms with a shorter replication cycle. In polymicrobic infections, the presence of nutritive material and delay in transit may so dramatically alter the proportions of species that the resultant culture will not reflect the actual individual concentrations of species at the infected site. Special transport formulations are available that preserve the viability of microorganisms and do not promote indiscriminant growth. Some are designed to select for survival or enhancement of only particular species.

In general, all specimens from infections located in normally sterile sites should be cultured at least for aerobic and anaerobic bacteria. Transport the specimens in an anaerobic transport device to preserve the viability of any anaerobic bacteria. Aerobic bacteria also survive well in anaerobic devices, and their numbers are somewhat more stabilized through this method than in aerobic transport. Use transport methods and devices designed especially for sexually transmitted organisms whenever these additional specimens are collected.

The remainder of this section describes selected special transport methods.

### *Anaerobic Transport*

Special tubes and vials containing oxygen-free gases should be used for transport of anaerobic organisms to prevent their exposure to oxygen and drying. Transport these devices at room temperature to arrive in the laboratory optimally within 30 minutes. In an anaerobic environment, microbial populations generally will remain nearly stable for 12 hours, and most microbes will survive for a longer period. Some examples of anaerobic transport devices include the following:

- Port-A-Cul vials (Becton Dickinson Microbiology Systems, Sparks, Maryland): Can be used for liquid specimens (body fluids or aspirated pus).
- Port-A-Cul tube (Becton Dickinson Microbiology Systems, Sparks, Maryland): Contains reduced transport media to receive a swab specimen.
- Vacutainer Anaerobic Specimen Collector (Becton Dickinson Microbiology Systems, Sparks, Maryland): Can be used for swab, liquid, or small pieces of tissue. A catalyst system removes oxygen.
- ACT I (Remel, Lenexa, Kansas): Can be used for liquid specimens.
- Anaerobic Transport Medium (Anaerobe Systems, San Jose, California): Can be used for liquid, tissue, or swab. *Caution*: If the top is removed, oxygen enters system.

### *Mycoplasmal Transport*

The genital mycoplasmas are seldom isolated in pure culture and are easily overgrown by competing microbes. Nevertheless, these organisms can be cultured from specimens delivered for aerobic/anaerobic culture in an anaerobic transport device if a sufficent sample is available and culture takes place within two to three hours. The special mycoplasmal transport broth contains antibiotics and therefore cannot be used for any other type of culture. Rapid delivery to the laboratory is best. If a delay occurs, however, the specimen can be maintained on wet ice for several hours. A3B Mycoplasmal Transport Broth (Remel, Lenexa, Kansas) is an example of this type of transport device.

## Laboratory Request Slip

On the laboratory requisition, provide at a minimum the specific collection site, the collection method, the time and date of collection, any antimicrobial therapy given, the clinical diagnosis, and the name of the physician to be consulted and to receive the report. If a specific organism is being sought (for example, *Actinomyces* in the presence of an IUD or *Listeria* in an appropriate perinatal setting), specifically note this requirement on the slip to alert the laboratory to employ appropriate culture techniques.

### Suggested Readings

Eschenbach DA. Bacterial vaginosis and anaerobes in obstetric-gynecologic infection. Clin Infect Dis 1993;16(suppl 4):S282–S287.

Hill GB. The microbiology of bacterial vaginosis. Am J Obstet Gynecol 1993;169(2 Pt 2):450–454.

Hillier SL, Krohn MA, Cassen E, et al. The role of bacterial vaginosis and vaginal bacteria in amniotic fluid infection in women in preterm labor with intact fetal membranes. Clin Infect Dis 1995;20(suppl 2):S276–S278.

Knuppel RA, Scerbo JC, Mitchell GW Jr, et al. Quantitative transcervical uterine culture with a new device. Obstet Gynecol 1981;57:243–248.

Martens MG, Faro S, Hammill HA, et al. Transcervical uterine cultures with a new endometrial suction curette: a comparison of three sampling methods in postpartum endometritis. Obstet Gynecol 1989;74:273–276.

Murray PR, Baron EJ, Pfaller MA, et al, eds. Manual of clinical microbiology. Washington, DC: ASM Press, 1995.

CHAPTER

# 67

# *Evaluation of the Infected Postoperative Patient*

*Joseph G. Pastorek II*
*Sebastian Faro*

## Background

The typical patient who receives care from an obstetrician-gynecologist is, as a rule, younger and healthier than the usual medical or general surgical patient. For this reason, infection-related mortality remains rare in ob-gyn practice. Nevertheless, infectious complications of such procedures as cesarean section and hysterectomy may prolong hospital stay, increase medical expense, and extend recovery time. As a result, the physician assessing the condition of a woman with suspected postoperative infection must be methodical and thorough to assure prompt and accurate diagnosis leading to the administration of appropriate and timely therapy.

## Patient Evaluation

Because most postoperative ob-gyn patients have a rather straightforward, obvious history—pregnancy, labor, cesarean section, fever—you must take care not to overlook important factors in these women's medical background. Illnesses such as viral infection, postpartal lupus flare, and drug fever, whose symptoms mimic postoperative infection, may mislead you.

The physical examination is paramount in evaluating the postsurgical ob-gyn patient. It is important not to concentrate exclusively on the abdomen and pelvis or to assume that the infection is always directly related to a surgical site such as the uterus or vaginal cuff. Although this relationship usually holds true, extrapelvic sources of postoperative symptoms also exist. A systemic head-to-toe survey is therefore necessary to exclude such entities as pneumonia, coincidental cold or flu, hepatitis (perhaps caused or aggravated by anesthetic agents), urinary tract infection, pyelonephritis, and puerperal mastitis.

Most sources of postoperative ob-gyn infection will lie in the pelvis, especially at the operative site. Therefore, the pelvic exam and the abdominal wound exam represent the most fruitful areas for investigation. When you suspect infection, follow a standard method for evaluating the abdomen and pelvis. Assess, by auscultation and then palpation, the entire abdomen, including the flanks and hypochondria. Look for and define tenderness, rebound tenderness, organomegaly, and abnormal masses or fluid collections. Investigate the abdominal wound, if present, for general appearance and texture, including the classic signs of rubor, dolor, calor, and abnormal drainage. Manually express or aspirate by needle any apparent abnormal fluid collections as you search for seroma, hematoma, or abscess.

In cases of puerperal fever, examine the uterine fundus for evidence of endomyometritis. Because the uterus projects out of the pelvis nearly to the level of the umbilicus, this step is easily accomplished after vaginal delivery in most cases. The fundus will be easy to palpate through the lax and attenuated abdominal wall. The inexperienced examiner, however, may experience some difficulty in distinguishing normal postoperative incisional pain from that due to infection. The experienced physician will palpate the fundus of the uterus from above the umbilicus, pressing in an inferior direction, while staying well above the most cephalad point of the usual lower abdominal incision. The adnexa of a woman who has had a bilateral tubal ligation after delivery may generate tenderness that may be mistaken for adnexitis.

After examining the abdomen, incision, and uterine fundus, perform a pelvic examination. To carry it out appropriately, arrange the patient optimally. A suitable pelvic examination table is a must. Insert the speculum, note the quantity and quality of the vaginal discharge or lochia, and check the amount of blood or pus contained therein. Inspect the vaginal barrel for evidence of inflammation, especially in proximity to vaginal lacerations or suture lines.

For patients with puerperal infection, especially those who have undergone cesarean section before ample cervical dilatation, gently dilate the cervix (for example, with a ringed forceps) to allow any "lochial block" to drain. In patients who have received a hysterectomy, visualize the vaginal cuff incision and pay special attention to any erythema, purulent discharge, or other signs of infection. Follow the speculum examination with a bimanual examination. When inserting the examining fingers, you may detect increased vaginal temperature in the patient with true pelvic infection. With this hand, palpate for abnormal fluid collections along the vagina, in the fornices, and even into the ischiorectal fossae. After hysterectomy, you may note induration and tenderness of the vaginal cuff incision, as well as fluctuance indicative of abscess or hematoma. Use the abdominal hand to delineate any unusual masses or loculations, as well as tenderness.

## Laboratory Evaluation

After the physical examination, perform a complete blood count and white blood cell differential, as well as general chemistry profile and urinalysis. Radiologic techniques are generally unnecessary if the pelvic examination is complete. In some cases of suspected pelvic infection—in particular, cases of salpingitis—ultrasonography or CT scanning may prove helpful. In general, reserve the more elaborate imaging techniques for especially difficult or unusual cases, or for patients who need preoperative evaluation before undergoing surgery for suspected abscess.

In any case of suspected infection, perform cultures of possible infected sites (see Chapter 66). Generally, in the patient who has moderate infection, you should perform blood, catheterized urine, and operative site cultures. Blood cultures are positive in only 5% to 10% of such patients, but the organisms found in the blood are frequently pathogens.

Controversy continues to swirl about the value of culturing specimens from the endometrium or vaginal cuff. The chance of vaginal contamination is high. The prudent course, however, calls for some type of genital culture, because the antibiotic sensitivity data generated can be used retrospectively. Although these genital cultures may not directly aid in treating a particular patient, knowledge of local bacterial isolation rates and antibiotic sensitivities may guide you in future choices of antibiotic therapy.

When taking cultures from sites of possible infection, be aware that most cases will yield a polymicrobial flora. You should therefore collect and transport specimens in media or tubes appropriate for both anaerobic and aerobic microorganisms. This recommendation applies whether the specimen comes from the vaginal cuff after hysterectomy, the endometrial cavity after parturition, or an abscessed wound. If fastidious organisms such as *Neisseria gonorrhoeae* are suspected, make sure that appropriate transport or culture media are available.

Collect the materials for bacterial processing before initiating antibiotic therapy. Specimens taken after the patient has received several doses of medication waste both time and money.

## Summary

Infection may manifest itself in the postoperative patient in a number of ways: unusual pain, leukocytosis, and loss of function (for example, paralytic ileus). The most common apparent indication of an infectious process is an elevated temperature, with an oral temperature of 38.0 °C (100.4 °F) or higher on two occasions, excluding the first 24 hours, or 38.3 °C (101.0 °F) or higher anytime. Not all febrile morbidity is infectious morbidity, however. It is incumbent upon the physician to evaluate every febrile postoperative patient and determine the most likely diagnosis. Only then can appropriate therapy be instituted to provide for the patient's ultimate cure, whether that therapy includes antibiotics or not.

## Suggested Readings

Cox SM, Gilstrap LC. Postpartum endometritis. Obstet Gynecol Clin North Am 1989;16:363–371.

Hemsell DL. Infections after gynecologic surgery. Obstet Gynecol Clin North Am 1989;16:381–400.

Hemsell DL, Nobles B, Heard MC. Recognition and treatment of post-hysterectomy pelvic infection. Infect Surg 1988;7:47.

Pastorek JG, Miller JM. Post-cesarean section infection. Infect Surg 1987;6:532.

CHAPTER
# 68

# *Prophylactic Antibiotics*

*William L. Ledger*

## Background and Pathophysiology

The pathophysiology of soft-tissue infection that occurs after obstetric and gynecologic operations is well known. These postoperative infections are caused by the overgrowth of the diverse bacterial flora of the genital tract. In the postoperative environment, bacteria invade tissue damaged by clamps and the emplacement of foreign body sutures in the wound. The response in the human to these multiple bacterial invaders mimics that reported by Bartlett and coworkers in the animal model of a mixed bacterial intraperitoneal infection.

In the animal, an early-onset phase of infection may be associated with bacteremia. In humans, a parallel phase occurs in women who develop endomyometritis and associated bacteremia after an emergency cesarean section. After hysterectomy, a vaginal cuff infection or a pelvic cellulitis can be seen early in the postoperative course.

In the human, as in the animal model, a late-onset phase of infection occurs in which abscesses form and anaerobic bacteria seem to be the dominant bacterial pathogens. An example is the formation of microabscesses in the uterus after cesarean section. The best parallel with the animal model, however, is adnexal abscess following vaginal hysterectomy. This serious problem arises late in the clinical course.

Fortunately, the frequency of these early and late events can be reduced by the use of prophylactic antibiotics. Prevention of postoperative-site infections via antibiotic administration is based on well-established scientific principles. When

Burke evaluated the role of systemic antibiotics in preventing local infections caused by bacteria, he found a measurable response after 24 hours to the injection of live and killed staphylococci at a skin site in animals. If he used IV penicillin effective against this strain of staphylococci, the timing of the antibiotic administration was important in determining response. If penicillin was given before or at the time of the injection of the bacteria, it effectively decreased the extent of the host response (that is, it reduced the area of induration). If penicillin administration was delayed three hours or more after the injection of bacteria, it was ineffective (that is, the area of induration was the same as when no antibiotics were given).

That critical timing has been the underlying principle of all successful studies of antibiotic prophylaxis in obstetric and gynecologic operations. Improved postoperative results with prophylactic antibiotics all have involved administration of these agents at the time of operation.

## Guidelines

The following eight principles can be applied to the use of prophylactic antibiotics in obstetric–gynecologic operations. If they fit a particular operation, a good case can be made for their use in that instance.

1. *Postoperative infections at the operative site create either short-term or long-term problems.* The important aspect of this guideline is the focus on operative-site infection. For the obstetrician–gynecologist, this criterion means postoperative infections such as vaginal cuff infection, pelvic cellulitis, adnexal abscess, abdominal wound infection following hysterectomy, or endomyometritis following cesarean section. If the postoperative infection centers on an organ system distant from the operative site (for example, lungs in a postoperative pneumonia), prophylactic antibiotics will not resolve the problem.

The significant risk in this guideline includes the frequency and severity of the infection at the operative site. Infections often follow hysterectomy and cesarean section, and they can have serious consequences. This type of infection is an important clinical problem for obstetrician–gynecologists. In contrast, infections after pregnancy termination and reconstructive tubal surgery are much less common. Even with these conditions, however, the outcome can be serious for the occasional patient who becomes infected, because the tubal damage can prevent future pregnancies.

2. *The operation should be associated with endogenous bacterial contamination.* One reality of any operation for an obstetrician–gynecologist is contamination of the operative field by the endogenous bacteria of the vagina and endocervix. These organisms may also cause bacterial contamination in vaginal hysterectomy, pregnancy termination, and cesarean section in the patient in labor.

Some novel ways to reduce this contamination have included hot conization of the cervix just before hysterectomy and antibiotic lavage of the uterine wound at the time of cesarean section. In Europe, lavage of the vagina of patients in labor with an antibacterial solution has been used to reduce the risk of newborn infection by group B streptococci (GBS).

Recent studies by a number of investigators have demonstrated the presence of *Chlamydia trachomatis* in the pelvic tissue of women with no gross evidence of inflammation. In addition, bacteria have been recovered from the lymph nodes of patients with a pelvic malignancy undergoing operation. Clearly, the potential for endogenous bacterial soiling exists in most obstetric–gynecologic operations. Careful prehysterectomy preparation of the vagina with an antiseptic solution can reduce the number of surface organisms, but it does not eliminate the problem. Bacteria can be recovered from the surface of the vagina at the end of the operation.

3. *The prophylactic antibiotic should have laboratory evidence of effectiveness against some of the contaminating microorganisms.* This guideline is the most controversial of all the recommendations. The controversy relates to the general success of prophylactic antibiotics in the most widely studied operations: cesarean section and vaginal hysterectomy.

**Table 68-1.** Results with Antibiotic Prophylaxis

| Operation | Outcome |
|---|---|
| Vaginal hysterectomy | Unequivocal |
| Cesarean section; patient in labor | Unequivocal |
| Radical hysterectomy | Unequivocal |
| Pregnancy termination | Unequivocal |
| Cesarean section; patient not in labor | Mixed results |
| Abdominal hysterectomy | Mixed results; the majority are successful |

Prophylactic antibiotics work, regardless of whether penicillin, tetracycline, a cephalosporin, or metronidazole is used. This seeming lack of difference, however, may reflect problems with study design in the evaluations reported to date.

Serious infections, such as postoperative adnexal abscesses, occur infrequently, and the small numbers of patients in many studies do not permit discrimination of differences in infrequently seen complications (a statistical problem of type II error). Thus far, all reports of postoperative adnexal abscesses after vaginal hysterectomy have dealt with occurrences in patients who received prophylactic antibiotics that showed little activity against gram-negative anaerobic bacteria. Similar concerns have been raised about the choice of antibiotics for prophylaxis in cesarean section. Antibiotics with gram-negative anaerobic activity have produced the best results. For pregnancy termination and reconstructive tubal surgery, the clinical concern is *C. trachomatis;* the best antibiotic to prevent infection with this organism is tetracycline. Although a wide range of possibilities exists, a preferred list of antibiotics for prophylaxis can be constructed for each operative procedure.

4. *There should be clinical evidence of effectiveness.* This recommendation is the most important guideline. Unless prophylactic antibiotics prevent postoperative infection, their use is unjustified. Table 68-1 lists the operative procedures in which prophylactic antibiotics are used. Reports give a wide variety of responses:

- Unequivocal success in operations with high rates of postoperative infection, such as vaginal hysterectomy, cesarean section for the patient in labor, and radical hysterectomy for genital malignancy
- General success in pregnancy termination, which has a much lower rate of infection
- Mixed results for elective cesarean section and abdominal hysterectomy

No study has shown an increase in the infection rate when patients receive prophylactic antibiotics. On the other hand, some studies have shown no benefit at all from the administration of these drugs.

5. *The prophylactic antibiotic should be present in the wound at some time during the operation.* The timing of administration of prophylactic antibiotics is crucial for success. For most operations, the antibiotic should be administered just before the operation begins so that it will be present in tissue as pedicles are clamped, cut, and ligated with a foreign body suture. If the operation lasts more than three hours and the patient has received a prophylactic antibiotic with a short half-life, then a second dose should be given intraoperatively. Antibiotics with a short half-life include ampicillin and cefoxitin. Agents with a long half-life include cefazolin, cefoperazone, tetracycline, doxycycline, and metronidazole.

A different clinical consideration exists with cesarean section. To avoid administering antibiotics to the baby, which could mask early signs of neonatal sepsis, the agents should be given only after the cord is clamped.

6. *A short course of antibiotic prophylaxis should be used.* This guideline attempts to provide for the rational use of prophylactic antibiotics. A short course has been shown to be just as effective as prolonged administration of antibiotics in vaginal hysterectomy and cesarean section. It reduces the risk that the patient will have an adverse reaction and lessens the risk of colonization with resistant organisms. If the patient becomes febrile after receiving prophylactic antibiotics, a different antibiotic should be used for treatment

because the failure might reflect the presence of resistant organisms.

With added knowledge, individual modifications may be necessary for a short-course strategy. It seems clear that a single dose of antibiotics is not always effective in the woman undergoing pregnancy termination who has been infected with *C. trachomatis*. To date, the most widely used protocol has called for screening for this organism and then treatment of women found to be colonized with effective antibiotics for 10 to 14 days. Alternatively, a drug that persists in tissue levels for longer periods, such as azithromycin, can be used, although the effectiveness of this strategy has not been studied.

An underlying concern with the widespread use of prophylactic antibiotics is that such strategies could lead to the appearance of resistant organisms. This concern has arisen, for example, with the new CDC guidelines for the prevention of perinatal GBS infection (see Chapter 5). Implementation of these guidelines will markedly increase the use of penicillin in preterm and term patients in labor. Past reports suggest that it often takes years of such use before resistant organisms are encountered on services. Careful microbiologic surveillance of obstetric and newborn services will be necessary because of these new guidelines.

7. *First-line antibiotics should be used for prophylaxis.* A number of studies have shown that antibiotics with gram-negative anaerobic bacterial coverage provide superior results in vaginal hysterectomy and the patient in labor undergoing cesarean section. In contrast, for the patient undergoing pregnancy termination or tubal reconstructive surgery, tetracycline should be employed to cover *C. trachomatis* for a protracted period of time in culture-positive patients. This serious pathogen can cause irreversible tubal damage even when the patient experiences only minimal symptoms.

8. *The benefits of antibiotic prophylaxis should outweigh the risks.* Prophylactic antibiotics are clearly indicated for vaginal hysterectomy, cesarean section in the patient in labor, radical hysterectomy, and pregnancy termination. On occasion, they may be employed for patients requiring abdominal hysterectomy and tubal reconstructive surgery. For the patient

undergoing elective cesarean section, more study is needed to confirm their appropriateness.

## Antibiotic Selection

Antiobiotic prophylaxis has clearly reduced the frequency and severity of postoperative infections. For vaginal hysterectomy, the author favors the use of cefoxitin, cefotetan, or metronidazole. In cesarean section, good results are achieved with cefoxitin, cefotetan, or mezlocillin. For radical hysterectomy, cefoxitin, cefotetan, mezlocillin, or metronidazole is helpful. For pregnancy termination and reconstructive tubal surgery, doxycycline should be administered because of its effectiveness against *C. trachomatis*. For elective cesarean section and abdominal hysterectomy, a first-generation cephalosporin such as cefazolin will probably suffice.

### Suggested Readings

Ledger WJ, Campbell C, Taylor D, et al. Adnexal abscess as late complication of pelvic operations. Surg Gynecol Obstet 1969;129: 973–978.

Levin DK, Gorschels C, Andersen R. Reduction of post-cesarean section infectious morbidity by means of antibiotic irrigation. Am J Obstet Gynecol 1983;147:273–277.

Livengood CH III, Addison WA. Adnexal abscess as a delayed complication of vaginal hysterectomy. Am J Obstet Gynecol 1982; 143:596–597.

Osborne NG, Wright RC, Dubay M. Preoperative hot conization of the cervix: a possible method to reduce postoperative febrile morbidity following vaginal hysterectomy. Am J Obstet Gynecol 1979;133:374–378.

Price DJ, Sleigh JD. Control of infection due to *Klebsiella aerogenes* in neurosurgical unit by withdrawal of all antibiotics. Lancet 1970;2:1213–1215.

CHAPTER

# 69

# *Prophylactic Antibiotics for Hysterectomy*

*Patrick Duff*

## Background and Incidence

Each year approximately 600,000 to 800,000 hysterectomies are performed in the United States. Two-thirds of these procedures are performed abdominally. Infection is the most common complication associated with hysterectomy. Because the frequency of infection after hysterectomy is relatively high, pelvic surgeons have evinced great interest in antibiotic prophylaxis. This chapter reviews the frequency and pathophysiology of postoperative infection and then evaluates the results of several clinical trials that investigated the use of prophylactic antibiotics in women undergoing vaginal and abdominal hysterectomy.

## Etiology

The principal microorganisms responsible for posthysterectomy infections are aerobic streptococci, mainly groups B and D; anaerobic gram-positive cocci; aerobic gram-negative bacilli, most notably *Escherichia coli*; and *Bacteroides* and *Prevotella* species. Although *Neisseria gonorrhoeae* and *Chlamydia trachomatis* are important factors in the pathogenesis of acute salpingitis, they are not commonly isolated from women with immediate postoperative infections. Likewise, the genital mycoplasmas do not appear to act as major pathogens in this clinical setting. Infection with particularly virulent aerobic gram-negative bacilli, such as *Pseudomonas*, *Enterobacter*, and *Serratia*, is distinctly uncommon except in immunocompromised patients.

## Pathophysiology

All of the organisms listed in the previous section can be normal inhabitants of the genital tract flora. During pelvic surgery, they may be introduced into the upper genital tract and, often, the bloodstream. Particularly high inoculation of bacteria takes place in women undergoing vaginal hysterectomy, because the entire procedure is performed through a contaminated surgical field. Other infection risk factors after both vaginal and abdominal operations include low socioeconomic status, premenopausal age, extended duration of surgery, excessive intraoperative blood loss, preoperative anemia, and concurrent debilitating systemic disease.

## Mechanism of Action

Before prophylactic antibiotics are routinely prescribed for pelvic surgery, three conditions must be met:

1. The operation must be performed through a contaminated surgical field.
2. In the absence of prophylaxis, the incidence of operative-site infection should be high.
3. It should be possible for serious sequelae, including bacteremia, septic shock, septic pelvic vein thrombophlebitis, and pelvic abscess, to develop from the primary infection.

These conditions are met in all patients having vaginal hysterectomy and in most patients having abdominal hysterectomy.

Prophylactic antibiotics exert their effect through four basic mechanisms. First, and of greatest importance, is their ability to reduce the size of the bacterial inoculum introduced into the pelvic cavity. Second, antibiotics alter the culture medium at the surgical site to prevent the growth of pathogenic bacteria. Third, they penetrate the genital tract's epithelial tissue and render it less susceptible to invasion by bacteria. Fourth, prophylactic antibiotics become concentrated in macrophages and polymorphonuclear leukocytes, thereby enhancing phagocytosis of microorganisms.

## Objectives

Four objectives apply when using prophylactic antibiotics for hysterectomy. First, the goal is to reduce the frequency of pelvic cellulitis, the most common posthysterectomy infection and the one that predisposes the patient to more serious sequelae. Patients who develop cellulitis usually have to spend one to two more days in the hospital than uninfected women. Second, this tactic is employed to prevent wound infection, which predisposes patients to such serious complications as dehiscence and evisceration and is likely to prolong hospitalization. Third, the aim is to decrease the use of more expensive therapeutic antibiotics. Fourth, an objective is to decrease the overall duration and expense of hospitalization, an endpoint that has become of increasing importance in the era of managed care, especially in health care systems that use capitated payments.

## Results of Clinical Trials

Clinical trials of prophylactic antibiotics for vaginal hysterectomy show that women who received these agents had significantly less pelvic cellulitis. This benefit is independent of the patient's age, menopausal status, phase of menstrual cycle, or requirement for concurrent adnexal, bladder, or rectal surgery. Also, single doses of antibiotics appear to be as effective as two- and three-dose regimens. In addition, limited-spectrum agents, such as cefazolin or ampicillin, are as effective for prophylaxis as are the more expensive, extended-spectrum cephalosporins or penicillins.

Individual trials of prophylaxis for abdominal hysterectomy have yielded less consistent results. Many trials have not documented a statistically significant decrease in the frequency of pelvic cellulitis in patients who received antibiotics. In most instances, this effect occurred because the baseline frequency of infection is lower after abdominal hysterectomy than after vaginal procedures. Most investigations, therefore, included an inadequate number of patients to enable researchers to detect a small difference in treatment effect.

In a recent meta-analysis, Mittendorf and coworkers did document a significant protective effect of antibiotic prophylaxis. Overall, in their combined trials, 21% of patients who did not receive prophylactic antibiotics developed serious infections, whereas only 9% of patients who received antibiotics developed such infections ($P = 0.00001$). In this analysis, "serious infections" included wound infection, pelvic or vaginal cuff cellulitis, pelvic abscess, postoperative pelvic inflammatory disease (PID), and bacteremia.

In individual studies that documented a beneficial effect of prophylaxis in patients undergoing abdominal hysterectomy, no advantage arose from using the more expensive, broader-spectrum cephalosporins and penicillins. Similarly, using more than two doses of antibiotic for prophylaxis did not confer any therapeutic advantage.

## Complications

One major complication that can develop from the administration of prophylactic antibiotics relates to adverse drug reactions. Isolated case reports reveal intraoperative deaths resulting from anaphylactic reactions to cephalosporins administered for prophylaxis. Although these fatal events have not been described in obstetric or gynecologic patients, you should nevertheless exercise extreme care by eliciting a history of drug allergy in any patient scheduled to receive prophylaxis.

Well-documented cases describe women who developed drug-induced diarrhea, and even pseudomembranous enterocolitis, after receiving prophylactic antibiotics for pelvic surgery. This problem seems particularly likely to occur when the patient receives multiple doses of extended-spectrum agents, but it can also arise with single-dose prophylaxis.

Another possible major complication with prophylactic antibiotics is alteration in the microbial flora of the genital tract. Although the specific alterations depend on which antibiotic is used, a consistent finding has been increased isolation of enterococci in women who received cephalosporins. Fortunately, no evidence suggests that patients who become infected despite prophylaxis will develop more severe infections or respond less readily to conventional treatment regimens.

## Guidelines

The following guidelines should be considered when prescribing prophylactic antibiotics:

1. Routine use of prophylactic antibiotics appears to be justified in all women undergoing vaginal and abdominal hysterectomy.
2. The most cost-effective antibiotics for prophylaxis are inexpensive, limited-spectrum agents, such as cefazolin (1 g) or ampicillin (2 g). In patients who have an immediate hypersensitivity reaction to ß-lactam antibiotics, doxycycline (100 mg), or trovafloxacin (200 mg) represents an acceptable alternative.
3. For most procedures, a single dose of antibiotic is enough for prophylaxis. This dose should be administered parenterally just prior to the start of surgery. When surgery is extended (that is, lasts for two or more hours), give a second dose four to six hours after the initial one.
4. A gynecologic service using prophylaxis must maintain surveillance to monitor for the emergence of drug-resistant microorganisms and the development of superinfections.

### Suggested Readings

Duff P. Antibiotic prophylaxis in abdominal hysterectomy. Obstet Gynecol 1982;60:25–29.

Duff P, Park RC. Antibiotic prophylaxis in vaginal hysterectomy. A review. Obstet Gynecol 1980;55(suppl):193S–202S.

Hemsell DL, Reisch J, Nobles B, et al. Prevention of major infection after elective abdominal hysterectomy: individual determination required. Am J Obstet Gynecol 1983;147:520–528.

Ledger WJ, Gee C, Lewis WP. Guidelines for antibiotic prophylaxis in gynecology. Am J Obstet Gynecol 1974;121:1038–1045.

Mittendorf R, Aronson MP, Berry RE, et al. Avoiding serious infections associated with abdominal hysterectomy: a meta-analysis of antibiotic prophylaxis. Am J Obstet Gynecol 1993;169:119–124.

Polk BF, Shapiro M, Goldstein P, et al. Randomized clinical trial of perioperative cefazolin in preventing infection after hysterectomy. Lancet 1980;1:437–440.

CHAPTER

# 70

# *Posthysterectomy Cuff and Pelvic Cellulitis*

*David L. Hemsell*

## Background and Incidence

Prior to the widespread use of antimicrobial prophylaxis for hysterectomy, the incidence of postoperative pelvic infection, excluding abscess, ranged from 5% to 70%. With the advent of routine prophylaxis, this incidence has fallen to approximately 5% or less, and abscess has become rare. Theoretically, all women undergoing vaginal hysterectomy fall into a "high risk" category because the entire surgical procedure takes place in a contaminated field. At abdominal hysterectomy, little risk of bacterial contamination exists until the vagina is transected. Individual risk factors must be used to identify patients considered to be at high risk after abdominal hysterectomy.

## Pathophysiology

Hysterectomy is classified as a clean-contaminated surgical procedure. It is the inoculation of species that constitute the normal flora of the lower genital tract into the vulnerable operative site that results in the postoperative pelvic infections observed after hysterectomy. If the anus is not carefully draped out of the field at vaginal hysterectomy, additional contamination may occur from that site as well. These factors, plus the duration of time that the cervical–vaginal junction remains open, may explain why reported infection rates without prophylaxis are higher after vaginal hysterectomy than after abdominal hysterectomy; they may also explain why antimicrobial prophylaxis is more effective for the former procedure. Preparing the vagina prior to surgery definitely decreases the bacterial inoculum of vaginal flora, but it has little effect on the endocervical bacteria.

## ETIOLOGY

Posthysterectomy pelvic infection comprises a polymicrobial pelvic soft-tissue infection. Infecting agents include predominantly gram-positive aerobes (*Enterococcus faecalis*, *Staphylococcus epidermidis*, and streptococci) and gram-positive and gram-negative anaerobes (*Peptostreptococcus* species, *Prevotella bivius*, and other *Prevotella* and *Bacteroides* species). Gram-negative aerobic organisms such as *Escherichia coli* and *Enterobacter* species are less commonly isolated.

Preoperative vaginal or endocervical and intraoperative cultures of the endocervix or cardinal ligaments have not proved useful in predicting which patients will develop postoperative pelvic infections. Key variables include the inoculum size and such bacterial virulence factors as ß-lactamase production, bacterial attachment, presence of a capsule, and ability to disseminate in tissues through production of proteases or collagenases. Cell-mediated and humoral immunity systems of the patient are important in preventing infection. Interactions between the inoculum of virulent bacteria and the host defense mechanisms ultimately determine who does and who does not develop a postoperative infection.

## DIAGNOSIS

Increasing pelvic and/or lower abdominal pain and tenderness at examination of the pelvis are the hallmarks of posthysterectomy cellulitis. Temperature elevation alone represents a poor indicator of clinically important infection. In Parkland

Memorial Hospital, as many as 17% of women undergoing vaginal hysterectomy and 35% of those undergoing abdominal hysterectomy have recurrent temperature elevations of 38 °C or higher on the second to third postoperative day, but have no symptoms and have a normal abdominal and pelvic examination. This temperature elevation disappears without therapy. Although temperature elevation cannot be ignored, it should be evaluated in conjunction with patient symptoms and signs of infection. It should never be employed as the sole indicator for infection or as an automatic indicator for antimicrobial administration.

## Cuff Cellulitis

An inflammatory response represents a normal development during wound healing. Surgical margins of the vagina will remain erythematous, edematous, and tender for several days after hysterectomy. These findings quickly subside in the absence of clinical infection, as do the purulent secretions that normally appear in the vagina immediately after hysterectomy. The occurrence of cellulitis of the vaginal "cuff" is a normal physiologic response to the incision occurring in a contaminated area. Usually, host defense mechanisms and antimicrobial prophylaxis quickly resolve this cellulitis, which can be identified in the absence of spontaneous pain and tenderness, and with or without temperature elevation. Whether it contributes to the asymptomatic temperature elevation frequently observed after hysterectomy remains unknown.

Perhaps 1% of patients will develop cuff cellulitis after hysterectomy that requires antimicrobial therapy. Most cases occur after the patient's discharge from the hospital, but usually not more than 10 days thereafter. Women may come to the emergency room or doctor's office for an unscheduled visit complaining of increasing spontaneous central lower abdominal or pelvic pain, and increased vaginal discharge associated with low-grade temperature elevation. Abdominal examination is usually normal, or the patient may show a slight suprapubic tenderness to deep palpation. Only the vaginal surgical margin is tender at bimanual examination, and no masses are palpable.

## Pelvic Cellulitis

Pelvic cellulitis is the most common infection after a hysterectomy, almost always being observed during the immediate postoperative period. Patients complain of increasing lower abdominal and pelvic pain that is usually accentuated on one side. Symptoms most commonly develop late on the second or during the third postoperative day, and the temperature usually exceeds 38.5 °C (101.3 °F).

At abdominal examination, gentle depression over the parametrial area elicits tenderness not previously present. The maximal tenderness usually appears where the symptoms originate. A Pfannenstiel incision makes it somewhat more difficult to locate the origin of the symptoms. Pain and tenderness are more marked with pelvic cellulitis than they are with cuff cellulitis; in addition, the patient's temperature is higher and she is more obviously ill.

The pelvis should be examined to confirm the abdominal examination findings of parametrial tenderness and to detect an infected cuff hematoma or abscess that can be drained. When evaluating a woman for infection after hysterectomy, the physician must exclude infections unrelated to the operative site.

## Laboratory Testing

History and physical examination will confirm the diagnosis of cellulitis in the pelvis after hysterectomy. Very little laboratory testing is necessary. A complete blood count with differential rarely proves helpful but may sometimes identify unsuspected blood loss indicating the presence of a hematoma. In the absence of site-specific symptoms and positive physical findings, it is not necessary routinely to order a chest X ray, a urinalysis with culture and sensitivity testing, or blood cultures.

The incidence of bacteremia is quite low. Its presence does not usually prolong antimicrobial therapy or predict initial antimicrobial therapy failure. Any patient who is suspected of having septicemia should have aerobic and anaerobic blood cultures obtained from at least two sites. A positive result mandates a repeat blood culture to confirm the absence of growth after antimicrobial therapy ends.

The use of a culture obtained with a sterile swab from the area cephalad to the vaginal surgical margin remains controversial. Obtaining the culture in a sterile fashion using a needle and syringe or a double- or triple-lumen brush is less likely to render contaminated results. Some physicians believe that culturing can help determine the species most likely to be responsible for the infection, especially when an infection does not respond to the initial antimicrobial regimen. It also allows for monitoring of resistance patterns if the laboratory performs sensitivity testing. Other clinicians believe that, because only a few patients will fail to respond to the initial therapy, culture is unnecessary for more than 90% to 95% of patients.

A culture performed when a treatment regimen fails should detect the true pathogen or pathogens, as other susceptible species will have been eradicated. Bacterial identification and sensitivity testing should be available from the hosptial laboratory for a culture to provide worthwhile information.

## Treatment

Women with postoperative pelvic cellulitis usually respond more promptly and more completely to the available treatment regimens than do women being treated for post-cesarean section endomyometritis. Combination antimicrobial therapy is effective but often unnecessary. Clinical trials have shown that single-agent therapy with a second- or third-generation cephalosporin, an expanded-spectrum semisynthetic penicillin, or a penicillin with a ß-lactamase inhibitor is as effective as combination therapy.

Successful single-agent intravenous regimens include cefotaxime, 1 g every 8 hours; cefotetan, 2 g every 12 hours; cefoxitin, 2 g every 6 hours; piperacillin, 4 g every 6 hours; and ampicillin/sulbactam, 3 g every 6 hours. Intravenous therapy should continue until the patient has been afebrile for 24 to 36 hours.

If a woman is truly allergic to ß-lactam antibiotics, then she should receive combination therapy. Choices include clindamycin, 900 mg every 8 hours, or metronidazole, 15 mg/kg loading dose followed by 7.5 mg/kg every 6 hours, combined with a 2 mg/kg loading dose of gentamicin, then 1 to 1.5 mg/kg of gentamicin every 8 hours. Recent data indicate that 5 or 7 mg/kg gentamicin given once daily is as effective, less toxic, and less expensive than the thrice-daily regimens. Ampicillin, 2 g every 6 hours, should be added to the metronidazole/gentamicin regimen and is optional for the clindamycin/gentamicin combination in non–penicillin-allergic patients. If therapy is necessary to eradicate gram-positive aerobes not covered by clindamycin, vancomycin, 500 mg IV every 6 hours, is the agent of choice for such patients with a true ß-lactam allergy. An alternative is the recently FDA-approved quinolone trovafloxacin, given 300 mg intravenously initially, then 200 mg intravenously or orally daily to complete therapy.

During therapy, the patient should be monitored at least twice daily to ensure the success of the treatment and to detect any adverse events resulting from it. Antimicrobials should never be administered for pelvic infection without a recent pelvic examination. An adequate and thorough pelvic examination may be uncomfortable for the patient, but it should nevertheless be performed both before initiation of therapy and prior to the patient's discharge from the hospital so as to detect any masses that might be present and to ensure treatment efficacy. Oral outpatient antimicrobial therapy is unnecessary after successful parenteral therapy.

Women with cuff cellulitis have been treated successfully on an outpatient basis with an oral antimicrobial. Some receive an initial intramuscular dose of one of the agents given for inpatient IV therapy. An oral agent providing a wide spectrum of antibacterial activity is amoxicillin with clavulanic acid. This drug is administered at a dose of 250 to 500 mg every 8 hours or 875 mg every 12 hours for five to seven days. Another agent is trovafloxacin, which would be dosed at 200 mg orally once daily. Patients should take their temperatures at home during treatment and should return if their symptoms become more severe or if the temperature elevation persists. All patients should be reevaluated in 72 hours.

## Treatment Failures

If women treated for cuff cellulitis do not respond to outpatient management, a parenteral therapy regimen becomes necessary. Women treated with either single-agent or combination regimens who fail initial therapy for pelvic cellulitis require altered therapy. In many women, *E. faecalis* can be isolated from the infection culture, as multiple-dose prophylaxis or therapy with a cephalosporin selects for that species. In most cases, the gram-positive aerobic or anaerobic species will be the organisms that require enhanced therapy. In many instances, anaerobic coverage can be accomplished with oral metronidazole rather than the parenteral form.

## Suggested Readings

Belliveau PP, Nicolau DP, Nightingale CH, et al. Once-daily gentamicin: experience in one hundred eighteen patients with postpartum endometritis. J Infect Dis 1995;1:11.

del Priore G, Jackson-Stone M, Shim EK, et al. A comparison of once-daily and 8-hour gentamicin dosing in the treatment of postpartum endometritis. Obstet Gynecol 1996;87:994–1000.

Faro S, Sanders CV, Aldridge KE. Use of single-agent antimicrobial therapy in the treatment of polymicrobial female pelvic infections. Obstet Gynecol 1982;60:232–236.

Hager WD, Pascuzzi M, Vernon M. Efficacy of oral antibiotics following parenteral antibiotics for serious infections in obstetrics and gynecology. Obstet Gynecol 1989;73:326–329.

Hemsell DL, Hemsell PG, Heard MC, et al. Piperacillin and a combination of clindamycin and gentamicin for the treatment of hospital and community acquired acute pelvic infections including pelvic abscess. Surg Gynecol Obstet 1987;165:223–229.

Ledger WJ. Prevention, diagnosis, and treatment of postoperative infections. Obstet Gynecol 1980;55(suppl 5):203S–206S.

Swenson RM, Michaelson TC, Daly MJ, et al. Anaerobic bacterial infections of the female genital tract. Obstet Gynecol 1973;42:538–541.

CHAPTER

# 71

# *Pelvic Abscess*

*Sebastian Faro*

## Background

Pelvic abscesses are classified by their location as either lower genital tract, which includes the vagina and vulva, or pelvic cavity, which includes the upper genital tract and the pelvic structures. Lower genital tract abscesses can occur at the following anatomic sites: Bartholin's gland, Skene's gland, a urethral diverticulum, Gartner's duct, and episiotomies. Abscesses can also form in the perirectal tissue or the ischiorectal fossa after a pudendal block, traumatic delivery, or complicating inflammatory bowel disease.

Pelvic abscesses frequently appear as a complication of pelvic inflammatory disease (PID) preceded by salpingitis, which can progress to a pyosalpinx, tubo-ovarian abscess, cul-de-sac abscess, or, infrequently, an ovarian abscess. Other common causes of a pelvic abscess include a ruptured appendix, rectosigmoid colon diverticulitis or perforation, and abscess of Meckel's diverticulum. Furthermore, pelvic abscesses can occur as a complication of hysterectomy or, occasionally, cesarean section. In postmenopausal women, these abscesses most commonly arise from diverticulitis, perforation, or malignancy.

## Pathophysiology

Abscesses of the lower genital tract are usually preceded by an acute infection of a gland or diverticulum. The duct draining the gland becomes inflamed and edematous, and opposing walls of the gland duct adhere, blocking egress of the gland's contents. If bacteria are present, growth will occur within the gland, causing it to swell and form an abscess as polymorphonuclear leukocytes, serum, and bacteria collect. The organisms most frequently initially involved are *Neisseria gonorrhoeae*, *Chlamydia trachomatis*, and the facultative and obligate anaerobes.

Initially, the host's defense mechanism will attempt to eliminate the infection. If the conditions prohibit a suitable response, however, the host will attempt to wall off the infected site so as to localize the infection. The resulting interaction between the infecting organisms and host will lead to the formation of an abscess. Often an extensive inflammatory response occurs involving adjacent structures such as the bowel. The inflamed bowel becomes edematous, peristalsis ceases, and gas and fluid collect within the lumen of the bowel, resulting in abdominal distention and pain.

Clinicians must take note of factors that could lead to an abscess during a surgical procedure. Pelvic infections following surgical procedures are not caused by sexually transmitted bacteria but rather by the endogenous vaginal microflora. Both vaginal hysterectomy and cesarean section are clean-contaminated surgical procedures. The vaginal hysterectomy is performed through a contaminated operative field, where bacteria from the vagina have ample opportunity to enter the pelvis, colonize it, and invade tissue. Necrotic tissue pedicles with suture are often left behind. These pedicles are placed retroperitoneally, leaving an area where blood and serum collect. The abdominal hysterectomy should be considered a clean-contaminated procedure when the vagina is opened and when suture is placed through the vagina.

Cesarean section performed after a patient has labored with ruptured amniotic membranes for more than 12 hours should be regarded as a contaminated procedure. Bacteria from the vagina may ascend into the uterine cavity, colonizing the amniotic membranes and the decidua, and invade the myometrium. An incision through the uterine musculature —either vertical (which involves the corpus and fundus) or transverse (in the lower segment)—or a low vertical incision (which involves the lower uterine segment and cuts through the uterine corpus but not the fundus) may be made through infected myometrial tissue. Closing the incision in a single or double layer can result in strangulation of the tissue because of the tendency to pull the suture tightly. This constriction, in effect, reduces the blood flow and oxygen supply in this area, possibly leading to tissue necrosis. Reduction in blood flow, oxygen concentration, tissue necrosis, and the presence of a foreign body (the suture) all contribute to infection.

## Etiology

The bacteria most frequently involved in postoperative pelvic infections are gram-positive and gram-negative facultative and obligate anaerobes. The facultative anaerobic bacteria probably play a significant role as initiators of the infectious process. Nevertheless, synergistic activity between the facultative and obligate anaerobes eventually results in abscess formation; for example, *Escherichia coli* and *Bacteroides fragilis* are abscessogenic.

Another potential source of bacteria is the rectosigmoid. Pelvic infection causes the bowel to become inflamed and edematous. Resulting microscopic breaks in the mucosal lining can allow bacteria to migrate across the bowel wall. This process is likely to be enhanced in the patient who is deprived of amino acids for an extended period of time. Such patients may include those who are unable to take suitable nutrients—that is, unable to take any food by mouth for more than seven days because of an ileus or pseudo-obstruction. Consequently, the bacterial inoculum may increase within the lumen of the rectosigmoid and sigmoid colon. The bacterial population contains large numbers of potentially abscessogenic combinations of bacteria.

## Diagnosis

A thorough review of the patient's history and operative procedure is required to determine whether any complications occurred during the operative procedure. Was antibiotic prophylaxis given? If so, which antibiotic was used and at what dosage? How many doses were administered? If the patient received a cephalosporin, an increased colonization in the lower genital tract by *Enterococcus faecalis* is possible. This bacterium, along with *B. fragilis* and *Prevotella bivia*, may act synergistically to produce abscesses.

Review of the fever curve may also indicate the presence of an abscess. Patients with an acute abscess typically exhibit high, spiking temperatures with marked variation throughout the day. The white blood cell (WBC) count is often in the 20,000/mm$^3$ range. If the patient's normal WBC count is 3000 to 5000/mm$^3$, however, a four- to fivefold increase is improbable; a threefold increase is more likely. The patient will also show an increase in immature polymorphonuclear neutrophil leukocytes.

The physical examination may reveal the presence of peritonitis. Bowel sounds tend to be infrequent, of low intensity, or even absent. Pelvic examination may reveal a pelvic mass that may be solid or cystic but is usually tender.

Ultrasonography, computed tomography (CT), or X ray of the pelvis may reveal characteristics of the mass that facilitate a diagnosis and treatment. Pelvic X ray, for example, may show gas within a mass. An intravenous pyelogram may reveal displacement of the ureter, a partial or complete obstruction, and the position of the abscess. Ultrasonography and CT scans will show the abscess's relationship to other intraperitoneal structures and help determine whether the mass is uniloculated or multiloculated, thin- or thick-walled, and drainable percutaneously.

## TREATMENT

If the abscess is located in the posterior cul-de-sac and colpotomy drainage can be attempted, ultrasonography should be employed to guide the drainage process. Initially, with ultrasound guidance, insert a needle through the posterior cul-de-sac, which may require general anesthesia or, at least, local infiltration of the epithelium overlying the cul-de-sac.

The aspirated fluid must be placed in an anaerobic transport medium. One aliquot of the aspirate should be tested via Gram's stain, and a second aliquot should be cultured for aerobic and anaerobic bacteria. Keep the needle in place to ensure proper placement of the incision, which should be made adjacent to the needle and simultaneously with entering the abscess.

The abscess cavity should be completely evacuated. Loculations often will be present and must be disrupted so that the patient will respond satisfactorily. Ultrasonography can assist in determining whether the entire abscess has been evacuated and all loculations disrupted. The abscess cavity must be irrigated with copious amounts of sterile normal saline until it is clear. Next, connect a Foley catheter or a Malecot or mushroom drain to suction the area, ensuring complete evacuation and preventing reaccumulation of fluid.

An abscess not located in the cul-de-sac may be drained percutaneously if it occurs adjacent to the abdominal wall or CT scan reveals that it is accessible. In such a case, a pigtail catheter or equivalent catheter can be placed into the abscess cavity. The catheters should remain in place until less than 30 mL of clear serous fluid is collected over a 24-hour period. Reexamine the abscess cavity by CT scan or ultrasound to confirm that no collections of fluid remain. Irrigate the cavity with bacteriostatic saline; then aspirate and culture the saline. If the Gram's stain results are negative, remove the drain.

If the patient is not taking antibiotics when the drainage procedure begins, administer them immediately after obtaining the initial aspirate. Because abscesses are likely to involve gram-negative and gram-positive facultative as well as obligate anaerobes, broad-spectrum antimicrobial therapy is indicated. Antibiotics should be administered intravenously.

Successful medicinal therapy depends on the delivery of adequate concentrations of antibiotic to the abscess. With a thick-walled abscess, the tissue adjacent to the abscess can be infected and the vessels supplying this area may be thrombosed. Antibiotic levels in the tissue will therefore be either absent or lower than the effective level. To treat this type of infection successfully, you must surgically remove the involved tissue. An example of this situation is encountered in women

**Table 71-1.** Antibiotic Choices for Treatment of Abscesses

| Agent | Dosage |
|---|---|
| Piperacillin/tazobactam | 3.375 g IV q6h |
| Ampicillin/sulbactam | 3 g IV q6h |
| Clindamycin plus gentamicin | 900 mg IV q8h |
| | 2 mg/kg loading dose followed with 1.5 mg/kg q8h |
| Metronidazole plus gentamicin | 500 mg IV q8h |

delivered by cesarean section who develop suppurative myometritis and necrosis of the lower uterine segment. In these patients, the vessels supplying blood to the uterus may become completely thrombosed. Similarly, patients who have tubo-ovarian abscesses, which have a thick abscess wall and are multiloculated, usually require surgical intervention.

If the patient is not receiving antimicrobial agents when an abscess is diagnosed, the treatment choice lies between a single antibiotic and combination therapy (Table 71-1). No large, prospective studies support the use of any specific antibiotic regimen; instead, limited published data support the use of single agents and combination therapy to treat abscesses. Because pelvic abscesses are predominantly polymicrobial, you must select an antibiotic or combination of antibiotics that show activity against a variety of bacteria, including streptococci, *Enterococcus*, members of the Enterobacteriaceae family, and obligate anaerobes, including the *B. fragilis* group. Several agents fulfill this requirement: ticarcillin/clavulanic acid, piperacillin/tazobactam, ampicillin/sulbactam, and imipenem/cilastatin. The penicillins have been combined with a ß-lactamase inhibitor that broadens the spectrum of piperacillin, ticarcillin, and ampicillin by inhibiting the activity of a variety of ß-lactamases. Imipenem, a carbapenem, is not affected by the activity of ß-lactamases. Other options include combinations such as ampicillin and gentamicin plus clindamycin or metronidazole.

If a patient fails to respond to therapy with one of the penicillin agents or imipenem, customary practice is to discontinue the agent and institute combination therapy. A more logical approach would be to build on the agent in use and expand the spectrum of activity. These agents offer good gram-positive coverage and anaerobic activity that is comparable to—and may exceed that of—clindamycin. The only weakness is coverage of the Enterobacteriaceae. The addition of an aminoglycoside enhances activity against facultative gram-negative anaerobes and provides synergistic activity against *Enterococcus*.

If the initial therapy consists of combinations of antibiotics (clindamycin or metronidazole plus ampicillin and an aminoglycoside) and the patient fails to improve, consider draining the abscess. Allow a trial of antibiotics for as long as 96 hours providing that the patient's condition does not worsen. Clindamycin shows activity against such gram-positive organisms as streptococci, staphylococci, and peptococci, whereas metronidazole does not have activity against the aerobic cocci. Neither of these agents is effective against *Enterococcus faecalis*. Patients who are allergic to penicillin should receive vancomycin if the enterococcus is known or strongly suspected of being present. If material can be aspirated from the abscess, place the fluid in an anaerobic transport vial. The fluid should be Gram-stained and cultured for aerobes and anaerobes. After the identification of specific bacteria and the elucidation of antibiotic sensitivities, you can modify antibiotic therapy.

Administer parenteral antibiotics until the patient becomes and remains afebrile for 72 hours. At this time, WBC should be normal, the patient should tolerate oral liquids, and signs and symptoms of peritonitis should resolve. Measure abscesses by ultrasonography; measurements should be obtained serially until resolution of the mass occurs. Typically, the abscess will not resolve within this initial treatment period. Once the patient's condition has improved, oral nourishment is well tolerated, and symptoms and signs of acute infection have resolved, the patient can be administered oral antibiotics. Agents such as oral metronidazole and ofloxacin, or clindamycin and ofloxacin, can be given for 10 to 14 days. Approximately 50% of patients will retain a residual mass, and many will ultimately require surgery.

A new quinalone, trovafloxacin, is now available for use as a parenteral and oral agent. Its spectrum covers aerobic, facultative, and obligate anaerobic bacteria, including *N. gonorrhoeae*, *C. trachomatis*, and *Mycoplasma hominis*. Other antibiotics that may be administered are amoxicillin/clavulanic acid and metronidazole plus trimethoprim/sulfamethoxazole.

Thick-walled and multiloculated abscesses are unlikely to respond to medical therapy and will require surgical intervention. In cases where an abscess has been surgically removed, antibiotic therapy should continue until the patient has been afebrile and clinically well for 48 to 72 hours. If the abscess has ruptured and free purulent material appears in the abdominal cavity, cleanse the abdomen with copious amounts of saline (at least 10 L). It is imperative to examine the subhepatic and subdiaphragmatic compartments for the presence of purulent material. Following the discharge from the hospital, the patient should be examined weekly for four weeks. If the clinician sees any indication that the patient's condition is not improving, a complete evaluation should be performed. In that event, the patient may require hospitalization and exploratory laparotomy.

## Suggested Readings

Aeder MI, Wellman JL, Haaga JR, et al. Role of surgical and percutaneous drainage in the treatment of abdominal abscess. Arch Surg 1983;118:273–280.

Graham D, Sanders RC. Ultrasound-directed transvaginal aspiration biopsy of pelvic masses. J Ultrasound Med 1982;1:279–280.

Hager WD, Pascuzzi M, Vernon M. Efficacy of oral antibiotics following parenteral antibiotics for serious infections in obstetrics and gynecology. Obstet Gynecol 1989;73:326–329.

Johnson WC, Gerzof SG, Robbins AH, et al. Treatment of abdominal abscesses: comparative evaluation of operative drainage versus percutaneous catheter drainage guided by computed tomography and ultrasound. Ann Surg 1981;194:510–520.

Loy RA, Gallup DG, Hill JA, et al. Pelvic abscess: examination and transvaginal drainage guided by real-time ultrasonography. South Med J 1989;82:788–790.

Martin EC, Karlson KB, Fankuchen EI, et al. Percutaneous drainage of postoperative intra-abdominal abscesses. Am J Roentgenol 1982;138:13–15.

CHAPTER

# 72

# *Incisional Surgical Site Infections (Wound Infections)*

*David A. Eschenbach*

## Incidence

Despite the use of prophylactic antibiotics, wound infections remain a common occurrence in postsurgical patients. Postoperative wound infections develop in 4% of patients following inpatient gynecologic surgery and in 5% to 7% of patients undergoing primary cesarean section. Surprisingly, few women develop infections after episiotomy. The wound infection rate depends largely on the degree of bacterial contamination, but also is influenced by local and systemic factors affecting the patient's resistance to infection and the time of the operation.

Wound infections are the most common cause of serious postoperative morbidity. They are also costly, adding approximately two days to the average hospital stay and an estimated $5000 to $10,000 in hospital charges.

## Definition of surgical site infection

Standard definitions of incisional surgical site infections (SSIs) are now available from the Centers for Disease Control and Prevention (CDC) (Table 72-1).

Incisional SSIs are classified as involving only the skin and subcutaneous tissue (superficial incisional SSIs) or deep soft tissues, such as fascial and muscle layers (deep incisional SSIs). Superficial incisional SSIs must occur within 30 days

**Table 72-1.** Classification of Wound Infections

**Clean**

*Uninfected operative wounds in which no inflammation is encountered and the respiratory, alimentary, genital, or uninfected urinary tracts are not entered.*

Clean wounds are primarily closed and, if necessary, drained with closed drainage. Operative incisional wounds that follow nonpenetrating (blunt) trauma should be included in this category if they meet the criteria.

**Clean-Contaminated**

*Operative wounds in which the respiratory, alimentary, genital, or urinary tract is entered under controlled conditions and without unusual contamination.*

Operations involving the biliary tract, appendix, vagina, and oropharynx are included in this category, provided that no evidence of infection or a major break in technique is encountered.

**Contaminated**

*Open, fresh, accidental wounds, operations with major breaks in sterile technique or gross spillage from the gastrointestinal tract, and incisions in which acute, nonpurulent inflammation is encountered.*

**Dirty-Infected**

*Old traumatic wounds with retained devitalized tissue and wounds that involve existing clinical infection or perforated viscera.*

This definition suggests that the organisms causing the postoperative infection were present before the operation.

SOURCE: Garner JS. CDC guideline for prevention of surgical wound infections, 1985. Infect Control 1986;7:195.

after the operative procedure and involve only skin or subcutaneous tissue of the incision. At least one of the following must be present:

- Purulent drainage from the superficial incision
- Organisms isolated from an aseptically obtained fluid or tissue from the superficial incision
- At least one of the following signs or symptoms of infection: pain or tenderness, localized swelling, redness, or heat
- A superficial incision that is deliberately opened by the surgeon (unless a culture of the incision is negative)
- A diagnosis of superficial incisional SSI by the surgeon or attending physician

The following are not reported as a superficial incisional SSI:

- A stitch abscess (minimal inflammation and discharge confined to the points of suture penetration)
- Infection of an episiotomy or a neonatal circumcision site
- An infected burn wound (specific criteria are used for infected episiotomy and circumcision sites and for burn wounds)
- An incisional SSI that extends into the fascial and muscle layers

Deep incisional SSIs must occur within 30 days after the operative procedure if no prosthetic implant is left in place or within one year if an implant is involved. The infection must appear related to the operative procedure and affect deep soft tissues (for example, fascial and muscle layers) of the incision. At least one of the following must be present:

- Purulent drainage from the deep incision but not from the organ or space component at the surgical site
- A deep incision that spontaneously dehisces or is deliberately opened by a surgeon when the patient has at least one of the following signs or symptoms: fever (>38 °C), localized pain, or tenderness, unless a culture from the incision is negative
- An abscess or other evidence of infection involving the deep incision found on direct examination, during reoperation, or by histopathologic or radiologic examination
- Diagnosis of a deep incisional SSI by a surgeon or attending physician

An organ and/or space SSI involves any part of the anatomy other than the incision that was opened or manipulated during the operative procedure. Specific sites are assigned to organ/space SSIs to identify the location of the infection. Organ/space SSIs are placed in a separate classification from incisional SSIs.

## Calculation of SSI Risk

Patients with *clean wounds* have the lowest rate of wound infection. In clean wounds, no inflammation is present in the operative field, no break occurs in aseptic technique, and the gastrointestinal, respiratory or vaginal tract is not entered.

In a *clean-contaminated wound*, the vagina or the gastrointestinal, respiratory, or uninfected urinary tract is entered, or minor breaks occur in sterile technique. Wound infection rates generally increase three- to fivefold in clean-contaminated wounds.

In a *contaminated wound,* gross spillage occurs from a hollow viscus or major breaks occur in sterile technique.

*Dirty and infected wounds* are associated with pus, acute inflammation, a perforated viscus, or a traumatic wound of more than four hours' duration.

The National Nosocomial Infection Surveillance (NNIS) System proposed by the CDC has been validated in more than 84,000 operations. The NNIS surgical patient risk index for each operation is determined by giving a 0 score for none and one point for any of the following risk factors:

- An American Society of Anesthesiologists (ASA) preoperative assessment score of 3 (severe systemic disease that limits activity but is not incapacitating), 4 (incapacitating systemic disease that is a constant threat to life), or 5 (not expected to survive the next 24 hours).
- A wound classified as either contaminated or dirty-infected.
- Surgery that exceeds the 75th percentile for mean duration. The 75th percentile duration of surgery is one hour for cesarean section and two hours for laparotomy, abdominal hysterectomy, and vaginal hysterectomy. Separate duration criteria for radical hysterectomies, cancer debulking procedures, and radical vulvectomies have not been established.

The patient's risk of SSI is calculated by combining her 0 to 1 points for the ASA score, the presence of a contaminated or dirty-infected wound, and the duration of surgery that exceeds the 75th percentile. The prevalence of SSIs is similar in contaminated and dirty-infected wounds (6% to 7%) and increases linearly with the ASA score. The ASA risk index score has a direct effect upon the wound classification categories. In combination, SSI rates are different in the four risk index categories.

## Additional Risk Factors for SSI

### *Surgeons*

The rate of incisional SSI in a clean wound varies among surgeons performing the same operation. It is quite possible to achieve incisional SSI rates of less than 1% in a clean wound. Concern should arise if an individual surgeon's incisional SSI rate exceeds 2% in these types of wounds. Regular publication and discussion of incisional SSI rates can serve as powerful inducements for surgeons to reduce rates of clean infection.

Incisional SSI rates reflect a complex interaction of surgical technique and attention to asepsis. Rates are lowest among surgeons with a strong interest in applying aseptic techniques and often rise dramatically with relaxed attention to these techniques. Other major factors contributing to wound infection by hospital personnel include failure to wash hands between patient examinations, moving freely from infected to noninfected patients, wearing soiled scrub clothes and shoes, and operating after cleaning an infected wound. As much as 25% of post-cesarean wound infection is caused by *Staphylococcus aureus* acquired from the skin of a member of the surgical team or the patient, possibly through failures in aseptic technique.

Antiseptic scrubs reduce counts of skin flora. Skin flora is adequately reduced after a 3- to 5-minute scrub for a first operation or a 2-minute scrub for a second consecutive one. Longer scrub times do not further reduce flora count. Hexachlorophene inhibits skin flora for at least one hour after application and is the scrub of choice. Povidone–iodine is also an adequate scrub antiseptic.

Between 25% and 50% of surgeons' gloves become perforated during an operation. Perforation rates are especially high for cesarean section. Preoperative hand scrubbing is therefore important for reducing skin contamination from surgeons in the event of glove perforation.

### *Patients*

Data showing that incisional SSIs occur in proportion to the number of days that the patient spends in the hospital before surgery suggest that the hospital environment itself increases colonization of the skin, vagina, urinary tract, and gut with virulent microorganisms. Clinical infection remote from the surgical site increases incisional SSI rates by a threefold level. Incisional SSIs are also associated with factors that reduce wound defenses, such as reoperation, increasing age after 50, malnutrition, diabetes, smoking, severe pulmonary disease, cirrhosis, uremia, and malignancy.

Skin scrubs used for patients ideally should comprise a two-step process: an initial scrub with soap or a fat solvent, followed by an antiseptic scrub with 1% iodine or 0.5% chlorhexidine in 70% alcohol. Mechanical friction is advised for the skin, to remove a layer of nonviable cells, and for the vagina, to thoroughly remove discharge from between vaginal folds. The importance of adequate vaginal preparation cannot be overemphasized. Despite the popular misconception, the vagina can usually be decolonized with an adequate prep. On the other hand, it is difficult to totally eliminate bacteria from the endocervix.

Superficial SSIs are more likely with shaving than with no shaving or with clipping. Shaving done more than two hours before surgery is particularly harmful because bacteria may colonize small nicks in the skin. Preoperative hexachlorophene showers may reduce the incidence of superficial SSIs.

Obesity resulting in a wound 4 cm or more in depth is associated with a threefold increased risk of superficial SSI following abdominal hysterectomy. Most bacteria recovered from SSIs in obese patients come from skin flora. Measures to reduce superficial SSI in obese patients include minimizing tissue damage, assuring strict hemostasis, and using closed drains.

Maintenance of body temperature is important for long operations. Low temperature may produce vasoconstriction, reduce oxygenation, and impair neutrophil function. In one study, patients whose body temperatures were maintained at 36.5 °C or higher with a fluid warmer and a forced-air cover had lower superficial SSI rates than patients whose body temperatures were allowed to reach 34.5 °C.

### *Surgical Wounds*

Experimentally, approximately 1 million bacteria per gram of tissue are required to produce infection in the normal wound.

The type of bacteria inoculated is not as important as the number of organisms present. The more abnormal the local wound condition, however, the fewer the bacteria needed to produce infection. Approximately 1000 times fewer bacteria are required to cause a wound infection when suture or shock decreases local wound resistance.

Devitalized tissue, hematomas, shock, and a foreign-body effect from suture all act to reduce local tissue resistance to infections. Wounds torn or opened with great force have increased areas of devitalized tissue. To minimize tissue devitalization, electrocoagulation currents should be kept at a minimum and blood vessels should be grasped with fine tissue forceps.

The tissue effect of electrocautery depends directly on the current's magnitude. Heat and the subsequent damage to tissue surrounding the blood vessel are markedly increased at high current settings. Compared with scalpel wounds, incisions made by electrosurgical knives have a threefold increased rate of wound infection.

It is important to avoid hematoma formation because blood collections allow bacteria to grow in fibrin spaces that are not accessible to white blood cell defenses. By reducing the local blood supply, shock weakens local defenses and markedly reduces the number of bacteria required to cause infection.

Sutures create a foreign-body effect by allowing bacterial attachment. For instance, bacteria may become buried on the surface of suture beneath a mucopolysaccharide covering. Sutures also devitalize tissue. Use of a large-size suture increases infection rates by increasing bacterial colonization and the volume of tissue devitalized. Nonabsorbable nonfilament nylon sutures have the least potential for causing infection, followed by Dacron braided-plain polyester sutures. Among absorbable sutures, polyglycolic material is the least likely to potentiate infection, perhaps because it inhibits bacterial growth in a low-pH environment. Silk, cotton, and chromic gut are the most likely candidates for potentiating infection. For skin closure, tape is least, staples next, and suture most likely to cause infection. Infection is least likely with an interrupted percutaneous technique and most likely with continuous subcutaneous skin sutures.

Drains remove harmful fluid collections but may also serve as sources of retrograde bacterial contamination. If drains are necessary, bring closed drains out away from the wound edge to assure the lowest superficial SSI rate. Penrose drains exiting through the wound should not be used: They not only promote high superficial SSI rates from retrograde bacterial contamination of skin bacteria into the wound, but also provide only limited drainage because particulate matter can become trapped within the fibrin deposits in the drain.

Each hour of surgery doubles the superficial SSI rate. This phenomenon undoubtedly results from time-related increases in bacterial contamination, wound injury, wound damage from suture and coagulation, and the difficulty of the operation at hand, particularly when it involves heavy blood loss.

### *Operating Room Personnel*

Surgical personnel need to adhere closely to aseptic techniques. Special training may be particularly necessary for labor and delivery nurses who act as scrub nurses or nurse circulators for cesarean section. The availability of personnel who are dedicated to practicing aseptic techniques can dramatically reduce SSI rates. Those with known skin infection—particularly staphylococci infection—should not participate in surgery. Finding staphylococcal infections among patients with clean wound categories should prompt further investigation in an attempt to identify asymptomatic (usually nares) staphylococcal carriers.

Use drapes that are impervious to fluids, because soaked drapes help absorb bacteria. Impervious cloth or disposable drapes are advised. Plastic adhesive drapes are associated with increased rates of superficial SSIs because bacteria proliferate underneath them; antiseptic solution on the skin should be removed before the application of such drapes. Neverthless, these drapes can help reduce the amount of contaminated fluid from sinuses and fistulas.

In summary, SSIs develop from contamination of a wound with bacteria and from systemic and, more important, local factors in the wound that reduce the patient's resistance to infection. Simply put, an increase in bacteria or a decrease in wound resistance creates the potential for infection.

## PREVENTION

### Mechanical Bowel Preparation

Mechanical bowel preparation reduces the bulk of stool and, more important, the number of bacteria present in stool. Use such preparation if the bowel may be entered. Traditionally, the patient underwent three days of low-residue diet, laxatives, and enemas. One of two preferable new techniques is a more comfortable whole-gut lavage with isotonic saline and potassium administered through a nasogastric tube. Rectal effluent usually becomes clear within three hours. The second method employs a commercially available, orally administered, balanced electrolyte GoLYTELY solution and polyethylene glycol taken in 250 mL increments every 10 minutes until 4 L are consumed.

### Oral Antibiotics

Nonabsorbable oral antibiotics can further reduce bowel flora. They should be given in conjunction with mechanical bowel preparation when bowel entry is likely. Administer 1 g each of neomycin and erythromycin base orally at 1 P.M., 2 P.M., and 11 P.M. the day before an operation scheduled at 8 A.M. the next day.

### Prophylactic Antibiotics

In patients with marked bacterial contamination, prophylactic antibiotics may reduce wound infections. Their benefits are only modest, however, and they offer little or no advantage for clean wounds. For the antibiotic to be effective, it must be given within one to two hours before the surgical incision. Cephalosporins are preferred for most obstetric and gynecologic procedures, except those involving colonic spillage. The most common errors in using prophylactic antibiotics include initiation only shortly before surgery and continuation beyond surgery, especially for more than 12 hours after completion of surgery.

## Delayed Primary Closure

Dirty wounds or those affecting patients with active infection, including foul-smelling amniotic fluid, are associated with an infection rate as high as 40%. As a result, these patients should be considered for delayed primary wound closure, which effectively reduces the infection rate. Do not close the wound until four to seven days later, when healthy granulation tissue develops. Other postoperative wound care does not significantly affect wound infection.

## Wound Irrigation

Saline irrigation of the abdomen and wound washes away debris and blood clots and may reduce bacterial contamination. Remove saline from the abdomen after irrigation so that leukocyte function is not inhibited. Soaking the wound after closure of the skin, however, increases infection by introducing bacteria from the skin.

## Surveillance

Periodic reports to surgeons combined with educational programs have a definite ameliorative effect on SSIs. Although costly, wound surveillance is a necessary part of surgical care, as corrective measures have been shown to markedly reduce infection rates.

# Clinical Infection

## Localized Wound Infection

Most superficial and deep incisional SSIs develop within four to six days of the operation. Rapid-onset incisional SSI (occurring within 6 to 24 hours of an operation) usually indicates an especially serious infection. The wound initially tends to develop a painful, red, and edematous area. The wide variety of bacteria recovered from such wounds can arise from either (1) the skin of a member of the surgical team or patient (in the case of staphylococci) or (2) patient body sites naturally contaminated with large numbers of indigenous flora (anaerobic or aerobic bacteria).

In patients already taking antibiotics for another postoperative infection, however, the first manifestation of SSI often consists of a secondary temperature spike without prominent findings in the wound. Fever and abdominal/uterine tenderness may resolve with the administration of antibiotics in patients treated for postpartum endometritis; the first sign of a late incisional SSI is therefore often only a secondary fever spike.

Exudate ranges from thick pus in staphylococcal infection to a thin, watery discharge in streptococcal infection. Abscess formation occurs with both odorless staphylococcal and foul-smelling anaerobic infection. Marked manifestation of cellulitis (sharp, red, edematous borders) beyond the wound's immediate vicinity should prompt suspicion of streptococcal infection or necrotizing fasciitis, especially in patients with prominent toxicity.

Infection usually remains localized to the subcutaneous tissue in the wound's immediate vicinity—that is, the area contaminated and damaged by the surgical incision. Surrounding areas of cellulitis tend to be limited. Open infected wounds to provide adequate wound debridement and drainage. Most patients should receive a general or regional anesthetic and sharp debridement, with removal of pus and necrotic and heavily contaminated tissue, to help control infection. After debridement, loosely pack the wound with fine gauze soaked in an isotonic saline solution and change this gauze two to three times daily. Gentle wound handling at this point promotes healing.

Use antibiotics only as adjunctive therapy for adjacent cellulitis. Well-localized infections—particularly those caused by staphylococci—do not require antibiotic therapy. Antibiotics are particularly helpful for treating cellulitis, lymphangitis, and septicemia; they are not effective in necrotic or pus-filled areas. Cephalosporins, vancomycin, or penicillinase-resistant penicillin should be considered first-line antibiotics unless anaerobes are suspected, in which case clindamycin, metronidazole, or ampicillin/sulbactam should be included.

## Necrotizing Fasciitis

Although an unusual complication, necrotizing fasciitis is a potentially lethal superficial incisional SSI. This infection of the superficial fascia (subcutaneous tissue) arises from a synergistic process whereby one bacterial agent causes an initial infection and a second causes tissue necrosis. Patients with necrotizing fasciitis are typically placed on antibiotic regimens sufficient to inhibit most aerobic and anaerobic bacteria. In these patients, however, the area of wound erythema and edema continues to increase. The wounds contain marked edema and are especially painful.

Patients with necrotizing facsiitis usually appear toxic and exhibit significant leukocytosis, often in the range of 30,000 to 60,000/mm$^3$. Anemia may result from hemolysis, but hemoconcentration also occurs when intravascular fluid extravasates into the area of the wound; indeed, hematocrits as high as 60% are common. Hypocalcemia is frequent because calcium binds to fat degraded by bacterial lipases to form soap.

The diagnosis of necrotizing fasciitis is often difficult to establish because the pus typical in incisional SSI is characteristically not found. Furthermore, the presence and extent of necrosis are not readily apparent in most cases. Discharge from the wound does not contain pus, but rather has a thin "dishwater" appearance. Necrotic fat appears edematous and without bleeding rather than black. Ecchymoses, bullae, crepitance, or gangrene of the skin indicate necrotizing fasciitis. Typically, skin changes occur only late in infection, when blood vessels transversing subcutaneous tissue become necrosed.

Because these clinical features are atypical of incisional SSI and because necrotizing fasciitis remains rare, misdiagnosis is common in such cases. Additionally, care givers may fail to appreciate the seriousness of infection. Necrotizing fasciitis has occurred in cesarean section, episiotomy, and laparotomy and laparoscopy wounds, as well as in superficial abrasions of the vulva and from Bartholin's gland infection.

If necrotizing fasciitis is suspected, the patient must undergo an exploration of the wound under anesthesia. Inadequate exploration and consequent missed diagnosis often occur because the wound is too tender to explore adequately without anesthesia. Necrosis of the superficial fascia (subcutaneous fat) can be diagnosed when cut subcutaneous tissue does not bleed and can be easily removed by blunt dissection. The mortality rate for necrotizing fasciitis is approximately 50% in surgically treated cases with adequate debridement, but it approaches 100% in patients treated medically without surgery. These patients usually die in septic shock. Septic shock, respiratory distress, or intravascular coagulopathy in patients with cellulitis should be considered to be caused by necrotizing fasciitis, clostridial gangrene, or toxic shock syndrome.

## Toxic Shock

A toxigenic strain of staphylococci can give rise to toxic shock, which has occurred in incisions after surgery, breast infection, clean abdominal wounds, and laparoscopy. Typical signs—high fever, hypotension, multisystem failure, and eventually skin peeling—may occur even before an incision exhibits obvious signs of infection.

Patients with a recent wound and manifestations of toxic shock should usually have the wound explored to exclude necrotizing fasciitis or clostridial gangrene before settling on a diagnosis of toxic shock syndrome (TSS). Debridement, IV fluid, and support of multisystem failure are usually sufficient treatment of TSS.

### Suggested Readings

Altemeier WA, Burke JF, Pruitt BA Jr, et al., eds. Manual on control of infection in surgical patients. Philadelphia: Lippincott, 1984.

Cruse PJ. Incidence of wound infection on the surgical services. Surg Clin North Am 1975;55:1269–1275.

Cruse PJ, Foord R. A five-year prospective study of 23,649 surgical wounds. Arch Surg 1973;107:206–210.

Culver DH, Horan TC, Gaynes RP, et al. Surgical wound infection rates by wound class, operative procedure, and patient risk index. Am J Med 1991;91(suppl 3B):152S–157S.

Horan TC, Gaynes RP, Martone WJ, et al. CDC definitions of nosocomial surgical site infections, 1992: a modification of CDC definitions of surgical wound infections. Am J Infect Control 1992;20:271–274.

Iffy L, Kaminetzky HA, Maidman JE, et al. Control of perinatal infection by traditional preventive measures. Obstet Gynecol 1979;54: 403–411.

Nichols RL, Condon RE, Gorbach SL, et al. Efficacy of preoperative antimicrobial preparation of the bowel. Ann Surg 1972;176:227–232.

CHAPTER

# 73

# *Necrotizing Fasciitis*

*Maurizio Maccato*

## Background and incidence

Necrotizing fasciitis is a potentially lethal infection of the subcutaneous tissue and fascial planes. Muscle tissue usually is not involved. Rapid diagnosis and prompt surgical and medical intervention are required to maximize the likelihood of recovery.

Necrotizing fasciitis has been described as a complication of vaginal delivery, cesarean section, postpartum tubal ligation, or any gynecologic surgery, including laparoscopy. In addition, it has been associated with soft-tissue trauma such as bites, burns, abscesses, or ulcerations. Finally, it has been reported in pregnant patients in the absence of recognizable foci of bacterial inoculation.

Predisposing factors include diabetes mellitus, compromised immunologic function, peripheral vascular disease, malnutrition, intravenous drug abuse, and malignancies. Incidence has been placed at 1.8 per 1000 cases in the post-cesarean section patient. Incidence in other settings is uncertain.

## Pathophysiology

Necrotizing fasciitis typically is a synergistic polymicrobial infection, with both aerobic and anaerobic organisms frequently being recovered. Cases caused by a single pathogen have been reported as well, with group A ß-hemolytic *Streptococcus* and *Staphylococcus aureus* being noted as the most common pathogens; their powerful exotoxins contribute to the tissue necrosis that is characteristic of this infection. The necrosis occurs secondary to vasculitis and thrombosis, and the histologic examination of the surgical specimen during debridement therefore will reveal vascular thrombosis with fasciitis, as well as lobular and septal panniculitis.

## DIAGNOSIS

Making a diagnosis of necrotizing fasciitis may prove difficult in the early stages of the disease. Therefore, because of the rapidity with which the infection spreads and the severity of this complication, a high index of suspicion must be maintained.

Although the early signs and symptoms of necrotizing fasciitis may be mild and nonspecific, the majority of patients will have pain, swelling, and erythema at the site of bacterial inoculation. Initially, pain appears out of proportion to the apparent involvement of the area. With progression of the infection, pain subsides and the area may become numb. The apparently normal skin overlying the infected fascia becomes ecchymotic, and bullae and crepitance develop as the disease progresses. Unfortunately, by the time skin changes have occurred, the infection is usually widespread.

The appearance of a surgical wound with necrotizing fasciitis will be remarkable for the absence of purulence and the presence of a brownish, thin discharge. The underlying fat layer will be edematous, and no bleeding will be elicited by exploration of the wound. Exploration of the involved site should not be delayed but may require anesthesia because of the discomfort involved.

Patients with necrotizing fasciitis commonly have severe systemic symptoms, such as hypotension, anemia or hemoconcentration, elevated white blood cell count, and possible hepatic or renal dysfunction. In the presence of streptococcal toxins, a toxic shock syndrome may be present. Some patients will develop hypocalcemia. Changes on X-ray films, CT scans, and MRIs have been described in cases of necrotizing fasciitis. Radiographic evaluation of the patient must not delay definitive diagnosis and therapy, however.

## Therapy

Treatment for necrotizing fasciitis should combine extensive, aggressive surgical debridement with antibiotic and supportive medical therapy. Because the infection may be polymicrobial, broad antibiotic coverage is necessary. After initiation of antibiotic therapy designed to cover both aerobic and anaerobic organisms, debridement of the infected area should be performed as expeditiously as possible. Adequate debridement may require multiple surgical procedures. Surgical therapy is indicated even for patients who are poor surgical candidates because failure to perform adequate debridement is associated with mortality in virtually all cases.

During debridement, the surgeon must excise all devitalized tissue. A frozen section obtained at the time of debridement may indicate the extent of debridement needed. Aggressive resuscitation efforts should be ongoing in conjunction with antibiotic therapy and surgical debridement.

Antibiotics used to treat necrotizing fasciitis include vancomycin or ampicillin, combined with a third-generation cephalosporin or an aminoglycoside, and clindamycin or metronidazole. Clindamycin appears to be more effective than penicillin for group A streptococcal infection. The use of hyperbaric oxygen or intravenous gamma globulin to treat severe group A streptococcal infection remains controversial. Penicillinase-resistant penicillins, penicillins plus ß-lactamase inhibitors, or fluorinated quinolones may also be part of the antibiotic regimen.

A frequent sequela of necrotizing fasciitis is development of large, open areas of debrided tissue that require reconstructive surgery.

## Summary

Necrotizing fasciitis is an uncommon but life-threatening complication that must be diagnosed early and treated aggressively to maximize the likelihood of recovery. A high index of suspicion for this condition and aggressive surgical exploration and confirmation of the diagnosis are the cornerstones of the successful therapy of this infection.

## Suggested Readings

Giuciano A, Lewis F Jr, Hadley K, et al. Bacteriology of necrotizing fasciitis. Am J Surg 1977;134:52–57.

Goepfert AR, Guinn DA, Andrews WW, et al. Necrotizing fasciitis after cesarean delivery. Obstet Gynecol 1997;89:409–412.

McHenry CR, Azar T, Ramahi AJ, et al. Monomicrobial necrotizing fasciitis complicating pregnancy and puerperium. Obstet Gynecol 1996;87:823–826.

Stamenkovic I, Lew PD. Early recognition of potentially fatal necrotizing fasciitis: the use of frozen-section biopsy. N Engl J Med 1984;310:1689–1693.

Stevens D. Necrotizing fasciitis: don't wait to make a diagnosis. Infect Med 1997;14:684–688.

CHAPTER

74

# Acute Respiratory Distress Syndrome

*Lindsay S. Alger*

## Background and Incidence

The term "adult respiratory distress syndrome" was first used by Ashbaugh and colleagues three decades ago to describe a pulmonary process categorized by noncardiogenic pulmonary edema, hypoxemia, shunting, and decreased compliance. This process often led to pulmonary failure and death. At a recent European–American consensus conference, the adult respiratory distress syndrome was renamed the acute respiratory distress syndrome (ARDS). The intent of the renaming was to emphasize that this condition represents an acute pulmonary response in any age group to a heterogeneous group of predisposing events, any of which can initiate a potentially lethal process of autodestructive inflammation.

Acute respiratory distress syndrome may result from direct lung injury, such as lung contusions, aspiration of gastric contents, or smoke inhalation. More frequently, it arises from indirect lung injury precipitated by processes originating outside the lung, such as bacterial sepsis, trauma, or pancreatitis. Any of these conditions can initiate both local and systemic inflammatory mediator release, a progressively dysfunctional host response, and, ultimately, multiple-organ failure and death. This process, called the systemic inflammatory response syndrome (SIRS), can affect any organ, including the kidneys, liver, brain, heart, and bone marrow. The first organ to become involved usually is the lung; thus ARDS represents the pulmonary manifestation of SIRS.

The consensus conference developed the following working definition of ARDS:

> A state of acute lung injury in which (1) the ratio of $Pao_2$ to $Fio_2$ is 200 or less, regardless of whether or how much positive end-expiratory pressure (PEEP) is used; (2) bilateral pulmonary infiltrates are seen on a frontal chest X ray; and (3) the pulmonary capillary wedge pressure (PCWP) is 18 mm Hg or less or the patient shows no clinical evidence of elevated left atrial pressure.

Previously, no accepted standard definition existed, making it very difficult to measure the incidence of ARDS. Recent reports indicate the incidence ranges from 1.5 to 7.1 persons annually per 100,000 of population.

Sepsis is the most common cause of ARDS, accounting for perhaps 50% of cases seen by the obstetrician–gynecologist. Approximately 25% of patients with gram-negative sepsis develop this syndrome. In the majority of cases, the abdomen represents the primary source of infection. Despite advances in respiratory therapy, many patients still progress to multiple-organ dysfunction syndrome, and mortality remains at approximately 50% (even higher in the presence of septic shock).

Although most frequently seen in association with endotoxin release from gram-negative organisms, ARDS can result from the release of exotoxins from gram-positive organisms. It may also develop in the setting of community- or hospital-acquired pneumonia caused by viral, parasitic, or fungal organisms. Alternatively, endotoxin release from the gut may result from altered bowel mucosal membrane function, following an ischemic insult of noninfectious origin, such as hemorrhagic shock.

## Pathophysiology

In ARDS, host exposure to bacterial cell wall products such as endotoxin and lipoteichoic acid generates a systemic inflammatory reaction. Cytokines and other mediators are released

**Table 74-1.** Mediators of ARDS

| |
|---|
| Coagulation cascade |
| Complement cascade (C5a) |
| Interleukins 1, 2, 4, 6, and 8 |
| Kinin cascade |
| Leukotrienes ($B_4$, $C_4$, $D_4$, $E_4$) |
| Macrophages |
| Angiogenesis factor |
| Macrophage-derived growth factor |
| Neutrophils and their proteases |
| Cathepsins |
| Collagenase |
| Elastase |
| Oxygen radicals, lipid peroxides |
| Platelets |
| Platelet-activating factor |
| Prostaglandins |
| Thromboxane $A_2$ |
| Tumor necrosis factor $\alpha$ |

from neutrophils, mononuclear cells, platelets, and endothelial cells (Table 74-1). The complement cascade is activated, which further promotes granulocyte aggregation and activation. Neutrophils contain a number of proteolytic enzymes that can damage lung tissue. In addition, release of oxygen radicals by neutrophils promotes local tissue damage. Because neutrophil-derived proteases enzymatically activate the clotting cascade, patients with ARDS frequently demonstrate evidence of a consumptive coagulopathy.

Platelet-activating factor serves as an important mediator in the acute phase. It has a negative inotropic effect on the heart and induces platelet aggregation, bronchoconstriction, and pulmonary hypertension. Macrophages initiate the inflammatory process through mediators similar to those associated with neutrophils. In addition, they have a major regulatory effect on healing of the lung. Macrophage-derived growth factor stimulates fibroblast proliferation and subsequent deposition of collagen. Excessive fibrosis in the late stages of ARDS may ultimately prove lethal.

Through the action of these mechanisms, both endothelial and epithelial damage occur early in the evolution of acute lung injury. This damage leads to severe alveolar flooding and both dilution and underproduction of surfactant. The alveolar space becomes filled with proteinaceous fluid and an inflammatory exudate of platelets, red blood cells, and leukocytes. Obliteration of the alveolar airspace causes shunting (perfusion of unventilated alveoli) and progressive hypoxemia; the latter condition responds poorly to oxygen therapy. Impaired surfactant activity results in the collapse of alveoli, loss of functional residual capacity, and decreased pulmonary compliance. Microvascular thrombosis contributes to the elevated pulmonary vascular resistance commonly seen in patients with ARDS. It also increases ventilation of dead space by creating areas of ventilated, but poorly perfused, lung.

After five to seven days, the process enters an organizing, or subacute, phase during which the airspaces become filled with granulation tissue. Neutrophils are gradually replaced with lymphocytes and plasma cells; type II pneumocytes replace injured type I cells, resulting in a diffusion defect related to their increased cellular thickness. This granulation tissue may obliterate air sacs, perpetuating the shunting of the acute phase. Activated myofibroblasts migrate through gaps in the epithelial basement membrane from the interstitium to the airspace and secrete matrix elements.

Finally, approximately three weeks after it started, the process enters a fibrotic phase. Rapid deposition of collagen —particularly nonelastic type I—leads to a very stiff lung. Areas of lung may consolidate and no longer be recoverable. Mechanical ventilation becomes difficult, requiring high inflation pressures that can, in turn, cause barotrauma. At this point, mortality rates may exceed 80%, with death usually caused by multiple-organ dysfunction, hemodynamic instability, or sepsis.

## Diagnosis

Clinical manifestations of lung injury develop rapidly in patients who ultimately develop ARDS, usually appearing within 24 hours of occurrence of the inciting factor. Initially, the patient experiences dyspnea, tachypnea, anxiety, and tachycardia. She soon becomes hypoxemic, as determined by pulse oximetry, and cyanotic. On auscultation, inspiratory crackles over both lung fields may be present. Although the chest X ray may be normal during the initial stages of injury, characteristic, diffuse, bilateral alveolar infiltrates—similar to those seen in congestive heart failure—soon develop while the heart is of normal size. Some authorities believe that the densities seen in ARDS tend to be more patchy and peripheral and less gravitationally oriented than those seen in heart failure, but this supposition is controversial. As alveolar filling continues, the radiographic changes progress until both lung fields may exhibit almost total white-out.

Measurement of gas exchange is essential for two reasons: to make the diagnosis and to care for patients with ARDS. Initially, hypoxemia is associated with respiratory alkalosis. The hypoxemia may prove relatively resistant to correction with oxygen by face mask, and intubation becomes necessary. No hemodynamic profile is diagnostic of ARDS, but a low PCWP (18 mm Hg or less) and high cardiac output in the presence of pulmonary edema is characteristic. If the $Pao_2/Fio_2$ ratio is equal to or less than 200, a diagnosis of ARDS can be made.

## TREATMENT

Management of ARDS has three goals:

- Establishing adequate tissue perfusion and oxygen delivery to prevent metabolic acidosis
- Identifying the source of infection and instituting appropriate antibiotic therapy
- Supporting and limiting damage to other involved organ systems

Unfortunately, few well-controlled clinical trials have supported the use of many of the current methods employed to treat ARDS. Placement of a flow-directed pulmonary artery catheter may prove helpful for fluid management when ARDS complicates sepsis. Fluid restriction and diuretics are advocated for treating the pulmonary edema of ARDS to keep the wedge pressure as low as possible while maintaining satisfactory oxygen delivery and urine output. This strategy, however, often cannot be used when the patient suffers from sepsis. Instead, volume expansion may be necessary to counteract the effects of vasodilation and extravasation of fluid into the extravascular compartment. The use of colloid generally is avoided in ARDS because it may exacerbate fluid leakage into the lungs, but blood products should be administered to keep the hematocrit above 30 (to improve oxygen-carrying capacity) and to correct any coagulopathy present.

## Mechanical Ventilation

Mechanical ventilation usually is required to improve oxygenation but has the potential to cause additional lung injury. Animal studies indicate that high peak airway pressures and overdistention because of large tidal volumes cause pulmonary injury (barotrauma) similar to that of ARDS.

Currently, most authorities recommend initiating treatment with a volume-cycled mechanical ventilator in the assist-control mode using an $Fio_2$ rate of 1.0 until it is clear that a lower value will provide adequate oxygenation. The lung volume that can be aerated in patients with ARDS is small. A low tidal volume of 6 to 10 mL/kg body weight will prevent overdistention and improve hemodynamics.

Positive end-expiratory pressure (PEEP) helps keep alveoli open and increases the functional residual capacity. On the other hand, PEEP increases intrathoracic pressure and the risk of barotrauma and, by impeding venous return, can decrease cardiac output. PEEP therefore is used routinely at low settings (5 cm $H_2O$). It can be increased by small increments of 3 to 5 cm $H_2O$ to a maximum of 15 cm $H_2O$ as necessary, while monitoring the effect that each increment has on oxygen delivery (cardiac output times the oxygen content of arterial blood).

The goal is to maintain arterial oxygen saturation at 0.9 or more using a nontoxic $Fio_2$ of 0.6 or less and acceptable peak inspiratory pressures of 40 cm $H_2O$ or less to prevent complications. Serial monitoring of arterial blood gases is essential; it is facilitated by placement of an arterial line. Because the ARDS patient has increased physiologic dead space and small aerated lung volumes, high ventilatory rates (more than 20 to 25 breaths/minute) may be necessary to eliminate carbon dioxide and maintain a normal pH. This action may result in intrathoracic gas trapping ("auto-PEEP") and excessive peak airway pressures.

Alternatively, the patient may undergo inverse-ratio ventilation (IRV), a technique that reverses the normal inspiratory-to-expiratory ratio and prolongs inspiration. With IRV, the increased inspiratory time increases mean airway pressures while maintaining acceptable peak pressures and improves alveolar recruitment. In this way, IRV reduces PEEP levels and decreases the ventilatory rate. This technique has not been tested in a prospective, randomized trial, however.

Cardiac performance may be impaired and the shortened expiratory phase also can cause auto-PEEP. In this situation, the preferred strategy relies on pressure-controlled ventilation and permissive hypercapnia. Tidal volume and respiratory rate are lowered to ensure that safe peak airway pressures are not exceeded, and the $Paco_2$ level is allowed to rise gradually. In the absence of intracranial lesions, levels below 100 mm Hg usually are well tolerated, and intravenous sodium bicarbonate can be used to correct marked acidosis ($pH < 7.25$). Alternatively, extracorporeal $CO_2$ removal has shown promise in several European centers, although no survival advantage was demonstrated in a recent study sponsored by the National Institutes of Health.

Because the lung is not uniformly affected by ARDS, repositioning the patient in the lateral decubitus or even the prone position may help in treating refractory hypoxemia. Most patients require at least 10 to 14 days of mechanical ventilation. Given that terminal airways remain unstable for long periods, once the patient shows improvement, weaning should take place slowly with PEEP being reduced by only 2 to 3 cm $H_2O$ every 12 hours.

## Other Therapeutic Considerations

ARDS patients often require paralysis or heavy sedation, particularly when the treatment involves unconventional ventilation techniques. In the presence of sepsis, until the causative organisms are identified, the patient should receive empiric coverage using a broad-spectrum antibiotic regimen (see Chapter 80). Pneumocystis infection should be treated empirically in the patient with AIDS presenting with infiltrates and ARDS. The patient's prognosis is directly related to finding, and then eradicating, the source of infection; at times this effort may require surgical intervention. Prompt curettage of infected uterine contents, debridement for necrotizing fasciitis, drainage of an abscess, or placement of stents to drain the urinary tract may save the patient's life.

Nosocomial pneumonia is a common complication that may arise after treatment of the initial source of sepsis. Catheter-related infections also can prove life-threatening. Early institution of enteral nutrition helps to maintain bowel integrity. Administration of sucralfate may prevent the development of stress-related gastrointestinal bleeding. Patients should also receive prophylaxis against deep venous thrombosis.

Corticosteroids offer no benefit in the acute phase of ARDS. Although they may help reduce pulmonary fibrosis in the late stages of the process, their use is controversial and all infection must be eliminated before their administration.

Additional agents that offer theoretical benefits have been used with varying degrees of success in small series of patients. These drugs include exogenous surfactant, antioxidants, nitric oxide, perfluorocarbon liquid ventilation, vasoactive agents, ketoconazole, ibuprofen, prostaglandin E, pentoxifylline, anti-endotoxin, and anticytokine therapy. Until additional information about their benefits becomes available, their use should be considered investigational.

## ARDS in Pregnancy

Infections associated with the development of ARDS in pregnancy include pyelonephritis, chorioamnionitis, endometritis, septic abortion, and pneumonia. When preterm labor occurs in association with infection, the use of tocolytic agents further predisposes the patient to pulmonary edema. Physiologic changes of pregnancy affect the development of ARDS in several ways:

1. Anemia slightly reduces oxygen delivery.
2. The fall in albumin concentration decreases osmotic pressure.
3. Uterine compression of the inferior vena cava can reduce venous return and, hence, cardiac output.
4. Functional residual capacity and extrathoracic lung compliance are reduced in late pregnancy.
5. Selective distribution of blood flow may preserve flow to some organs at the expense of others, thereby increasing the pregnant woman's vulnerability to multiple-organ dysfunction syndrome.

Delivery will not necessarily facilitate management of ARDS. In the absence of fetal distress or an intrauterine infectious process, the pregnancy remote from term should be allowed to continue. If delivery is indicated, vaginal delivery is preferred and often gives successful results in mechanically ventilated women. Cesarean section should be reserved for the usual obstetric indications.

## Suggested Readings

Demling RH. Adult respiratory distress syndrome: current concepts. New Horizons 1993;1:388–401.

Kollef MH, Schuster DP. The acute respiratory distress syndrome. N Eng J Med 1995;332:27–37.

Levy PC, Utell MJ, Sickel JZ, et al. The acute respiratory distress syndrome: current trends in pathogenesis and management. Compr Ther 1995;21:438–444.

Mabie WC, Barton JR, Sibai BM. Adult respiratory distress syndrome in pregnancy. Am J Obstet Gynecol 1992; 167(4 Pt 1):950–957.

Marinelli WA, Ingbar DH. Diagnosis and management of acute lung injury. Clin Chest Med 1994;15:517–546.

Sessler CN, Bloomfield GL, Fowler AA III. Current concepts of sepsis and acute lung injury. Clin Chest Med 1996;17:213–235.

CHAPTER

# 75

# *Osteomyelitis Pubis*

*Udo B. Hoyme*

## Background and Incidence

Osteomyelitis of the pubis is a rare but serious infection that can result from bacteremia or occur secondary to a contiguous focus of infection. Parenteral drug abuse and insulin-dependent diabetes have been described as predisposing conditions for bacteremia-related pubis infection. Most cases, however, have arisen after surgical procedures, such as bladder resection, urethral suspension, herniorrhaphy, pelvic exenteration, or radical vulvectomy. On rare occasions, they have originated after obstetric procedures, such as forceps or complicated delivery. In addition, a few cases have been seen following small bowel fistula, renal transplantation, or hematoma around the femoral artery after cardiac catheterization.

## Pathophysiology

Most cases of postoperative infection arise in an area of surgical trauma that becomes contaminated with bacteria. In vesicourethral suspension, the exposed retropubic space can be traumatized by electrocoagulation or during placement of suture into the periosteal space behind the symphysis. Also, pelvic exenteration or radical vulvectomy can injure the os pubis through the pressure of retractors, direct trauma of sharp dissection, or use of electrocautery for hemostasis. Long operation time, a possibly large blood loss, and frequent contamination of the wound and retropubic space by urine may affect the local environment of the symphysis as well.

Besides trauma and impaired blood circulation, irradiation may deprive the bone or synchondrosis of vascular supply. This effect is most prominent after a patient receives high-dose, poorly fractionated, or repeated courses of low-energy radiation.

Most patients enrolled in recent studies of osteomyelitis pubis received perioperative antibiotics that showed activity against the facultative and part of the anaerobic bacterial flora. Despite receiving these agents, all patients who developed osteomyelitis of the pubis initially had a postoperative wound infection. Regardless of whether infection of the bone or necrosis occurs first, postoperative osteomyelitis of the pubis results in an infected necrotic area of the pubic bone at the interpubic disk.

Several teams of investigators have suggested that a noninfectious inflammatory process—osteitis pubis—may have pathogenic, clinical, and radiologic characteristics identical to those of osteomyelitis of the pubis. Osteitis pubis has been described as a self-limited disease of unknown etiology that occurs after pelvic surgery or trauma, vigorous physical exercise, or childbirth. Some have attributed it to unrecognized anaerobic infection, although its actual source remains uncertain.

## Etiology

Documentation of an infectious process in a woman suspected of having osteitis pubis by blood culture or by culture of a bone biopsy specimen or aspirate allows specific treatment. In most cases, bacteria recovered from the bone infection have been previously isolated from wound and soft tissue infections. In approximately one-half of all such patients, multiple bacterial species cause the infection.

*Staphylococcus aureus* is present in 60% of these infections. Gram-negative bacteria account for some 40% of the cases, half of them in mixed infections with *Pseudomonas aeruginosa* predominating. In a few case reports, *Streptococcus anginosus*, *Streptococcus agalactiae*, or *Mycobacterium tuberculosis* has been seen. Anaerobes are rarely isolated in these infections but must be considered potential pathogens, especially in chronic bone infections secondary to contiguous septic foci. Use of suboptimal anaerobic transport and culture techniques in published reports may explain the rarity of anaerobic isolates.

## Diagnosis

Symptoms related to osteomyelitis pubis do not usually appear until at least eight weeks after the initial procedure, and it can take several months and an aggressive approach to establish the correct diagnosis. The manifestations of the disease are frequently very subtle and commonly first attributed to wound infection. Extensive destruction of the bones may occur without obvious external signs of bone infection.

Pelvic bone tenderness and pain, avoidance of ambulation, pain of the adductor muscles, and severe pain on abduction are typical of osteomyelitis of the pubis. Many patients have drainage from the wound or from a fistula. In addition, low-grade fever, moderate leukocytosis, an increased erythrocyte sedimentation rate, and elevated alkaline phosphatase may be present.

An X ray or computed tomographic scan of the pubic bone often shows rarefaction, erosion, osteolytic lesions, or irregularities of the bone margins with separation of the symphysis. These abnormalities can be misdiagnosed as metastasis from malignancy.

Later in the course of the disease, evidence of bone repair becomes apparent, with new bone formation from the periosteum or sclerosis of the symphysis. Further evidence of these changes appears in the form of increased activity in the gallium scan.

## Treatment

Various methods have been recommended for therapy of noninfectious osteitis pubis, including bed rest, immobilization in a spica body cast, irradiation, vitamin B, antibiotics, diathermy, surgical debridement, and injection of local anesthetic, adrenocorticotrophic hormone, or cortisone. Classic noninfectious osteitis pubis should be self-limiting, however, and the effectiveness of these measures is uncertain.

Start treatment of the lesion early in the course of infectious osteomyelitis with an antibiotic that has been selected according to antibiotic susceptibility data and its ability to concentrate in bone. Obtain an adequate culture before beginning therapy. If a causative organism cannot be identified in a patient with suspicious clinical findings, start empiric antibiotic treatment to cover both *S. aureus* and aerobic gram-negative bacteria. The minimum course of therapy is two to four weeks of IV antibiotics followed by oral antibiotics (for example, quinolones) for two to three additional weeks.

If blood flow to the bone is compromised, the antibiotic will not achieve a therapeutic level in the infected area. In these patients, effective treatment includes surgical decompression and evacuation of pus and infected tissue.

## Suggested Readings

Grace JN, Sim FH, Shives TC, et al. Wedge resection of the symphysis pubis for the treatment of osteitis pubis. J Bone Joint Surg [Am] 1989;71:358–364.

Hoyme UB, Tamimi HK, Eschenbach DA, et al. Osteomyelitis pubis after radical gynecologic operations. Obstet Gynecol 1984;63: 47S–53S.

Jenkins FH, Raff MJ, Florman LD, et al. Pubic osteomyelitis due to anaerobic bacteria. Arch Intern Med 1984;144:842–843.

Sexton DJ, Heskestad L, Lambeth WR, et al. Postoperative pubic osteomyelitis misdiagnosed as osteitis pubis: report of four cases and review. Clin Infect Dis 1993;17:695–700.

CHAPTER

# 76

# *Septic Pelvic Thrombophlebitis*

*Neil S. Silverman*

## Background and Incidence

Although the use of peripartum antibiotics, particularly after cesarean section, has decreased the incidence of postdelivery infection, the management of the patient with persistent febrile morbidity despite presumed adequate antimicrobial therapy remains problematic. In the absence of a clear source of infection, such as an infected hematoma or an abscess, the diagnosis of septic pelvic thrombophlebitis (SPT) is commonly made presumptively, with the majority of patients responding clinically to therapeutic anticoagulation plus antibiotics.

Septic pelvic thrombophlebitis has been reported to occur after approximately 1 in 2000 deliveries, with one recent series demonstrating a markedly higher rate after cesarean section than after vaginal delivery (0.24% versus 0.01%). Although the debate historically centered on medical versus surgical management of this condition, SPT is now treated medically almost exclusively, even in the infrequent case where imaging studies reveal the presence of a clot.

## Etiology

The conditions surrounding delivery, especially those related to obstetric surgery, meet the criteria commonly known as Virchow's triad for venous thrombosis: increased coagulability, altered venous integrity, and venous stasis. Even in the absence of surgery, pregnant women are at increased risk for venous thrombosis; the coexistence of pregnancy and the potential for an operative site infection place the pelvic venous anatomy particularly at risk. Moreover, in the face of post-delivery endometritis, a rate as high as 2% for SPT has been reported. It is unclear whether the currently accepted practice of administering antibiotics after cord clamping in cesarean section has, by decreasing the incidence of infected operative sites, also diminished the incidence of postcesarean SPT.

To date, studies have not found a typical, or even most common, bacteriologic agent that causes the infectious morbidity attributed to SPT. In addition, because patients who carry the diagnosis rarely have symptoms associated with clinical sepsis and commonly do not have a clot demonstrated on a variety of suggested diagnostic studies, some authors have suggested the name "enigmatic fever" for the clinical syndrome commonly described as SPT. In contrast, a clinically distinct postpartum syndrome, termed "ovarian vein thrombosis," although treated similarly, is associated with a very different symptom complex and demonstrable anatomic and radiologic abnormalities.

## Clinical Presentation and Diagnosis

With ovarian vein thrombosis, patients present with worsening abdominal or flank pain, spiking fevers, and general malaise, usually two to four days after delivery. A recent series of 11 patients treated for ovarian vein thrombosis after vaginal deliveries included no women who returned for care because of symptoms earlier than 72 hours postpartum.

In contrast with enigmatic fever, a palpable midabdominal mass commonly is present in 50% to 70% of SPT patients and more frequently is noted on the patient's right side, probably because of the dextrorotation of the gravid uterus. The most common misdiagnosis in this subset of patients is appendicitis, which reflects the severely ill appearance of many women with SPT. Because of the lateralizing symptoms common with ovarian vein thrombosis, the differential diagnosis also includes pyelonephritis, ureterolithiasis, broad ligament hematoma, ovarian torsion, and degenerating fibroid, along with pelvic abscess. The diagnosis is particularly difficult and often not considered in patients who have had vaginal deliveries, for whom the incidence of endometritis is much lower.

In patients with "enigmatic" SPT, an operative—usually abdominal—delivery almost always precedes their illness, with evidence of an antecedent chorioamnionitis or endometritis. These patients are rarely acutely ill; in fact, they usually remain clinically asymptomatic except for the impressive "picket fence" fever curve typical of the syndrome, with temperature peaks as high as 106 °F as well as episodic tachycardia. These patients may have been clinically ill with endometritis before receiving appropriate antibiotics to cover a polymicrobial pelvic infection; typically, those symptoms resolve but the febrile state persists.

For both subsets of patients, the diagnostic workup includes investigation of other sources of infection, including—especially in postoperative patients—the urinary and pulmonary systems. Urinalysis (urine culture) and chest X ray are, by definition, negative in patients given the diagnosis of SPT but are a required component of the evaluation of puerperal fever. Transabdominal or endovaginal sonography may reveal an infected, undrained collection but typically fails to show a pelvic clot in this clinical setting. In general, ventilation–perfusion scans are reserved for patients who exhibit evidence of pulmonary compromise; screening by measuring arterial blood gas levels or performing capillary pulse oximetry seems reasonable in the absence of such symptoms.

Small series have described the diagnosis of pelvic and ovarian vein thrombosis by means of ultrasound, computed X-ray tomography (CT), and magnetic resonance imaging (MRI). As yet, however, the sensitivity and specificity of these methods has not been proven in any controlled fashion to be better than clinical exclusionary diagnosis. In recent reports, the yield appears to be somewhat better for the diagnosis of ovarian vein thrombosis, where the criteria for diagnosis are (1) enlargement of the thrombosed vein, (2) a low-density lumen, and (3) a sharply defined vessel wall. An inflammatory reaction consisting of a dense mass surrounding a thrombosed ovarian vein has been described in one case report. Interestingly, in cases where CT has revealed venous thrombosis prior to instituting anticoagulation therapy for SPT, use of that same imaging modality in follow-up appears to be helpful in documenting resolution of the clot.

## Treatment

For more than 30 years, anticoagulation has served as the mainstay of treatment for SPT. It should be kept in mind, however, that no randomized clinical trials have been conducted to determine the optimal duration of therapy, the length of time that the combination of antibiotic therapy and anticoagulation should continue, or the length of time necessary to consider surgical management of the condition. Earlier studies also failed to distinguish between patients with ovarian vein thrombosis and enigmatic fever.

Nevertheless, all authors accept that once a diagnosis of SPT is entertained, intravenous heparin should be added to an adequate antibiotic treatment regimen in doses sufficient to achieve therapeutic anticoagulation with a partial thromboplastin time (PTT) of 1.5 to 2 times control values. As more experience is gained with the use of low-molecular-weight heparin for initial therapy of venous thrombosis in general, this approach may play a role in the treatment of SPT; at present, however, the use of intravenous heparin for this indication is preferred. Infusion of heparin is begun with a bolus of 2500 to 5000 U, followed by a maintenance infusion of 1000 U/hour, which is then titrated to reach the PTT target. Patients almost uniformly reach appropriate PTT levels within 24 to 36 hours of initiating therapy.

Antibiotic therapy, including anaerobic coverage, should continue along with IV heparin until the patient remains afebrile and clinically well for 48 hours. This recommendation is supported by retrospective review and experience rather than clinical trials. In the uncommon case of the patient who remains febrile despite therapeutic heparinization, consider a diagnosis of antibiotic drug fever and discontinue antibiotics while maintaining heparin administration. One group of investigators has recently reported a median time to defervescence after heparinization of five days for women with either ovarian vein thrombosis or SPT. In either case, heparin therapy should continue for a total of five to seven days of apyrexia.

In the absence of data supporting its use, conversion of patients to oral anticoagulation is not recommended, except in rare cases where pulmonary emboli or extension of clotting into the iliac veins or vena cava is demonstrated. In those patients, three to six months of treatment with warfarin sodium is recommended.

## Outcomes and Sequelae

Even when the diagnosis of SPT is made on clinical grounds alone, treatment with anticoagulation therapy has been reported to be successful in approximately 90% of cases. Surgical treatment is reserved for patients who fail to respond to heparin therapy (although no absolute endpoint for failure has been defined) or for women whose clinical course deteriorates despite therapeutic heparinization. Almost all of these patients will prove to have ovarian vein syndrome rather than enigmatic fever.

Operative techniques have consisted of ligation of one or both ovarian veins; ligation of the vena cava is reserved for cases where a clot is clearly demonstrated in that vessel. Patients who have had pulmonary emboli despite therapeutic anticoagulation also represent candidates for vena cava ligation. Published series have demonstrated that surgical cure can be achieved without excision of the involved vessel. Ligation, in conjunction with subsequently continuing heparinization, prevents clot propagation and allows the patient's thrombolytic system to resolve the problem. Patients receiving this therapy will require conversion to oral anticoagulation.

Recovery from SPT, once defervescence has occurred, takes place rapidly, and proceeds with few significant sequelae. Only one small recent series has evaluated the risk for subsequent pregnancies in the face of SPT in an index pregnancy. Among 29 patients successfully treated for SPT, 13 pregnancies were evaluated in nine women. None was found to have a recurrence of either SPT or any thromboembolic phenomena, and none received prophylactic anticoagulation with subsequent pregnancies.

## Suggested Readings

Brown CE, Lowe TW, Cunningham FG, et al. Puerperal pelvic thrombophlebitis: impact on diagnosis and treatment using x-ray computed tomography and magnetic resonance imaging. Obstet Gynecol 1986;68:789–794.

Collins CG. Suppurative pelvic thrombophlebitis. Am J Obstet Gynecol 1970;108:681–687.

Duff P, Gibbs RS. Pelvic vein thrombophlebitis: diagnostic dilemma and therapeutic challenge. Obstet Gynecol Surv 1983;38:365–373.

Dunnihoo DR, Gallaspy JW, Wise RB, et al. Postpartum ovarian vein thrombophlebitis: a review. Obstet Gynecol Surv 1991;46:415–427.

Gibbs RS, Jones PM, Wilder R. Antibiotic therapy of endometritis following cesarean section. Obstet Gynecol 1978;52:31–37.

Josey WE, Staggers SR Jr. Heparin therapy in septic pelvic thrombophlebitis: a study of 46 cases. Am J Obstet Gynecol 1974;120: 228–233.

Munsick RA, Gillanders LA. A review of the syndrome of puerperal ovarian vein thrombophlebitis. Obstet Gynecol Surv 1981;36:57–66.

Rozier JC Jr, Brown EH Jr, Berne FA. Diagnosis of puerperal ovarian vein thrombophlebitis by computed tomography. Am J Obstet Gynecol 1988;159:737–740.

Witlin AG, Mercer BM, Sibai BM. Septic pelvic thrombophlebitis or refractory postpartum fever of undetermined etiology. J Matern Fetal Med 1996;5:355–358.

Witlin AG, Sibai BM. Postpartum ovarian vein thrombosis after vaginal delivery: a report of 11 cases. Obstet Gynecol 1995;85: 775–780.

CHAPTER

# 77

# *Infections in the Oncology Patient*

*Paul Nyirjesy*
*W. David Hager*

## BACKGROUND AND INCIDENCE

Each year, gynecologic malignancies are diagnosed in more than 70,000 women in the United States. The majority of these women require surgery for staging or treatment of their cancer.

Postoperative febrile morbidity is common following most gynecologic procedures. In this situation, however, temperature does not correlate well with infection. In fact, an infectious etiology is documented in fewer than 30% of gynecologic patients with postoperative fever. Because the febrile morbidity rate is approximately 50% after radical surgery in gynecology, infectious morbidity is calculated as approximately 15%. Infection following radical vulvar procedures is significantly higher.

The etiology and techniques for diagnosis of postoperative infections are discussed elsewhere in this book (see Chapters 66 and 67). In both normal and immunocompromised women undergoing treatment for gynecologic malignancy, prevention is the key to minimizing infection-related morbidity. Many variables related to the disease process, coexisting disease, and treatment exist. The surgeon must attempt to alter or modify these associated variables, regardless of the degree of immunocompromise, in a manner that reduces infectious risk.

Each year, more than 4 million women—including the majority of those with gynecologic cancer—undergo a surgical procedure. Regardless of their preoperative immunologic status, the operative procedure adversely affects the host defenses of these patients. The trauma of incision itself interrupts multiple epithelial or mucosal barriers. Most gynecologic operations that require vaginal entry are associated with significant bacterial contamination. In fact, the unprepared vagina has as many as $10^9$ organisms per gram of vaginal fluid, with anaerobic organisms outnumbering aerobes by 10 to 1. Each sutured pedicle leaves necrotic tissue distal to the suture and forms a potential nidus for postoperative infection, at a time characterized by suppression of phagocytic activity. All of these factors combine to place the gynecologic cancer patient at risk for postoperative infection.

## Risk Factors and Preventive Measures

Many factors influence the risk of infection in a given patient. Cruse and Foord have described several risk factors for infection in surgery and detailed ways to alter these factors so as to decrease postoperative morbidity. Other textbooks also describe these factors in detail. This chapter lists these factors and applicable preventive measures.

A significant number of hospitalized women have evidence of an existing nutritional deficiency. At least 10% of women with early-stage endometrial or cervical cancer have abnormal nutritional parameters, for example. The need for adequate preoperative nutrition must be emphasized.

Older women, obese women, and women with coexisting medical illness such as diabetes are at increased risk of developing postoperative infection. For example, gynecologic cancer patients are typically older women. Obesity—a common finding among women with endometrial cancer—is associated with longer operative times, increased surgical blood loss, poor healing, and increased risk of surgical wound infection. Adequate control of ancillary medical illnesses is essential in operative patients. In addition, prolonged preoperative hospitalization increases the risk of postoperative infection.

The risk of surgical site infection, even in short operations such as appendectomy, increases linearly with surgical exposure. The experienced surgeon strives to decrease manipulation of tissue and operative time.

Preoperative patient preparation is important in minimizing both intraoperative and postoperative morbidity. Most patients can tolerate mechanical bowel preparation with liquids and cathartics and compliant patients can complete this step at home. In contrast with bowel preparation, preoperative douching has not been shown to have a significant benefit in reducing postoperative infection. Removal of hair from the operative site is preferred by most surgeons. As compared with shaving, clipping of hair or use of a depilatory is associated with lower wound infection rates.

Electrocautery used in the cutting mode to maintain intraoperative hemostasis is associated with significant thermal damage and a potential increase in wound culture media. It also has an adverse effect on wound healing strength. Suture material should be of the smallest caliber possible for the procedure at hand. Because suture materials vary in terms of their reactivity, the least reactive material should be used (see Chapter 72). To avoid tissue necrosis, sutures should not be tightly cinched down.

Intraoperative irrigation of the abdomen or incision theoretically decreases the amount of necrotic tissue, fibrin, and other materials that can potentially serve as culture media. Any irrigation fluid placed into the abdomen or pelvis should be removed in its entirety, as excess intra-abdominal fluid may interfere with normal macrophage function. If the surgeon deems that a drain would decrease the amount of residual fluid in or near the operative site, closed suction drains should always be employed.

Antibiotic prophylaxis to prevent postoperative infectious morbidity is discussed in Chapters 68 and 69 of this book. The antibiotic selected should be an agent that would not be used to treat serious infections. It should have a low toxicity and low cost, and it should be given in a single dose. If operative time extends beyond two hours, the dose should be repeated.

## ETIOLOGY

Like most pelvic infections, those occurring in oncology patients are polymicrobial in origin. Many cancer patients are immunocompromised because of their disease or the effects of chemotherapy on neutrophils. Approximately 80% of organisms responsible for neutropenic infection are a part of the endogenous human flora, and almost 50% of cancer-related infections involve hospital-acquired organisms. The latter tend to have been selected out by antibiotic pressure for their virulence and resistance.

Within several days of hospitalization, the normal skin and mucosal flora may shift from penicillin-sensitive, coagulase-negative staphylococci and *Corynebacteria* to methicillin-resistant *Staphylococcus epidermidis*, as well as other resistant organisms. For patients in intensive-care units, the flora may reflect an increase in resistant aerobic gram-negative bacilli such as *Pseudomonas* species or other nosocomial pathogens. These changes in flora increase the risk and severity of infections and suggest that decreasing the frequency and duration of hospitalization may confer a benefit on preoperative patients and patients receiving chemotherapy.

## Treatment

Success in treating any infection can be correlated with index of suspicion, rapidity of diagnosis, appropriate antibiotic therapy, and timely use of surgical or percutaneous drainage. Depending on the extent or location of the infection, other system support—such as mechanical ventilation, vasopressor administration, hyperalimentation, or transfusion—may play a crucial role. The clinician must evaluate each process and the given clinical situation before instituting appropriate treatment. In cases such as those involving postoperative abdominal wound infection, simple drainage may be the only treatment necessary. In other instances, such as soft tissue infections in neutropenic patients, extensive debridement, antibiotic treatment, and other support may be necessary and life-saving.

The availability of a variety of antibiotics sometimes makes treatment decisions difficult or almost impossible, as each new drug or drug combination offers potential or reported benefits. Antibiotic therapy for intra-abdominal infection in the postoperative patient should be directed toward the mixed pattern of pathogens usually present. Anaerobic bacteria alone or in combination with aerobes will be isolated in approximately 88% of infections. Rarely is there an initial need for drugs directed toward enterococci or *Pseudomonas* sp., unless the patient has been in the intensive-care unit or is neutropenic. The physician should not reinstitute therapy with a drug given for prior, recent prophylaxis. Fortunately, fungal, viral, and protozoan infections are rare in this patient population.

The gold standard regimen for antibiotic coverage of postoperative intra-abdominal infection combines an aminoglycoside (gentamicin, 1.5 mg/kg IV every 8 hours) with clindamycin (900 mg IV every 8 hours) or metronidazole (500 mg IV every 6 hours). Although extremely successful, this regimen requires multiple drug administrations and has significant potential toxicity. More recently, aminoglycosides have been given in large doses at extended intervals. For example, a woman with normal renal function can receive 5 to 7 mg/kg daily. Such an approach is less expensive because it entails fewer administration costs and because only serum trough levels need to be obtained. In studies of different populations, clinical outcomes have been equivalent. In animal studies, the ototoxicity and nephrotoxicity of the aminoglycosides have been less severe.

In part because of concerns about aminoglycoside toxicity, monotherapy with broad-spectrum antibiotics has become a popular option in oncology patients. Monotherapy proponents cite the advantages of decreased toxicity, lower cost, and less need for drug toxicity monitoring. Unfortunately, the majority of the studies of these single-agent treatments involve only small numbers of patients and fail to report their diagnostic criteria for patient inclusion or even drug failure. In many cases, they intermix patients with multiple diagnoses and coexisting illness. Despite these shortcomings, most reports suggest that treatment of a postoperative intra-abdominal infection with a single broad-spectrum antibiotic or a combination is successful approximately 90% of the time. Additional drugs and surgical or percutaneous drainage are rarely necessary.

At this time, no single antibiotic or drug combination appears to be ultimately superior for broad-spectrum (aerobic and anaerobic) coverage. The choice of drug or drug regimen must be guided by local antibiotic sensitivities, local and reported experience, and potential toxicities. Culture results should guide the antibiotic treatment of specific infections (pulmonary or urinary infections, for example).

Antibiotic selection and treatment principles change dramatically in the febrile neutropenic patient (polymorphonuclear [PMN] leukocytes < 500/mm$^3$). In these cases, the infecting pathogens differ because of the patient's antecedent hospitalization, and unusual problems such as perineal soft tissue infections become more common. If the neutrophil count is less than 100/mm$^3$, 20% or more of febrile epsiodes will have an associated bacteremia. Most importantly, higher mortality is observed when the start of antibiotic therapy is delayed to search for the cause of the fever. Evaluation of these patients should be thorough, with attention paid to all potential infectious sites. Because the lack of an inflammatory response may mask the signs of an infection, however, most febrile neutropenic patients will have no localized findings. Empirical therapy therefore serves as the standard of care for such patients.

In selecting antimicrobial therapy for febrile neutropenic patients with no clear or suspected source of infection, the clinician should choose drugs that are bactericidal, synergistic, and of low toxicity. The spectrum of antibacterial activity should cover gram-positive and gram-negative organisms, including more resistant nosocomial gram-negative bacilli such as *Pseudomonas*. The current trend calls for single-drug therapy with third-generation cephalosporins such as ceftazidime or carbapenems, although many clinicians prefer to combine these agents with an aminoglycoside. Some 40% to 50% of patients may require later modification of their antibiotics to fully resolve their fever. In many cases, this step will involve the addition of vancomycin to treat a suspected methicillin-resistant *Staphylococcus aureus* infection. Beginning vancomycin earlier in the febrile course does not seem to affect survival rates, however, and it may contribute to the emergence of vancomycin-resistant enterococcal strains.

If a site of infection is found or a culture permits identification of the infecting organism, antibiotic therapy can be tailored to suit the agent's susceptibility profile. Even if the patient defervesces, antibiotic therapy should generally continue until the neutropenia resolves completely. Discontinuing antibiotics earlier results in a recrudescence of fever (40%) and hypotension (12%) in a significant number of patients.

Evaluation and treatment of fungal infections continue to be problematic in granulocytopenic patients. Although they occasionally occur as primary infections, these infections commonly are seen in persistently febrile granulocytopenic patients. Amphotericin B remains the drug of choice, despite the availability of a number of antifungal medications. Although its toxicity prohibits empiric use, early therapy with this agent is essential in patients who are persistently febrile and granulocytopenic despite four to seven days of antibiotic treatment or who have a positive blood culture for fungi.

## Suggested Readings

Cruse PJ, Foord R. A five-year prospective study of 23,649 surgical wounds. Arch Surg 1973;107:206–210.

Cunningham FG, Gilstrap LC III, Kappus SS. Cefamandole for treatment of obstetrical and gynecological infections. Scand J Infect Dis 1980;25(suppl):75–82.

Deitch EA. Infection in the compromised host. Surg Clin North Am 1988;68:181–187.

Orr JW Jr. Sutures and closures. Ala J Med Sci 1986;23:36–41.

Orr JW Jr, Shingleton HM. Importance of nutritional assessment and support in surgical and cancer patients. J Reprod Med 1984;29: 635–650.

Orr JW Jr, Taylor PT. Reducing postoperative infection in the patient with gynecologic cancer. Infect Surg 1987;12:666–675.

Pizzo PA. Management of fever in patients with cancer and treatment-induced neutropenia. N Engl J Med 1993;328:1323–1332.

Shapiro M, Munoz A, Tager IB, et al. Risk factors for infection at the operative site after abdominal or vaginal hysterectomy. N Engl J Med 1982;307:1661–1666.

CHAPTER

# 78

# *Prevention of Bacterial Endocarditis*

*Philip B. Mead*

## Background

Bacterial endocarditis continues to cause serious morbidity and mortality despite advances in diagnosis and treatment. Because of this fact, prevention remains the most important goal. No randomized, controlled trials have as yet established the efficacy of endocarditis prophylaxis definitively, but most authorities agree that prophylaxis should be offered to susceptible patients during procedures known to be associated with bacteremia. In 1997, the American Heart Association (AHA) published its updated guidelines for prevention of bacterial endocarditis. Although these recommendations are specific and authoritative, they have not resolved all controversy about when to employ prophylaxis.

## Individuals at Risk

Endocarditis usually affects individuals with underlying structural cardiac defects who develop bacteremia with organisms likely to cause endocarditis. Certain cardiac conditions are more commonly associated with the occurrence of endocarditis—and poorer outcomes—than others. Table 78-1 stratifies cardiac conditions into high- and moderate-risk categories.

**Table 78-1.** AHA Risk Stratification of Cardiac Conditions Associated with Endocarditis

**Endocarditis Prophylaxis Recommended**

***High-Risk Category***

Prosthetic cardiac valves, including bioprosthetic and homograft valves
Previous bacterial endocarditis
Complex cyanotic congenital heart disease (e.g., single-ventricle states, transposition of the great arteries, tetralogy of Fallot)
Surgically constructed systemic pulmonary shunts or conduits

***Moderate-Risk Category***

Most other congenital cardiac malformations (other than those listed above and below)
Acquired valvar dysfunction (e.g., rheumatic heart disease)
Hypertrophic cardiomyopathy
Mitral valve prolapse with valvar regurgitation and/or thickened leaflets

**Endocarditis Prophylaxis Not Recommended**

***Negligible-Risk Category (Risk No Greater Than That of the General Population)***

Isolated secundum atrial septum defect
Surgical repair of atrial septal defect, ventricular septal defect, or patent ductus arteriosus (without residua beyond 6 months)
Previous coronary artery bypass graft surgery
Mitral valve prolapse without valvar regurgitation
Physiologic, functional, or innocent heart murmurs
Previous Kawasaki disease without valvar dysfunction
Previous rheumatic fever without valvar dysfunction
Cardiac pacemakers (intravascular and epicardial) and implanted defibrillators

SOURCE: Dajani AS, Taubert KA, Wilson WW, et al. Prevention of bacterial endocarditis. JAMA 1997;277:1795.

Mitral valve prolapse deserves special mention because it is common and because the need for prophylaxis for this condition continues to inspire controversy. The AHA has developed a clinical algorithm for determining the need for prophylaxis in patients with suspected mitral valve prolapse (see Dajani in Suggested Readings list).

Although endocarditis may develop in any individual, including persons with no underlying cardiac defect, the negligible-risk category encompasses cardiac conditions in which the risk of developing endcarditis is not higher than that of the general population.

## Risk Related to Surgical Procedure

Bacteremia is known to be associated with certain surgical procedures; consequently, antimicrobial prophylaxis is recommended for individuals with underlying structural cardiac defects undergoing these procedures. Table 78-2 lists the AHA recommendations for endocarditis prophylaxis by surgical procedure. Note that endocarditis prophylaxis is optional for high-risk patients undergoing vaginal delivery and that, in the absence of infection, it is not recommended for patients delivering by cesarean section.

Because only 1% to 5% of patients develop bacteremia after a vaginal delivery, the AHA does not recommend prophylaxis for normal vaginal delivery except as an option for patients with high-risk cardiac conditions. The recommendations also state, "If an unanticipated bacteremia is suspected during vaginal delivery, intravenous antibiotics can be administered at that time." The American College of Obstetricians and Gynecologists (ACOG) advises that susceptible patients who are febrile at delivery, and therefore already potentially bacteremic, should receive endocarditis prophylaxis.

Boggess and coworkers have recently reported on bacteremia during cesarean delivery. They detected bacteremia in 14% of women undergoing cesarean section after labor or rupture of membranes compared with 0% of women not in labor. Many of the isolates were capable of causing endocarditis. These investigators concluded that women who deliver by cesarean section after labor or rupture of membranes are at an intermediate risk of bacteremia. They departed from the AHA guidelines in recommending that these women be considered for endocarditis prophylaxis if they have predisposing cardiac conditions.

Bacteremia has not been detected after cervical biopsy or manipulation of an IUD in the absence of obvious infections. The AHA recommends the administration of endocarditis

**Table 78-2.** AHA Recommendations for Endocarditis Prophylaxis in Susceptible Patients by Surgical Procedure

**Endocarditis Prophylaxis Recommended**

***Respiratory Tract***
Tonsillectomy and/or adenoidectomy
Surgical operations that involve respiratory mucosa
Bronchoscopy with a rigid bronchoscope

***Gastrointestinal Tract****
Sclerotherapy for esophageal varices
Esophageal stricture dilation
Endoscopic retrograde cholangiography with biliary obstruction
Biliary tract surgery
Surgical operations that involve intestinal mucosa

***Genitourinary Tract***
Cystocopy
Urethral dilation

**Endocarditis Prophylaxis Not Recommended**

***Respiratory Tract***
Endotracheal intubation
Bronchoscopy with a flexible bronchoscope, with or without biopsy†
Tympanostomy tube insertion

***Gastrointestinal Tract***
Transesophageal echocardiography†
Endoscopy with or without gastrointestinal biopsy†

***Genitourinary Tract***
Vaginal hysterectomy†
Vaginal delivery†
Cesarean section
In uninfected tissue:
  Urethral catheterization
  Uterine dilatation and curettage
  Therapeutic abortion
  Sterilization procedures
  Insertion or removal of intrauterine devices

***Other***
Cardiac catheterization, including balloon angioplasty
Implanted cardiac pacemakers, implanted defibrillators, and coronary stents
Incision or biopsy of surgically scrubbed skin

* Prophylaxis is recommended for high-risk patients; optional for medium-risk patients.
† Prophylaxis is optional for high-risk patients.
SOURCE: Dajani AS, Taubert KA, Wilson WW, et al. Prevention of bacterial endocarditis. JAMA 1997;277:1797.

prophylaxis after removal of an infected IUD as well as for other genitourinary procedures where infection is present.

## Antimicrobial Regimens for Endocarditis Prophylaxis

Organisms isolated from obstetric and gynecologic patients with infective endocarditis are similar to those that cause endocarditis in other patient groups. Viridans streptococci are the most common culprits, followed by enterococci, *Staphylococcus aureus*, and group B streptococci. Table 78-3 lists the current AHA recommendations for susceptible individuals undergoing genitourinary or gastrointestinal procedures.

If a patient is already taking an antibiotic normally used for endocarditis prophylaxis, a drug from a different class should be selected. In particular, antibiotic regimens used to prevent the recurrence of acute rheumatic fever are inadequate for the prevention of bacterial endocarditis.

Incision and drainage or other procedures involving infected tissues may result in bacteremia involving the same organism that caused the initial infection. In individuals at risk for endocarditis, it is advisable to administer antimicrobial prophylaxis before the procedure. Prophylaxis should be directed at the pathogen that is most likely to cause the infection.

## Summary

The AHA has provided guidelines for the use of endocarditis prophylaxis. According to these guidelines, the clinician should consider the degree to which the patient's underlying cardiac condition creates a risk for endocarditis (see Table 78-1), as well as the apparent risk of bacteremia with the proposed procedure (see Table 78-2), before deciding whether to institute endocarditis prophylaxis. These guidelines are not intended as the standard of care or as a substitute for clinical judgment. Moreover, controversy persists over the use of endocarditis prophylaxis in susceptible women undergoing cesarean section after labor.

**Table 78-3.** AHA Prophylactic Regimens for Susceptible Patients Undergoing Genitourinary or Gastrointestinal Procedures

| Situation | Agents* | Regimen† |
|---|---|---|
| High-risk patients | Ampicillin plus gentamicin | Adults: Ampicillin, 2 g IM or IV, plus gentamicin, 1.5 mg/kg (not to exceed 120 mg) within 30 minutes of starting the procedure; 6 hours later, ampicillin, 1 g IM/IV, or amoxicillin, 1 g orally |
| | | Children: Ampicillin, 50 mg/kg IM or IV (not to exceed 2 g), plus gentamicin, 1.5 mg/kg within 30 minutes of starting the procedure; 6 hours later, ampicillin, 25 mg/kg IM/IV, or amoxicillin, 25 mg/kg orally |
| High-risk patients allergic to ampicillin/ amoxicillin | Vancomycin plus gentamicin | Adults: Vancomycin, 1 g IV over 1 to 2 hours, plus gentamicin, 1.5 mg/kg IV/IM (not to exceed 120 mg); complete injection/infusion within 30 minutes of starting the procedure |
| | | Children: Vancomycin, 20 mg/kg IV over 1 to 2 hours, plus gentamicin, 1.5 mg/kg IV/IM; complete injection/infusion within 30 minutes of starting the procedure |
| Moderate-risk patients | Amoxicillin or ampicillin | Adults: Amoxicillin, 2 g orally 1 hour before procedure, or ampicillin, 2 g IM/IV within 30 minutes of starting the procedure |
| | | Children: Amoxicillin, 50 mg/kg orally 1 hour before procedure, or ampicillin, 50 mg/kg IM/IV within 30 minutes of starting the procedure |
| Moderate-risk patients allergic to ampicillin/ amoxicillin | Vancomycin | Adults: Vancomycin, 1 g IV over 1 to 2 hours; complete infusion within 30 minutes of starting the procedure |
| | | Children: Vancomycin, 20 mg/kg IV over 1 to 2 hours; complete infusion within 30 min of starting the procedure |

* Total children's dose should not exceed the adult dose.

† No second dose of vancomycin or gentamicin is recommended.

Source: Dajani AS, Taubert KA, Wilson WW, et al. Prevention of bacterial endocarditis. JAMA 1997;277:1799.

## Suggested Readings

American College of Obstetricians and Gynecologists. Antimicrobial therapy for obstetric patients. Educational Bulletin No. 245. March 1998.

Boggess KA, Watts DH, Hillier SL, et al. Bacteremia shortly after placental separation during cesarean delivery. Obstet Gynecol 1996;87:779–784.

Dajani AS, Taubert KA, Wilson W, et al. Prevention of bacterial endocarditis. Recommendations by the American Heart Association. JAMA 1997;277:1794–1801.

Payne DG, Fishburne JI, Rufty AJ, et al. Bacterial endocarditis in pregnancy. Obstet Gynecol 1982;60:247–252.

CHAPTER

# 79

# *Toxic Shock Syndrome*

*Roger Bawdon*

## Background and Incidence

During the peak of the toxic shock syndrome (TSS) outbreak in 1980, the case rate was 3 for every 100,000 menstruating women; in California, this rate reached 9.1 for every 100,000. Women with TSS who had used high-absorbency tampons had a recurrence rate as high as 30%. Even after removing certain brands of tampons from the market, some states reported no change in the TSS case rate. Subsequent studies have shown no difference exists in the amount of toxic shock syndrome toxin (TSST) produced in cotton or rayon tampons.

Because other diseases mimic TSS, as many as 53% of reported cases did not meet the criteria for TSS, suggesting marked overdiagnosis. Clinicians probably failed to uncover cases of TSS because they tried to relate TSS to menstruation and tampon use. Menstrual-related TSS, however, is merely one aspect of this clinically challenging disease. Other manifestations of the disease or similar diseases include postoperative TSS and streptococcal toxic shock syndrome (STSS).

Recent data indicate that the incidence of menstruation-associated TSS is about 1 case per 1 million women and of postoperative TSS about 0.7 cases per million U.S. women. Because of the failure to apply the strict definition of TSS, STSS, although uncommon, may be confused with staphylococcal TSS, which was prevalent between 1987 and 1989. Even when strict guidelines are followed during taking of the patient history, physical examination, and evaluation of preliminary laboratory data, the initial differentiation between TSS and STSS may be clinically challenging.

Although fewer cases have been noted since 1980, both menstrual and nonmenstrual cases continue to be reported. They may be associated with vaginal infections, vaginal delivery, cesarean section, spontaneous abortion, diaphragm use, postpartum endometritis, $CO_2$ laser treatment of condyloma acuminatum, complications of salpingitis, or any surgical or accidental tissue trauma. Generally, STSS is more related to trauma or underlying disease; if a patient does not have a rash or skin lesions postinfection, however, she does not meet the strict definition of a TSS case. Although most cases of STSS do not involve the pelvic cavity, neither do some cases of postoperative TSS.

## ETIOLOGY

TSS is caused by a microbial infection or colonization with bacteriophage-specific strains of *Staphylococcus aureus* in a wound, in a body cavity, or on a foreign object in a body orifice associated with the production of an epidermal toxin, toxic shock syndrome toxin-1 (TSST-1). This toxin and staphylococcal enterotoxin B (SEB)—and perhaps other staphylococcal toxins—generate the clinical symptoms. TSST is generally associated with the group I bacteriophage, which is found in approximately 10% of all *S. aureus* strains.

STSS is related to a genetic shift in the presence of group A streptococcus, with an increase of certain M proteins and the number of strains producing streptococcal pyrogen exotoxin A.

## PATHOPHYSIOLOGY

The pathogenesis of TSS and host defense involve a number of complex variables. The following factors have been implicated:

- Most TSS patients have little or no preexisting antibody to TSST-1.

- *S. aureus* strains that do not produce TSST-1 are isolated from 40% of patients with non-menstrual-associated TSS, suggesting that other toxins produce TSS.
- The antibody titer to TSST-1 is variable and may not be elevated even in convalescent patients who develop TSS.
- Some patients may be antibody (IgG)-deficient for TSS, and TSST–1 may suppress the B-cell response in vitro.
- Patients can have a high TSST-1 antibody titer but have never developed the disease or been carriers of the toxin-producing strain of *S. aureus*.
- Patients with a usually low hormonal state who are menstruating, postpartum, or young are at greater risk for TSS.

The toxic response mechanism activates macrophages and produces interleukin. In the acute phase, white blood cell (WBC) counts drop, plasma fibronectin levels rise, and C-reactive protein appears. Other usual clinical responses to small quantities of TSST-1 and SEB also become evident.

Although the pathophysiology of STSS is complex, all cases have had group A streptococci isolated from normally sterile sites, were hypotensive, and had multiorgan system failures. All streptococcal isolates were serotyped and screened for streptococcal pyrogenic exotoxin B and species A, B, and C toxin-producing genes by DNA probes.

## Diagnosis

In 1980, the Centers for Disease Control and Prevention (CDC) compiled the most commonly used diagnostic criteria for TSS. These include the following clinical signs:

- Temperature exceeding 38.9 °C (102 °F);
- Erythematous rash during acute illness
- Desquamation of the palms and soles one to two weeks after onset of the illness
- Hypotension
- Negative blood, throat, and cerebrospinal fluid (CSF) cultures
- Negative serologic tests for Rocky Mountain spotted fever, leptospirosis, and measles

- Three or more of the following: (1) vomiting or diarrhea during acute illness; (2) severe myalgia or elevated creatine phosphokinase; (3) vaginal, oropharyngeal, or conjunctival mucous membrane hyperemia; (4) elevated blood-urea nitrogen, elevated creatinine, or more than five WBCs in a high-power field in the absence of a urinary tract infection; (5) a platelet count of less than 100,000/$mm^3$; (6) elevated serum glutamic pyruvic transaminase; and (7) disorientation or alteration in consciousness without focal neurologic signs

These findings, complicated by shock and multisystem failure, can result in death.

If TSS is suspected, look for changes in the vagina, cervix, kidneys, liver, and lungs. The cervical mucosa may show desquamation and ulceration. Pulmonary changes consist of congestion, alveolar hemorrhage, and possibly hyaline membrane formation. Kidney pathology is consistent with tubular necrosis. Liver findings include variable periportal inflammation and microvesicular fatty changes.

Because most of the preceding laboratory findings mimic STSS, it is very important to perform a Gram's stain and blood, throat, and CSF culture collection before administering antibiotics. In some infections caused by trauma, a rapidly progressing tissue infection occurs and results in fasciitis of that area. These tissue infections and lack of skin desquamation on recovery suggest group A streptococcal infection; cultures and assays for toxins produced by group A streptococcus and *S. aureus* are critical for the final diagnosis.

## Treatment

Hospital management of TSS and STSS cases associated with vaginal infection includes close observation for erythema and, less frequently, ulcerations. Instruct the patient to discontinue tampon use. You must also take culture specimens from the vagina, cervix, blood, and lesions (whether inflamed or not) to search for foci of *S. aureus* and group A streptococci infection elsewhere in the body. In nonmenstrual TSS, perform wound and blood cultures.

The most important treatment is fluid replacement with crystalloid solutions. Carefully monitor the patient's pulmonary, cardiovascular, and renal systems. Although antibiotics cannot shorten the duration of acute disease, they may prevent its recurrence. Include penicillinase-resistant penicillins, such as methicillin or nafcillin, for TSS—and give these agents early in case the diagnosis of TSS is incorrect. Similarly, if the diagnosis of STSS is unconfirmed, it may be necessary to employ empirical treatment with vancomycin, metronidazole, gentamicin, ciprofloxacin, and dopamine. Antimicrobial therapy generally does not dictate patient survival. The mortality rate for STSS, although variable, is approximately 30%; in TSS, it is about 10%. Recurrence rates in patients with a previous episode of menstrual-related TSS approach 30%; however, they may drop to 5% if the patient is treated with ß-lactamase-resistant antibiotics. Recurrence of STSS is usually not significant.

## Prevention

Steps for preventing recurrence of TSS include parenteral antibiotic treatment of first episodes as described in the previous section, patient education, and avoidance of tampon use. To prevent first episodes, advise patients to minimize their use of high-absorbency tampons.

### Suggested Readings

Centers for Disease Control and Prevention. Summary: cases of specified notifiable diseases, U.S. MMWR 1989;38:392–399.

Centers for Disease Control and Prevention. Toxic shock syndrome: U.S. 1970–1982. MMWR 1982;31:201–204.

Davis JP, Chesney PJ, Wand PJ, et al. Toxic shock syndrome: epidemiologic features, recurrence, risk factors and prevention. N Engl J Med 1980;303:1429–1435.

Graham DR, O'Brien M, Hayes JM, et al. Postoperative toxic shock syndrome. Clin Infect Dis 1995;20:895–899.

Nyirjesy P, Jones RS, Chatwani A, et al. Streptococcal toxic shock-like syndrome as an unusual complication of laparoscopic tubal ligation. J Reprod Med 1994;39:649–651.

Petitti D, D'Agostino RB, Oldman MJ. Nonmenstrual toxic shock syndrome: methodologic problems in estimating incidence and delineating risk factors. J Reprod Med 1987;32:10–16.

Schlievert PM. Comparison of cotton and cotton/rayon tampons for effect on production of toxic shock syndrome toxin. J Infect Dis 1995;172:1112–1114.

Stevens DL. Invasive group A streptococcal infections. Clin Infect Dis 1992;14:2–11.

Todd JK. Toxic shock syndrome. Clin Microbiol Rev 1989;1:432–446.

Todd JK, Ressman M, Caston SA, et al. Corticosteroid therapy for the patients with toxic shock syndrome. JAMA 1984;252:3399–3402.

CHAPTER

# 80

# *Bacteremia and Septic Shock*

*Bernard Gonik*

## Background, Incidence, and Definition

The incidence of bacteremia in obstetric and gynecologic infections is 8% to 10% and that of septic shock in bacteremic ob-gyn patients is 0% to 12%—quite low overall. Conditions that predispose a woman to septic shock include chorioamnionitis, postpartum endometritis, upper urinary tract infection, septic abortion, cuff cellulitis, pelvic inflammatory disease and pelvic abscess, and toxic shock syndrome. Fortunately, in obstetrics and gynecology, unlike in other medical and surgical fields, the risk of death from septic shock is low in the otherwise healthy patient. Incidence of death from sepsis is estimated as 0% to 3%.

The systemic inflammatory response syndrome (SIRS) is a recently popularized classification that describes the general inflammatory response to a variety of insults. Its etiology is not limited to infection—indeed, burns, trauma, and pancreatitis can elicit a similar clinical picture. SIRS is characterized by two or more of the following:

- Body temperature less than 36 °C or more than 38 °C
- Pulse greater than 90 beats per minute
- Tachypnea manifested as respiratory rate exceeding 20 per minute or $Paco_2$ less than 32 mm Hg
- Leukocyte count less than 4000/mm$^3$, greater than 12,000/mm$^3$, or with more than 10% immature forms in the differential count

SIRS that results from documented infection is termed "sepsis." A diagnosis of severe sepsis is made when SIRS is associated with organ dysfunction, hypoperfusion, or hypotension. Useful indicators of hypoperfusion include lactic acidosis, oliguria, or acute alterations in mental status. If blood pressure and perfusion abnormalities persist despite adequate fluid resuscitation, the patient is deemed to be suffering from septic shock. Multiple-organ system dysfunction syndrome (MODS) is the terminal phase of this spectrum; it involves the progressive physiologic deterioration of interdependent organ systems such that homeostatis cannot be maintained. Commonly affected organ systems include pulmonary and renal dysfunction with adult respiratory distress syndrome (ARDS) and acute renal failure, respectively.

## Pathophysiology

Most studies related to septic shock have focused on gram-negative sepsis. Endotoxin—a complex lipopolysaccharide present in the cell walls of gram-negative bacteria—appears to be a critical factor in producing the pathophysiologic derangements associated with septic shock. Shock, which is apparently closely related to release of a variety of exotoxins, can also develop in patients with gram-positive sepsis.

The series of events initiated by bacteremia or endotoxemia is complex. Local activation of the immune system and its effector cells is important at the site of infection. If the body loses its ability to regulate this response locally, systemic activation of effector cells will promote the release of pro-inflammatory cytokines with widespread systemic effects. At the cellular level, lipopolysaccharide (LPS) bound to a carrier protein interacts with the CD14 receptor on cells of the monocyte line. The resulting monocyte activation leads to production of tumor necrosis factor $\alpha$ (TNF$\alpha$) and interleukin-1 (IL-1). The production of TNF$\alpha$ stimulates the secretion of additional interleukins, prostaglandins, leukotrienes, and other inflammatory mediators. These inflammatory products, in turn, cause the clinical symptoms associated with sepsis as well as capillary leak, hypotension, and activation of the coagulation system.

TNFα and complement fragments attract neutrophils, whose products exacerbate the endothelial injury. Neutrophil activation stimulates a respiratory burst, characterized by increased production and release of lysosomal enzymes and toxic oxygen species such as superoxide, hydroxyl, and peroxide radicals.

Leukocyte migration and activation promote the release of vasoactive substances such as histamine, serotonin, and bradykinin. Direct effects of bacterial immunologic complexes are also thought to play an important role in tissue injury. Immune complex precipitants have been identified within the lung vasculature and may contribute to the development of ARDS. Likewise, focal areas of acute tubular necrosis seen in the kidney have been associated with the deposition of these inflammatory infiltrates.

## Clinical Presentation and Diagnosis

In early septic shock, the patient experiences a shaking chill, sudden rise in temperature, tachycardia, and warm extremities ("warm" shock). Although she appears "infected," a diagnosis of septic shock may elude the clinician who neglects a careful evaluation for hypotension or other signs of reduced organ perfusion.

Laboratory findings vary substantially during this early phase. The white blood cell count may show marked leukocytosis or it may be somewhat depressed. Transient hyperglycemia, caused by catecholamine release and tissue underuse of glucose as a substrate, sometimes appears. Early evidence of disseminated intravascular coagulation (DIC) may take the form of decreased platelet count and fibrinogen levels and elevated fibrin split products and thrombin time. Initial arterial blood gas determinations tend to reflect a mild respiratory alkalosis.

As shock progresses, intact neuronal reflex responses (transmitted by sympathetic activation) produce profound vasoconstriction in all organ systems. This vasoconstriction further reduces tissue and organ perfusion. Clinical manifestations of this later stage include cold extremities, oliguria, and peripheral cyanosis ("cold" shock). The resultant cellular hypoxia and acidosis disrupt the ability of individual cells to use oxygen. This effect produces capillary bed dysfunction, with marked reductions in peripheral vascular resistance due to extensive capillary pooling of blood.

The classic complex of hypotension, cardiovascular collapse, and hypoxia is usually referred to as secondary or "irreversible" shock. A central feature of this stage is profound myocardial depression related to systemic release of a myocardial depressant factor. Subsequent widespread end-organ failure is invariably followed by coma and death.

In most cases, the approach to diagnosis should include microbiologic evaluation of specimens from blood, urine, sputum, and the wound. Even though mixed flora is usually identified in transvaginal cultures, the clinician should carry out careful sampling of the endometrial cavity if this area is the suspected source of infection. In patients thought to have chorioamnionitis, transabdominal amniocentesis or cultures taken from a free-flowing internal pressure transducer catheter may prove useful.

## Appearance in Pregnancy

Physiologic adaptations to pregnancy occur in practically every organ system. These changes can theoretically influence the presentation and course of septic shock. In experiments by Beller and coworkers involving endotoxin-induced septic shock, pregnant animals showed a much more pronounced metabolic acidosis and earlier cardiovascular collapse than did controls.

Interestingly, the fetus and newborn are much more resistant to the direct deleterious effects of endotoxin than is the mother. Fetal and newborn lambs, for example, have been shown to be capable of tolerating endotoxin doses 10 times larger than those lethal to adult pregnant sheep. On the other hand, Morishima and coworkers, after giving endotoxin to pregnant baboons, reported profound asphyxia and rapid deterioration in the fetus. These effects were thought to result primarily from maternal factors, such as hypotension and increased myometrial activity, that reduce placental perfusion.

## TREATMENT

Initial intervention for septic shock strives to accomplish the following goals:

- Improvement of functional circulating intravascular volume
- Establishment and maintenance of an adequate airway to facilitate management of respiratory failure
- Determination of the septic focus through diagnostic evaluation
- Institution of empiric antimicrobial therapy to eradicate the most likely pathogens

When dealing with a pregnant patient, the clinician should strive foremost to maintain maternal well-being, as fetal compromise results primarily from maternal cardiovascular decompensation. Improvements in maternal status will have positive effects on fetal condition. Furthermore, attempts at delivering the fetus of a hemodynamically compromised mother may increase the risk of fetal distress and create a need for more aggressive surgical intervention.

An exception is the case when the fetal compartment is the source of sepsis (for example, in case of chorioamnionitis). In such circumstances, therapy includes stabilizing the mother while initiating antibiotic therapy and beginning attempts at delivery.

### Fluid Management

The mainstay of acute management of septic shock involves volume expansion to correct absolute or relative hypovolemia. At times, considerable fluid is needed because of profound vasodilation, increased capillary permeability, and extravasation of fluid into extravascular spaces. The best monitoring approach is to use a flow-directed pulmonary artery catheter, which also allows for the determination of cardiac output and oxygen-related variables.

One method of monitoring fluid is to administer up to 200 mL IV over 10 minutes. If pulmonary capillary wedge pressure increases by more than 7 mm Hg, withhold additional fluid. Otherwise, administer a repeat dose. Isotonic crystalloid solutions, such as normal saline, are the most popular option. Some authors, however, have recommended the use of colloid solutions, such as 5% normal human albumin, to maintain a normal colloid osmotic–pulmonary artery wedge pressure gradient (more than 4 mm Hg), thereby reducing the risk of pulmonary edema.

## Vasopressor Therapy

If fluid resuscitation alone proves inadequate for restoring optimal cardiovascular function, administer vasoactive agents. Traditionally, dopamine hydrochloride has been the most popular agent, although increasing attention is being focused on the early use of norepinephrine in septic shock.

Dopamine has dose-dependent effects on dopaminergic, alpha-adrenergic, and beta-adrenergic receptors. It is administered as a continuous infusion, starting at 2 to 5 μg/kg/min and being titrated according to clinical and hemodynamic responses.

In one recent study of septic shock, norepinephrine was found to reverse hypotension and oliguria more reliably than dopamine. Likewise, oxygen delivery and consumption were more favorably improved with norepinephrine. Dopamine has also been demonstrated to adversely affect the balance between splanchnic oxygen delivery and utilization, as compared with norepinephrine. Both agents comparably increased mean arterial pressure, but dopamine decreased gastric intramucosal pH, suggesting detrimental effects on splanchnic perfusion. Some investigators have therefore encouraged the use of norepinephrine as a primary agent for inotropic support in septic shock.

## Assessment of Tissue Oxygenation

Oxygenation at the lungs can be assessed easily by arterial blood-gas measurements. In contrast, oxygen consumption or use is more difficult to gauge. The patient with septic shock frequently exhibits reduced peripheral tissue use of oxygen. An indirect measurement of poor tissue oxygen extraction is a finding of a high mixed-venous oxygen saturation or determination of a reduction in arteriovenous oxygen content difference. Actual peripheral oxygen consumption can be calculated using the Fick equation: the normal indexed nonpregnant range is 120 to 140 mL $O_2/min/m^2$. Clinical improvement in the patient's condition should be accompanied by an increase or normalization of peripheral oxygen consumption.

## Adult Respiratory Distress Syndrome

A common complication encountered in the septic shock patient is adult respiratory distress syndrome (ARDS). Its diagnosis is made on the basis of progressive hypoxemia, a normal pulmonary capillary wedge pressure, diffuse infiltrates on chest X ray, and decreased pulmonary compliance. Treatment involves intubation and ventilatory support to maintain adequate gas exchange at nontoxic levels of inspired oxygen. Positive end-expiratory pressure (PEEP) is often necessary to accomplish this goal. Serial monitoring of arterial blood gases is essential.

### Antibiotic Therapy

Because the course of septic shock can be short and fulminant, the clinician should perform a diagnostic workup without delay and immediately start empiric antimicrobial therapy.

In the obstetric patient, empiric therapy should provide coverage for a wide variety of aerobic and anaerobic bacteria, including both gram-negative and gram-positive organisms. Parenteral therapy combining aqueous penicillin (3,000,000 U every 4 hours) or ampicillin (2 g every 6 hours), an aminoglycoside (loading dose of 2 mg/kg, followed by maintenance doses of 1.5 mg/kg every 8 hours for patients with normal renal function), and clindamycin (900 mg every 8 hours) is recommended. If you suspect a *Staphylococcus aureus* infection, a semisynthetic penicillin may be substituted for the aqueous penicillin agent.

Because nephrotoxicity is a well-established complication of aminoglycoside usage, monitor peak (6 to 10 μg/mL) and trough (less than 2 μg/mL) aminoglycoside levels. When available, use culture results and organism sensitivities to guide subsequent therapy, which can be chosen more selectively. Newer broad-spectrum monotherapeutic antimicrobial regimens may be substituted for those listed previously, depending on the individual clinician's experience, hospital resistance patterns, and toxicities encountered.

## Surgical Therapy

In patients with septic abortion, attempt to evacuate the uterus promptly after initiating antibiotics and stabilizing the patient. Likewise, septic shock in association with chorioamnionitis in a gestationally viable fetus is treated best by expeditious evacuation of the uterus. Evacuation can be accomplished vaginally if maternal hemodynamic parameters are stable and labor is progressing adequately.

In the postpartum patient, hysterectomy may be necessary if microabscess formation occurs within the myometrial tissue or if clinical evidence indicates deterioration despite appropriate antibiotic therapy. Similarly, when overwhelming sepsis is associated with PID, suspect abscess formation. Under these circumstances, an operative approach is frequently needed to drain the abscess and effect stabilization.

## Additional Supportive Measures

Supportive measures include managing electrolyte imbalances, correcting metabolic acidosis, stabilizing coagulation defects, and monitoring renal function. Monitor lactic acidosis stemming from anaerobic metabolism by measuring serial arterial blood gas and serum lactate levels. Administer normal saline infusions with one to two ampules of sodium bicarbonate periodically to help correct severe acidosis.

Laboratory coagulation abnormalities tend to reflect generalized DIC. Unless the patient shows clinical evidence of bleeding or a need for surgical intervention, do not aggressively attempt to correct DIC. Spontaneous amelioration will occur once the patient's overall clinical status improves.

Renal function is best monitored with an indwelling Foley catheter and serial creatinine and blood urea nitrogen determinations. In cases of acute renal failure, tests of tubular function show increased fractional excretion of sodium (urinary sodium greater than 40 mEq/L) and impaired concentrating ability (urine osmolality less than 400 mOsm/kg $H_2O$). Provided irreversible acute tubular necrosis has not occurred, correction of underlying hemodynamic and perfusion deficits should restore renal function.

## Suggested Readings

Beller FK, Schmidt EH, Holzgreve W, et al. Septicemia during pregnancy: a study in different species of experimental animals. Am J Obstet Gynecol 1985;151:967–975.

Blanco JD, Gibbs RS, Castaneda YS. Bacteremia in obstetrics: clinical course. Obstet Gynecol 1981;58:621–625.

Bone RC, Balk RA, Cerra FB, et al. Definitions for sepsis and organ failure and guidelines for the use of innovative therapies in sepsis. Chest 1992;101:1644–1655.

Bryan CS, Reynolds KL, Moore EE. Bacteremia in obstetrics and gynecology. Obstet Gynecol 1984;64:155–158.

Gonik B. Intensive care monitoring of the critically ill pregnant patient. In: Creasy RK, Resnik R, eds. Maternal-fetal medicine: principles and practice, 3rd ed. Philadelphia: WB Saunders, 1994: 865–890.

Lee W, Clark SL, Cotton DB, et al. Septic shock during pregnancy. Obstet Gynecol 1988;159:410–416.

Morishima HO, Niemann WH, James LS. Effects of endotoxin on the pregnant baboon and fetus. Am J Obstet Gynecol 1978;131: 899–902.

Parrillo JE. Mechanisms of disease: pathogenetic mechanisms of septic shock. N Engl J Med 1993;328:1471–1477.

Rackow EC, Astiz ME. Pathophysiology and treatment of septic shock. JAMA 1991;266:548–554.

# Index